BRAUNER

Published

RADIOLOGY OF THE PANCREAS AND DUODENUM
S. Boyd Eaton, Jr., M.D., and Joseph T. Ferrucci, Jr., M.D.

THE HAND IN RADIOLOGIC DIAGNOSIS
Andrew K. Poznanski, M.D.

RADIOLOGY OF THE ILEOCECAL AREA
Robert N. Berk, M.D., and Elliott C. Lasser, M.D.

FUNDAMENTALS OF ABDOMINAL AND PELVIC ULTRASONOGRAPHY
George R. Leopold, M.D., and W. Michael Asher, M.D.

RADIOLOGY OF THE ORBIT
G. A. S. Lloyd, B.M., B.Ch. Oxf., F.F.R., D.M.R.D.

SPECIAL PROCEDURES IN CHEST RADIOLOGY
Stuart S. Sagel, M.D.

RADIOLOGY OF RENAL FAILURE
Harry J. Griffiths, M.D.

PEDIATRIC RADIOLOGY OF THE ALIMENTARY TRACT
Edward B. Singleton, M.D., Milton L. Wagner, M.D., and Robert V. Dutton, M.D.

RADIOLOGIC DIAGNOSIS OF RENAL PARENCHYMAL DISEASE
Alan J. Davidson, M.D.

RADIOLOGY OF THE GALLBLADDER AND BILE DUCTS
Robert N. Berk, M.D., and Arthur R. Clemett, M.D.

RADIOLOGY OF THE LIVER
James G. McNulty, M.B., F.R.C.R.

GASTROINTESTINAL ANGIOGRAPHY — 2nd Edition
Stewart R. Reuter, M.D., and Helen C. Redman, M.D.

CLINICAL RADIOLOGY OF THE EAR, NOSE AND THROAT — 2nd Edition
Eric Samuel, M.D., and Glyn A. S. Lloyd, M.D.

PEDIATRIC ORTHOPEDIC RADIOLOGY
Michael B. Ozonoff, M.D.

THE RADIOLOGY OF JOINT DISEASE — 2nd Edition
D. M. Forrester, M.D., J. C. Brown, M.D., and John W. Nesson, M.D.

THE RADIOLOGY OF VERTEBRAL TRAUMA
John A. Gehweiler, Jr., M.D., Raymond L. Osborne, Jr., M.D., and R. Frederick Becker, Ph.D.

RADIOLOGY OF THE ADRENALS
Harold A. Mitty, M.D., and H. C. Yeh, M.D.

Volume 18 in the Series
SAUNDERS
MONOGRAPHS
IN CLINICAL
RADIOLOGY

Forthcoming Monographs

TECHNIQUES OF THERAPEUTIC ANGIOGRAPHY
Robert I. White, M.D., S. I. Kadir, M.D., Klemmens Barth, M.D., and Stephen L. Kaufman, M.D.

RADIOLOGY OF ORTHOPEDIC PROCEDURES
Martin I. Gelman, M.D.

PLAIN FILM APPROACH TO ABDOMINAL CALCIFICATIONS
Steven Baker, M.D., and Milton Elkin, M.D.

ARTHROGRAPHY OF THE KNEE
Richard Wolfe, M.D.

CARDIAC IMAGING IN ADULTS
C. Carl Jaffe, M.D.

CARDIAC IMAGING IN INFANTS AND CHILDREN

MICHAEL J. KELLEY, M.D., F.A.C.C.

Associate Clinical Professor of Radiology
University of California
San Diego School of Medicine
Co-Director, Cardiac Catheterization Laboratory
Anaheim Memorial Hospital
Anaheim, California
Formerly, Associate Professor of Radiology and Medicine
and Chief of Cardiac Radiology
Yale University School of Medicine
New Haven, Connecticut

C. CARL JAFFE, M.D.

Associate Professor of Radiology and Medicine
Yale University School of Medicine
New Haven, Connecticut

CHARLES S. KLEINMAN, M.D.

Assistant Professor of Pediatrics and Diagnostic Radiology
Yale University School of Medicine
New Haven, Connecticut

1982

W. B. SAUNDERS COMPANY
Philadelphia   London   Toronto   Mexico City   Rio de Janeiro   Sydney   Tokyo

W. B. Saunders Company: West Washington Square
Philadelphia, PA   19105

1 St. Anne's Road
Eastbourne, East Sussex BN21 3UN, England

1 Goldthorne Avenue
Toronto, Ontario M8Z 5T9, Canada

Apartado 26370 — Cedro 512
Mexico 4, D.F., Mexico

Rua Coronel Cabrita, 8
Sao Cristovao Caixa Postal 21176
Rio de Janeiro, Brazil

9 Waltham Street
Artarmon, N.S.W. 2064, Australia

Ichibancho, Central Bldg., 22-1 Ichibancho
Chiyoda-Ku, Tokyo 102, Japan

Library of Congress Cataloging in Publication Data

Kelley, Michael J., 1942–

Cardiac imaging in infants and children.

1. Heart — Radiography.   2. Pediatric cardiology — Diagnosis.
   3. Pediatric radiography.   4. Ultrasonic cardiography.
   5. Radioisotopes in cardiology.   I. Jaffe, C. Carl.
   II. Kleinman, Charles S.   III. Title. [DNLM: 1. Heart —
   Radionuclide imaging.   2. Heart — Radiography.
   3. Heart diseases — In infancy and childhood.   4. Heart
   diseases — In adolescence.   5. Echocardiography — In
   infancy and childhood.   6. Echocardiography — In
   adolescence. WS 290 K29c]

RJ423.5.R33K44   618.92′1207572   81–40563

ISBN 0–7216–5361–8   AACR2

Cardiac Imaging in Infants and Children   ISBN   0-7216-5361-8

Last digit is the print number: 9   8   7   6   5   4   3   2   1

This book is dedicated with love to
our wives and children
Loretta, Maureen, Ryan, Michelle and Kathleen Kelley
Toini Lefren, Peter and Judson Jaffe
Jessica, Ari and Joshua Kleinman

ACKNOWLEDGMENTS

Preparation of this volume has involved three institutions, a good deal of transcontinental communication, and the efforts of a great number of people. It is difficult to express adequately our appreciation to the many individuals who have contributed time, effort, and those certain intangibles necessary for the completion of this task.

Departmental chairmen and clinical directors have given support, encouragement, and the necessary freedom required to "finish the book." Our thanks go to Drs. Norman S. Talner and Richard H. Greenspan at Yale; to Drs. Charles Putman and Carl Raven, formerly at Yale, now at Duke University; and to Drs. Robert N. Berk, Donald Resnick, and Jack Forrest at the University of California, San Diego.

We are indebted to many of our colleagues and associates in pediatric radiology, cardiac radiology, pediatric cardiology, and ultrasound who have provided the necessary environment for a beneficial interchange of ideas. Our gratitude is extended to Drs. Kenneth J. Taylor, Ronald Ablow, Nancy Rosenfield, William E. Hellenbrand, and Michael Berman at Yale, and to Drs. David Edwards, Charles Higgins, William Friedman, and Stan Kirkpatrick at San Diego. The friendship and skilled collaboration of Dr. John Hobbins and Diana C. Lynch, R.N., of Yale have made our studies in fetal echocardiography possible.

The illustrations for many of the radiographs and angiocardiograms used here were printed from radiographs filed in the incredible Hewlett Radiology Library at Yale University School of Medicine. Miss Viola Jacobs, the head librarian, provided untiring enthusiasm and dedication in helping us gather this material. Many of these radiographs were submitted by Dr. Gerald Fishbone. Most of the fine quality prints were the work of Tom McCarthy and his staff at Yale. Other photographs were the work of Ms. Susan Brown at San Diego, and Ernie Rodriquez, Gary Greene, and Ed Lovell of Anaheim Memorial Hospital.

Special affection and recognition go to Mrs. Kathleen Finn, chief pediatric echocardiographic technician at the Yale–New Haven Medical Center, and to Mrs. Eileen Gallagher, whose efforts resulted in the many superb echocardiographs included here.

The numerous rewrites and drafts of this text are the work of three wonderful, cheerful, dedicated individuals: Sandra Sudac at Yale, and Kathy Nancarrow and Marilyn Johnson at San Diego.

The senior author has had the pleasure of working closely with two cardiac radiology fellows at San Diego and gratefully acknowledges the warm friendship and numerous contributions of Drs. Curtis Green and John Newell.

The senior author also wishes to thank his new colleagues at Anaheim Memorial Hospital for their understanding and acceptance: Drs. Raymond

Berk, William Birnbaum, Robert Cimini, William Grandolpho, Russell Ludwig, Richard Penfil, and especially Neil Siegel (who provided both physical and mental space when it was needed).

Additionally, we wish to express our gratitude to former fellows and medical students in pediatric cardiology and radiology who provided many stimulating and useful insights during the completion of their studies: Drs. John C. Werner, Michael H. Gewitz, Raymond R. Fripp, Richard L. Donnerstein, Ellen M. Weinstein, Kirk Wang, Steven Shoum, and Anita Montez.

The authors wish to give special thanks to Ms. Lisette Bralow, associate medical editor at W. B. Saunders, for prodding at the right moments and for "laying back" at others, but most importantly for her friendship and guidance in seeing this transcontinental project through to completion.

Finally, we would all like to acknowledge our most valued teachers, our parents.

MICHAEL J. KELLEY, M.D.
C. CARL JAFFE, M.D.
CHARLES S. KLEINMAN, M.D.

SPECIAL ACKNOWLEDGMENT

Although this work was originally conceived while the senior author was chief of cardiac radiology at the Yale University School of Medicine, the seeds of the idea were planted many years before while I was a sophomore medical student at Washington University. There I had the privilege of taking an elective course in cardiac radiology given by Dr. Larry P. Elliott. Although the knowledge gained during that short six weeks was to provide a stimulus for my future studies, it became secondary to learning Dr. Elliott's logical approach to the diagnosis of heart disease utilizing the electrocardiogram and the chest radiograph. Thereafter, this approach continued to provide the framework for new knowledge gained in angiocardiography, echocardiography, and nuclear medicine. It also became my chief tool for sharing this knowledge with medical students, residents, and fellows. It should not be surprising then that Dr. Elliott's approach to the diagnosis of heart disease using radiographic methods provides the framework for much of the organization of this book. It seems appropriate that I acknowledge my debt to him and that I recognize his valuable contribution to the field of cardiac radiology.

M.J.K.

CONTENTS

INTRODUCTION

The incidence of congenital heart disease in infants varies from 3.2 to 7.6 babies in one thousand live births.[1-4] It is estimated that over half of infants born with congenital heart disease die before one year if proper diagnosis is not made and treatment is not instituted.[1] In several series of cases diagnosed at catheterization, operation, or postmortem, ten lesions comprised approximately 90 per cent of the defects (Table 1).[5-7] In other large series,[6-9] ten additional lesions (most associated with cyanosis) make up an additional 10 per cent of congenital cardiac anomalies (Table 2).

Acquired heart disease in infants and children is rare. It may involve conditions that present shortly after birth (endocardial fibroelastosis) or in late childhood (rheumatic heart disease). In one study, it was estimated that ten times as many new patients with congenital heart disease were admitted to the hospital as were new patients with rheumatic fever.[5]

In evaluating children with suspected heart disease, the clinical history, physical examination, and electrocardiogram are the time-honored ways of arriving at a differential diagnosis. If these modalities constitute the diagnostic foundations, then the chest radiograph and the M-mode echocardio-gram must be considered the walls and support structure, since an objective evaluation of both can further focus and narrow the differential diagnosis. Recently, two-dimensional (real-time) echocardiography and various radionuclide methods have been added to the diagnostic armamentarium. Facts obtained from these "cardiac imaging" examinations have helped bridge the gap between the clinical data and the cardiac catheterization and angiocardiographic examination. Rather than acting as a substitute for the more invasive procedures, noninvasive imaging data may aid in planning such exams, especially in the severely ill infant. In the child with an established diagnosis, these methods have been of value in clinical management and timing of repeat cardiac catheterizations, in planning for future surgery, and in the follow-up of patients in the postoperative period.

Although the lesions listed in Tables 1 and 2 involve a variety of malformations of the heart and great vessels, their clinical and radiographic presentations are often quite simple. Generally, patients with significant congenital heart disease are either acyanotic or cyanotic. Children with rheumatic heart disease and other acquired conditions are acyanotic. Although the chest

TABLE 1. Incidence of the Ten Most Common Congenital Heart Defects[5-7]

Ventricular Septal Defect	20%
Pulmonic Stenosis with VSD	15
Patent Ductus Arteriosus	12
Pulmonic Stenosis	12
Atrial Septal Defect	10
Aortic Stenosis	6
Coarctation of the Aorta	5
Transposition of the Great Vessels	4
Endocardial Cushion Defects	4
Tricuspid Atresia	1
	89%

TABLE 2. Other Lesions Making Up Approximately 10 Per Cent of Congenital Heart Defects[6-9]

Left Heart Outflow Obstruction (other than AS)
Anomalous Pulmonary Venous Connections
Left Heart Inflow Obstruction
Severe Pulmonary Stenosis or Atresia
Ebstein's Anomaly of the Tricuspid Valve
Truncus Arteriosus
Single Ventricle
Double Outlet Right Ventricle
Aortic Insufficiency
Coronary and Arch Anomalies

TABLE 3. Clinical-Radiographic Classification of Congenital Heart Defects

LESION	CLINICAL-RADIOGRAPHIC CATEGORY
1. Ventricular Septal Defect	Acyanotic with shunt vascularity
2. Pulmonary Stenosis with VSD	Cyanotic with decreased vascularity
3. Patent Ductus Arteriosus	Acyanotic with shunt vascularity
4. Pulmonary Valve Stenosis	Acyanotic with normal vascularity
5. Atrial Septal Defect	Acyanotic with shunt vascularity
6. Aortic Valve Stenosis	Acyanotic with normal vascularity
7. Coarctation of the Aorta	Acyanotic with normal vascularity
8. Complete Transposition of the Great Vessels	Cyanotic with shunt vascularity
9. Endocardial Cushion Defect	Acyanotic with shunt vascularity
10. Tricuspid Atresia	Cyanotic with (decreased)* vascularity
11. Left Heart Outflow Obstruction (other than AS)	Acyanotic with normal vascularity or pulmonary venous hypertension
12. Anomalous Pulmonary Venous Connections	(A)cyanotic with shunt vascularity or pulmonary venous obstruction
13. Left Heart Inflow Obstruction	Acyanotic with pulmonary venous hypertension
14. Severe Pulmonary Stenosis or Atresia	Cyanotic with decreased vascularity
15. Ebstein's Anomaly of the Tricuspid Valve	Cyanotic with decreased vascularity
16. Truncus Arteriosus	Cyanotic with shunt vascularity
17. Single Ventricle	Cyanotic with (shunt) vascularity
18. Double Outlet Right Ventricle	Cyanotic with (shunt) vascularity
19. Aortic Insufficiency	Acyanotic with normal vascularity
20. Coronary Artery and Arch Anomalies	Acyanotic with normal vascularity

*Parentheses indicate vascular pattern may vary depending on presence or absence of obstruction to pulmonary flow.

radiograph provides the first step in the imaging work-up of these patients, it is uncommon to find an approach to its use in current textbooks of "cardiac imaging." This is unfortunate, for in the day-to-day labors of evaluating children with suspected heart disease, the chest radiograph is unique in its ability to contribute information. Since the echocardiogram, especially the two-dimensional exam, can provide an accurate "inside" view of the heart and since radionuclide methods may add functional as well as anatomic information, it is not surprising that quantification of chamber size by chest x-ray has taken a back seat. However, the chest radiograph continues to be extremely valuable in providing certain "outside" information. Its most important use is in assessing the state of the pulmonary vasculature. The effects of the lesions listed in Tables 1 and 2 on pulmonary blood flow result in four vascular patterns seen on the plain chest film: normal vascularity, "shunt" vascularity, pulmonary venous hypertension pattern, or decreased vascularity. These patterns will be dealt with in the section on the analysis of the plain chest film. Using clinical information regarding the presence or absence of cyanosis and radiographic findings regarding the

state of the pulmonary vascularity, one can evolve a clinical-radiographic classification of the 20 lesions listed in Tables 1 and 2. Such a clinical-radiographic categorization is given in Table 3. The chest radiograph is perhaps the most accurate method for rapidly defining the situs of the patient and for determining cardiac malpositions in the presence of normal situs. It can often give clues as to great vessel relationships (for example, L-transposition of the great vessels) and define the position of the aortic arch as well as the presence or absence of certain vascular anomalies. In addition, unusual bumps on the cardiac silhouette may provide useful information (for example, left atrial appendage enlargement in rheumatic heart disease). Finally, the chest film may prove virtually diagnostic in certain conditions for which other imaging modalities have limited value (for example, coarctation of the aorta and the unobstructed variety of total anomalous pulmonary venous return). The information available from the chest radiograph when used in conjunction with M-mode and two-dimensional echocardiographic and nuclear medicine data will almost always result in a reasonable and relatively short list of diagnostic possibilities. Not infrequently, the definitive diagnosis will be made. As is the case in many institutions, however, we use this combined approach as a "road map" for subsequent angiocardiographic and hemodynamic evaluation.

In the first section of this text, the reader will be given an overview of the various cardiac imaging modalities: the plain chest film, the echocardiogram, nuclear medicine procedures, and the angiocardiogram. In this section, an approach to the performance and interpretation of each modality will be developed along with an overview of cardiac anatomy as seen from the vantage point of each imaging modality. A special section on clinical applicability will be included in the nuclear medicine chapter. Having established this foundation of information, certain pathophysiologic states existing in infants and children with congenital or acquired heart disease will be coupled with the appearance of the pulmonary vascularity on the chest film to present a clinical-radiographic classification of the various disease states (Section II). The lesions within each clinical-radiologic category will then be presented in four separate chapters. After a brief pathologic-clinical definition of the lesion, the radiographic and echocardiographic features will be reviewed. Finally, the typical angiographic findings will be demonstrated.

Although the organization used in this text tends to simplify a very complex topic in which crossovers from one category to another may occur, it is hoped that it will provide the reader with a logical approach to the utilization and interpretation of the imaging modalities used in assessing the variety of cardiac lesions that may present in infants and children. The authors also hope that nuances and exceptions to this approach will be appreciated with further study and experience.

New developments in cardiac imaging in infants and children are occurring at a rapid rate. Real-time echocardiography is but one of these areas, with nuclear cardiography and computerized tomographic techniques looming on the horizon. In terms of imaging, however, the plain chest radiograph will remain a valuable portal of entry for the assessment of these children. It is hoped that this book will provide a logical approach to current modalities of imaging the heart and will help bring together pediatric cardiologists, cardiovascular radiologists, and residents and fellows training in both areas to the ultimate benefit of the pediatric patient.

REFERENCES

1. MacMahon, B., McKeown, T., Record, R. G.: The incidence and life expectation of children with congenital heart disease. Br Heart J 15:121, 1953.
2. Richards, M. R., Merritt, K. K., Samuels, M. H., Longmann, A. G.: Congenital malformations of the cardiovascular system in series of 6053 infants. Pediatrics 15:12, 1955.
3. Mustacchi, P., Sherins, R. S., Miller, M. J.: Congenital malformation of the heart and great vessels. JAMA 183:241, 1963.
4. Carlgren, L.: The incidence of congenital heart disease in children born in Cothenburg 1941–1950. Br Heart J 21:40, 1959.
5. Nadas, A. S.: Pediatric Cardiology, 2nd ed. W. B. Saunders Co., Philadelphia, 1963.
6. Keith, J. D., Rowe, R. D., Vlad, P.: Heart Disease in Infancy and Childhood, MacMillan Co., New York, 1979.
7. Gasul, B. M., Arcilla, R. A., Leo, M.: Heart Disease in Children: Diagnosis and Treatment, J. B. Lippincott, Philadelphia, 1966.
8. Krovetz, L. J., Gessner, I. H., Schiebler, G. L.: Handbook of Pediatric Cardiology, Hoeber Harper, New York, 1981.
9. Perloff, J. K.: The Clinical Recognition of Congenital Heart Disease, W. B. Saunders Co., Philadelphia, 1978.

Section I

CARDIAC IMAGING MODALITIES IN INFANTS AND CHILDREN

Chapter 1

THE CHEST RADIOGRAPH

"Not invisible but unnoticed, Watson. You did not know where to look, and so you missed all that was important."

Sherlock Holmes
(A.C. Doyle, "Case of Identity")

As Sherlock Holmes suggests, there are many valuable clues that can be obtained by a meticulous visual assessment of a subject. This applies to the evaluation of chest films. Many cardiac disorders in children leave telltale clues on the chest radiograph that are often seen only in retrospect. The following approach offers a step-wise method of evaluating the chest film that should help to eliminate "retrospective calls." Using this format, the reader should be able to (1) arrive at a proper physiologic diagnosis (for example, cyanosis is due to diminished pulmonary blood flow), (2) be able to offer a reasonable differential diagnosis (tetralogy of Fallot; pulmonary atresia with intact ventricular septum; Ebstein's anomaly of the tricuspid valve; tricuspid-pulmonary atresia), and (3) often suggest the final diagnosis prior to further noninvasive and invasive diagnostic tests.

By using this approach and taking a clue from Holmes, one will hopefully realize that the art of chest film interpretation in children with suspected congenital heart disease involves taking meager clinical information (that is, the presence or absence of cyanosis) and looking *sequentially* at the film. In doing so, one must not only know *where* to look, but also know which structure takes *precedence* over another in the analysis. Underlying this approach is the importance of the *pulmonary vascularity* in determining the physiology of the cardiac lesion. Finally, structures that make up the cardiomediastinal silhouette can then be evaluated and abnormalities found there can be interpreted in light of the pulmonary vascular findings. When one adds additional information regarding chamber size, great vessel relationships, and valve location and function obtained by echocardiography to the above analysis, a final physiologic-anatomic diagnosis should result.

Individuals interpreting chest films often begin with an assessment of the most obvious (the heart), while failing to evaluate other less obvious but equally essential structures (the aortic arch, stomach position, lung fields, and so on). The following approach to the chest film has been developed in an attempt to steer the neophyte in the right direction and to remind the seasoned practitioner of his errant ways. If this sequence of analysis is applied seriously to each "unknown" chest film, it will lead to a surprising amount of physiologic and anatomic information.

TECHNICAL CONSIDERATIONS

Children wiggle and children breathe. Radiologic technologists overexpose and underexpose chest films. Therefore, when evaluating a chest film of a child, it is important to decide whether one is dealing with a technically adequate film. A poor technical examination may lead to erroneous conclusions (as outlined below) and

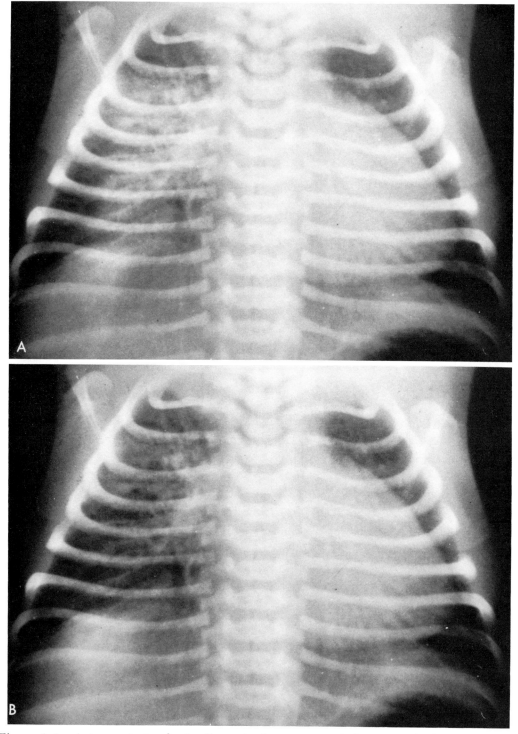

Figure 1-1. Anteroposterior chest radiograph of a neonate with dyspnea and a heart murmur. The initial film (*A*) shows underexposed technique with a white area of opacification in the right lung field. This suggests pulmonary edema. A repeat examination (*B*) shows that this is due to a technical error of the underexposed film. The patient does have shunt vascularity and was found to have a large ventricular septal defect at cardiac catheterization.

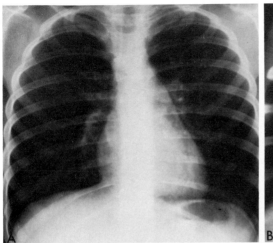
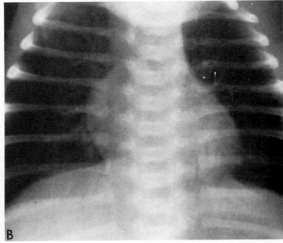
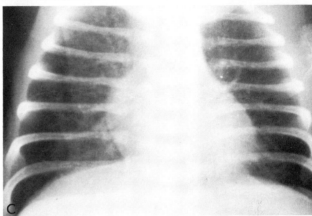

Figure 1–2. Overexposed chest films in a child (A) and a neonate (B). The technical quality of these films makes it difficult to interpret the pulmonary vascularity and to evaluate the lung parenchyma; however, one can use a high intensity light (bright light) to obtain this information. Repeat examination in the neonate (C) shows bilateral perihilar infiltrates.

should be repeated. Good communication between the radiologist and the technologist regarding technique and a quick review of films before a patient leaves the x-ray department should alleviate many of these problems.

Exposure and Motion

In individuals with suspected heart disease, the chest film makes perhaps its greatest contribution by allowing one to assess the pulmonary vascularity. Therefore, the optimum chest film is one that shows the pulmonary vessels and lung parenchyma to best advantage. Usually, this is a film with exposure factors just sufficient to allow visualization of the intervertebral disc spaces of the thoracic spine through the cardiome-

diastinal silhouette. A film that is too light (underexposed) may suggest pulmonary edema or pneumonia (Fig. 1–1). Information lost by this technical route is irretrievable and the film should be repeated. Another technical faux pas, but one that can be salvaged, is the overexposed (too dark) film. This error may cause one to "undercall" pulmonary vasculature, or to overlook infiltrates, nodules, or a pneumothorax (Fig. 1–2). Fortunately, a bright light can usually be used to assess the pulmonary vascularity and lung parenchyma when one is confronted with such a film.

Patient motion may also affect interpretation of the vascularity. This is manifested by blurring of the cardiac silhouette or the hemidiaphragms (Fig. 1–3). An impression of "ill-defined" vessels may result if this problem is not recognized (Fig. 1–3).

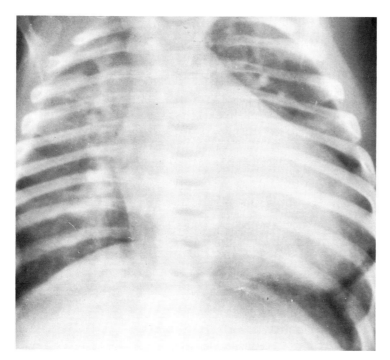

Figure 1–3. Anteroposterior chest film in a neonate with a suspected cardiac lesion. The infant was crying during the examination and there is motion as evidenced by slight blurring of the hemidiaphragms and ill-defined pulmonary vascular markings. If this technical problem goes undiscovered, one may over-read the presence of interstitial edema and congestive failure. This patient did have a large left-to-right shunt at cardiac catheterization.

Respiratory Phase

The degree of inspiration should always be assessed when evaluating pediatric chest films. A film obtained in expiration may suggest edema, atelectasis, or pneumonia (Fig. 1–4). An expiratory film affects interpretation of vascularity, since resultant crowding of lung vessels causes them to look fuzzy (Fig. 1–4A). In addition, the more horizontal position assumed by the heart makes estimation of heart size difficult (Fig. 1–4A).

Since it is the cardiac size that is most affected by poor inspiratory effort, and since most of the heart is in continuity with the left hemidiaphragm, the left ribs are most useful in the assessment. A good inspiratory effort in an infant or child is one in which the anterior sixth rib (or posterior eighth rib) is visualized above the apex of the left hemidiaphragm (Fig. 1–4B). An expiratory film is indicated when the dome of the left hemidiaphragm is at the level of the fifth anterior rib (seventh posterior rib) or higher (Fig. 1–4A). A lateral film taken in inspiration accompanying an expiratory frontal film may help one to evaluate pulmonary vascularity viewed as possibly abnormal on the frontal film. When doubt exists, the frontal film should be repeated.

Rotation and Angulation

It is not uncommon to obtain a rotated film on a squirming child. Since rotation to the right or the left of the central axis of the

Figure 1–4. A, Anteroposterior chest radiograph obtained in a cyanotic infant. If one were to mistakenly interpret this film, conclusions that might be reached would be that there is pulmonary edema, possible pneumonia, and cardiomegaly. Pulmonary vascularity would be extremely difficult to evaluate. Note that there are only seven posterior ribs and five anterior ribs above the right hemidiaphragm.

B, A repeat examination with good inspiratory effort shows that nine posterior ribs and five to six anterior ribs are clear of the right hemidiaphragm. One can now readily assess the pulmonary vascularity and lung parenchyma. The lung fields are clear and the pulmonary vascularity appears slightly diminished. Overall heart size is normal and there is a right aortic arch (arrows). These findings along with the clinical history of cyanosis are consistent with the diagnosis of tetralogy of Fallot.

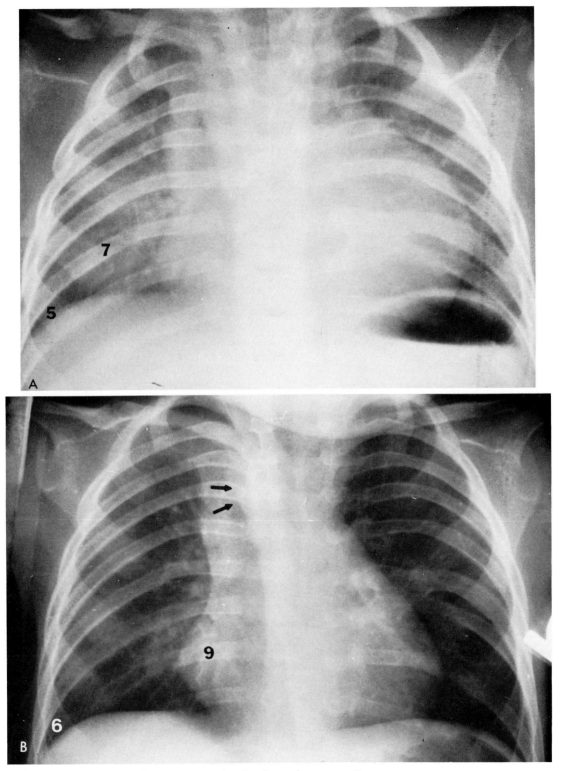

Figure 1–4. See legend on opposite page

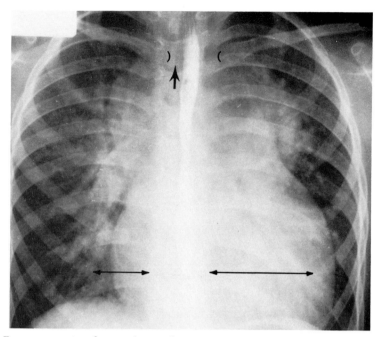

Figure 1–5. Posteroanterior chest radiograph in a patient with total anomalous pulmonary venous return to the supracardiac position (note the "snowman" appearance to the cardiovascular silhouette). Rotation to the left is indicated by the relationship of the medial aspects of the clavicles to the spinous process of the third thoracic vertebral body (arrow). In addition one can see that the anterior rib to lateral spinous distance is shorter on the right than on the left (arrows). Both methods may be applied to delineating rotation in children, but the latter method is perhaps most useful in the very young child or infant.

body may significantly distort cardiac and great vessel anatomy, it is important to evaluate the degree of rotation on the frontal film. The most common method of assessing rotation is to compare the medial aspects of the clavicles with the spinous process of the upper thoracic vertebral bodies (Fig. 1–5). Unfortunately, children can fix their shoulders and upper thorax (and, therefore, their clavicles) in a straight anterior-posterior position while still rotating their lower thorax. If one compares the anterior portions of the ribs with the lateral aspects of the vertebral bodies, one can eliminate this problem and obtain the same information (Figs. 1–5, 1–6). This method also accomplishes an evaluation of the whole thorax from anterior (ribs) to posterior (vertebrae). The nonrotated lateral film is indicated by the presence of a small distance between the posterior rib margins (Fig. 1–7). Significant rotation in this projection may lead to incorrect impressions regarding the hilar structures.

When a child rotates to the left, the resulting radiograph will show a prominence of the left superior mediastinal structures (especially the pulmonary trunk), while making it difficult to visualize the right-sided structures (Fig. 1–6A). Conversely, rotation to the right will result in prominence of the right heart border, superior vena cava, and ascending aorta and will diminish the size of the aortic knob, pulmonary trunk, and the left heart border (Fig. 1–6B).

Newborn chest films are often slightly lordotic (clavicles higher than first rib arc) (Fig. 1–8A). A more exaggerated lordotic film in which the anterior ribs are superior to the posterior ribs should be repeated, since it causes an increase in the cardiac diameter, results in an upturned cardiac apex, and may give the appearance of a prominent pulmonary trunk (Fig. 1–8B).

EXTRACARDIAC EVALUATION

It is useful, especially when dealing with possible congenital heart disease, to evaluate the bony thorax, the great vessel–

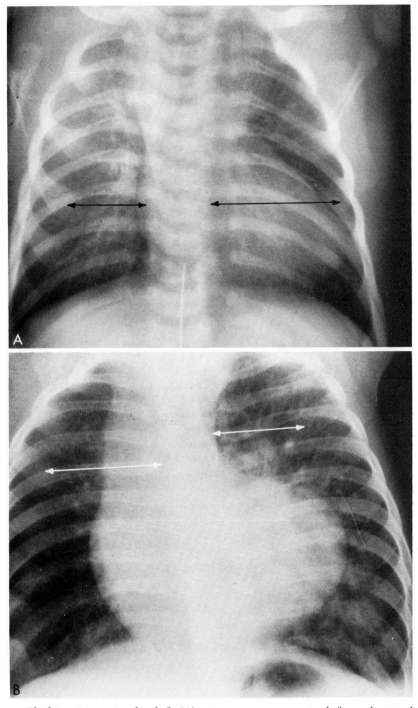

Figure 1–6. Slight rotation to the left (A) gives prominence to left mediastinal and cardiac structures, while slight rotation to the right (B) gives prominence to right mediastinal and right heart structures. Both of these patients had significant congenital heart disease: the patient in A, a double outlet right ventricle with a right aortic arch and pulmonic stenosis; and the patient in B, a hemitruncus with a right aortic arch.

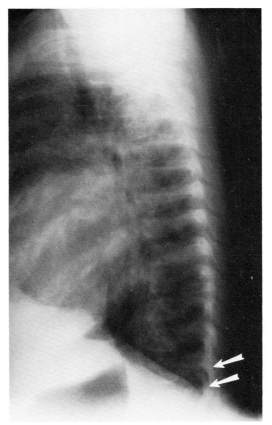

Figure 1–7. A nonrotated lateral film is indicated by the presence of a small distance between the posterior margins of the right and left ribs (arrows).

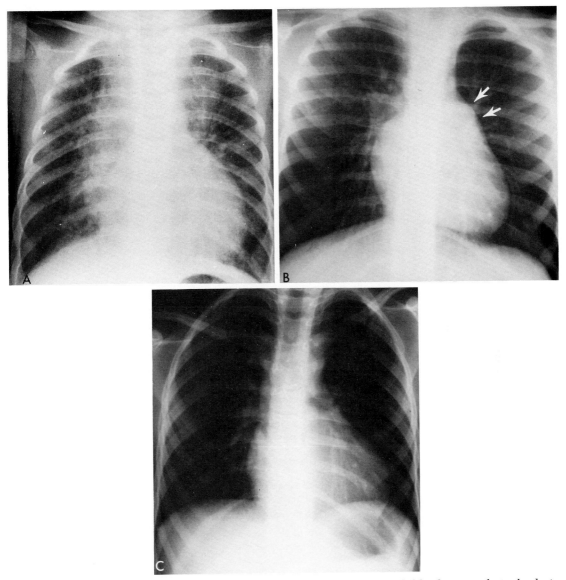

Figure 1–8. A, Chest films obtained in the neonate or young child often result in lordotic positioning with the clavicles projected higher than the arch of the first rib. B, A lordotic film in an older child may result in erroneous interpretations regarding cardiac size and contour. The pulmonary trunk (arrows) appears prominent and the cardiac apex upturned. C, Repeat chest film of the patient shown in B at a slightly later date, shows normal pulmonary trunk and cardiac apex.

mediastinal region, and the abdomen before proceeding to evaluate the pulmonary vascularity and cardiac anatomy. Information gleaned from these areas will often provide significant clues to the final radiographic diagnosis in children with heart disease. Determination of a patient's situs is also part of this extracardiac evaluation and will be discussed in the next section.

Skeletal Structures

One reason to consider the bones of the thorax early in chest film analysis is that certain bone abnormalities are associated with specific cardiac conditions. These are listed in Table 1–1. Scoliosis occurs in 0.4 per cent of the general population, 0.8 per cent of patients with acyanotic congenital heart disease, and 6 per cent of those with cyanotic congenital defects.[1] In addition, since this deformity is often progressive and may lead to pulmonary disability, it is important for the radiologist and pediatrician to evaluate the spine on serial chest films. If the film has been properly analyzed and a particular abnormality of the thoracic cage identified, a proper radiographic diagnosis may be suggested and supporting clues sought when evaluating the pulmonary vascularity and mediastinal and cardiac structures.

It is of interest that extracardiac anomalies occur in 25 per cent of infants seen during the first year of life for significant cardiac disease.[2] The most frequent anomalies involve the musculoskeletal system or are associated with a specific syndrome. Some of these abnormalities involve the thorax or upper skeleton and may be detected on the chest film. The more common syndromes, with their skeletal abnormalities and associated cardiac lesions, are listed in Table 1–2. In children with musculoskeletal defects and congenital heart disease, simple left-to-right shunts make up one third of the cardiac lesions[2] (Fig. 1–9A and B). Fusion of the manubrial sternal joint occurs in approximately 16 per cent of patients with congenital heart disease (as opposed to 2 per cent of the normal population). Fusion of the body of the sternum is also quite frequent.[3] Both of the sternal abnormalities occur more commonly in cyanotic as opposed to acyanotic congenital heart disease.[3] This finding in a cyanotic infant may occasionally prove helpful in distinguishing cardiac from pulmonary causes of respiratory distress (Fig. 1–9C).

In children with severe cyanotic heart disease, skeletal abnormalities may be provoked by the hypoxemia and secondary polycythemia.[4] These changes include bone marrow expansion (thin cortices, decreased metaphyseal mineralization), periosteal new bone formation (pulmonary osteoarthropathy), cortical sclerosis, and rib notching (due to dilated intercostal arteries collateralizing the lungs).

TABLE 1–1.   Bone Abnormalities Related to Cardiac Disease

BONE ABNORMALITY	CARDIAC DISEASE
Rib notching or hyperostosis of inferior rib margins	Aortic coarctation
Double manubrial center, 11 ribs	Down's syndrome (endocardial cushion defect)
Scoliosis	6% of patients with cyanotic CHD
"Straight back," pectus, scoliosis	Mitral valve prolapse
Prominent superior sternum	Atrial septal defect
Prominent inferior sternum	Ventricular septal defect
Bone marrow expansion (coarsening of trabecular pattern and thinning of cortical bone)	High output states (thalassemia, sickle cell anemia, other anemias) and cyanotic CHD
Bone infarcts	Sickle cell anemia, other high output states, cardiomyopathy
Scoliosis Manubrial-sternal fusion Mesosternum (fusion of the body of sternum) Retarded bone age Reduced cortical bone formation	Favors cyanotic CHD vs. acyanotic CHD

Perhaps the most important reason for giving close scrutiny to the bony structures in patients with heart disease relates to the fact that some children have had previous surgery. Although the clinician ordering the chest radiograph may be aware of previous surgery, the radiologist may not. In the ideal world this information will be transmitted to the consulting radiologist. In reality, this information is frequently lacking and the radiologist must be aware of the characteristic radiographic appearance and variety of cardiothoracic surgical procedures. These procedures may alter both the thoracic cage and the cardiomediastinal anatomy as well. Clues to the presence of a thoracotomy on the chest film may be as subtle as mild pleural reaction on the side of surgical intervention or as obvious as a missing portion of a rib (Fig. 1–10A and B). Often there will be eccentric separation between the anterior ribs in the region of the first five thoracic segments. The subtle finding of an "inset" rib may also signal a previous thoracotomy (Fig. 1–11A). Acutely, soft tissue swelling or irregularity or subcutaneous emphysema may be present.

The types of surgery and the surgical approach used for common congenital heart defects are listed in Table 1–3. Additional clues that a specific type of surgery has been performed reside in various changes in the bones, mediastinum, and pulmonary vascularity. If the patient has had a right superior vena cava to right pulmonary artery anastomosis (Glenn shunt), the superior vena cava will often be prominent (Fig. 1–11A and B). The patient who has had a subclavian artery to pulmonary artery anastomosis (Blalock-Taussig shunt), a procedure that can be performed through either the right or left chest (but is usually performed on the side opposite the aortic arch), will often demonstrate rib notching on the side of the surgery (Fig. 1–12). This is due to enlarged intercostal arteries that serve as collaterals to the axillary artery and maintain circulation to the arm. The pulmonary vascularity in a patient who has had a Blalock-Taussig anastomosis will usually be uniform. Occasionally, one may visualize a density in the superior mediastinum that represents the subclavian artery "turned down" to achieve this shunt (Fig. 1–12). The ascending aorta to pulmonary artery anastomosis (Waterston-Cooley shunt) performed through a right thoracotomy often results in unilateral prominence of the right pulmonary artery and vasculature. The descending aorta to left pulmonary artery anastomosis (Potts' shunt) may be associated with a prominent bulge at the junction of the proximal descending thoracic aorta and left pulmonary artery (Fig. 1–13). Because of difficulty encountered in taking down this anastomosis, it is rarely performed today.

In the child with a history of cyanosis, a thoracotomy is performed for palliation, while a median sternotomy is performed for definitive repair of various congenital defects. An easy way to remember the types of surgery performed through the median sternotomy is that either the semilunar valves (pulmonary and aortic) or the septum (atrial and ventricular) can be repaired from this approach (Table 1–3). When faced with a chest film that shows evidence of a thoracotomy and a median sternotomy, the patient most likely has had early palliation and later definitive repair of a lesion associated with cyanosis. A typical example of this would be a patient with a right thoracotomy and median sternotomy. This could be a patient with tetralogy of Fallot who was palliated with a Blalock-Taussig or Waterston-Cooley shunt (right thoracotomy) and had repair of the ventricular septal defect and pulmonary stenosis through the sternum. Alternatively, it could be a patient with complete transposition who had an atrial septectomy (to increase atrial mixing), followed later by a Mustard procedure (interatrial baffle to redirect systemic and pulmonary venous blood into an appropriate great vessel). In other words, the combination of a right or left thoracotomy and a median sternotomy often indicates initial palliation followed by repair of cyanotic congenital heart disease. It should be mentioned that the palliation-repair approach is being supplanted by earlier and earlier definitive repair of cyanotic lesions, especially tetralogy of Fallot. A knowledge of the various types of procedures that can be performed and their radiographic manifestations should frequently allow one (after an assessment of the vascularity and the cardiac silhouette) to predict the nature of the initial cardiac lesion.

Text continued on page 25

TABLE 1–2. Syndromes Associated With Thoracic Cage Abnormalities and Cardiac Lesions

SYNDROME	THORACIC ABNORMALITIES	CARDIAC LESION
Congenital rubella	Coarsening of metaphyseal trabeculae with longitudinal areas of radiolucency and sclerosis; poorly defined provisional zones of calcification; "celery stalk" long bones	Patent ductus arteriosus, valvar pulmonary stenosis and peripheral pulmonary stenosis
DiGeorge	Absent thymic tissue	Conotruncal malformations, interrupted aortic arch
Ellis-van Creveld (Chondroectodermal dysplasia)	Short and heavy tubular bones, small thorax	CHD 50%, ventricular septal defect, and others
Goldenhar	Oculovertebral abnormalities	Tetralogy of Fallot
Holt-Oram	"Digitalized" thumb and radial abnormalities; hypoplasia of upper limbs and shoulder girdle; short clavicles	Atrial and ventricular septal defects
Homocystinuria	Kyphoscoliosis; pectus carinatum	Coronary occlusions
Hurler (Mucopolysaccharidosis I-H)	Dorsal gibbus with small vertebral bodies and hook-shaped anterior surface	Cardiomyopathy
Klinefelter (XXY)	Brachycephaly; radioulnar synostosis	Ventricular septal defect

Marfan	Kyphoscoliosis; pectus excavatum and carinatum; long, thin bones	Cystic medial necrosis of ascending aorta, mitral valve prolapse, sinus of Valsalva, and ascending aortic aneurysms
Noonan (XX, XY) (Pseudo-Turner)	Webbed neck, short stature	CHD 30 to 50%, pulmonary valve stenosis, also atrial and ventricular septal defects and cardiomyopathy
Osteogenesis imperfecta tarda	Osteoporosis within cortices; recent and old fractures	Valvular heart disease (especially aortic valve)
Pierre Robin	Various skeletal abnormalities; micrognathia	Patent ductus arteriosus, atrial septal defect
Trisomy 13–15 (Patau)	Hypoplasia of the ribs; "trigger" thumbs	CHD 80 to 90%, ventricular septal defect, tetralogy of Fallot, aortic coarctation, patent ductus arteriosus, double outlet right ventricle
Trisomy 16–18 (Edward)	Thin ribs; elongated and tapered clavicles; hypoplastic or absent sternal ossification centers	CHD approaches 100%, ventricular septal defect, patent ductus arteriosus, aortic coarctation, pulmonic stenosis, double outlet right ventricle
Trisomy 21 (Down's syndrome)	Double manubrial center; 11 ribs	CHD 40 to 50%, endocardial cushion deformity, ventricular septal defect, tetralogy of Fallot, patent ductus arteriosus
Turner (XO) (Gonadal dysgenesis)	Webbed neck; cubitus valgus	Aortic coarctation, also aortic and pulmonic stenosis, tetralogy of Fallot, Ebstein's anomaly
Williams (Idiopathic hypercalcemia)	Osteosclerosis with "celery stalking" of metaphyses; ectopic calcification	Supravalvular aortic stenosis, peripheral pulmonary stenosis

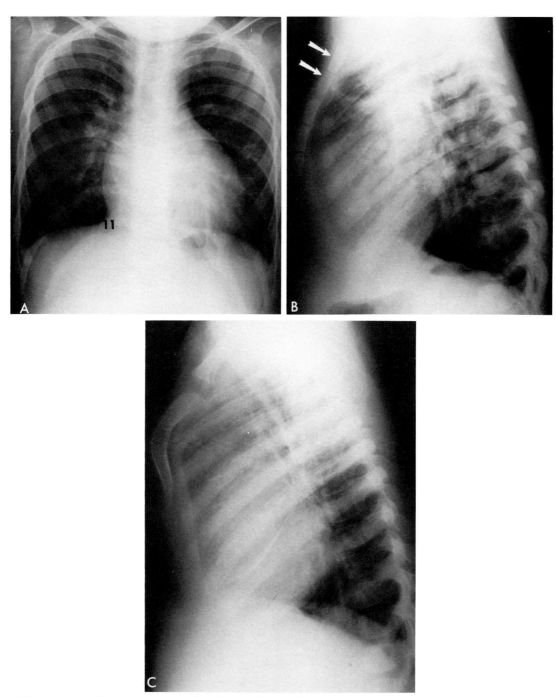

Figure 1–9. Posteroanterior (A) and lateral (B) chest radiographs show 11 ribs and a double manubrial center (arrows) as separate anomalies in this child with Down's syndrome and an endocardial cushion defect. In C, fusion and hypoplasia of the body of the sternum is noted in this patient with tetralogy of Fallot. Sternal anomalies occur more commonly with cyanotic, as opposed to acyanotic, congenital cardiac defects.

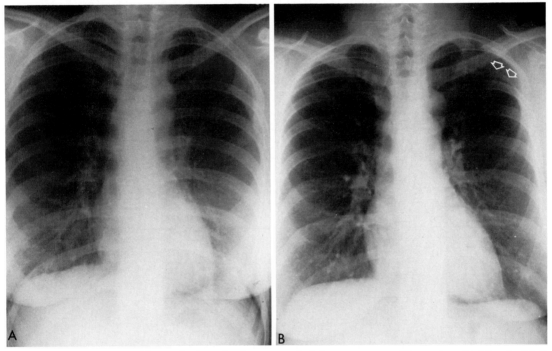

Figure 1–10. Two children who have had previous left thoracotomies. The patient in *A* has had left thoracotomy for coarctation of the aorta. The missing left fourth rib and pleural thickening are obvious. An explanation for the deformed aortic arch in the patient shown in *B* is suggested by the left thoracotomy (partially regenerated left fourth rib — arrows). This patient has also had coarctation repair.

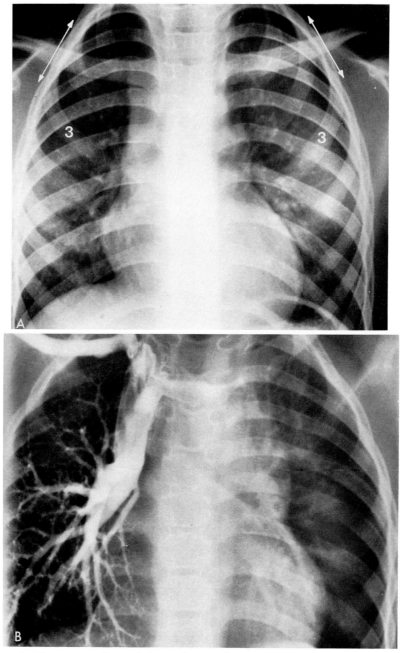

Figure 1–11. *A,* This patient has subtle evidence of a previous right thoracotomy. Note that the third rib (3) on the right is "inset," as compared with the second and fourth ribs above and below (double arrow). If one compares the right and left sides, one can see that the third rib on the left maintains a smooth arch with its neighbors above and below (double arrow). *B,* Right subclavian venogram in the patient shown in *A* demonstrates the presence of anastomosis between the superior vena cava and right pulmonary artery — a so-called Glenn shunt. This palliative shunt was performed in this patient with tricuspid atresia through a right thoracotomy. Note that the chest radiograph shows an unusually prominent superior vena cava.

TABLE 1–3. Surgical Approaches for Common Congenital Heart Lesions

LEFT THORACOTOMY

1. Patent Ductus Arteriosus (ligation)
2. Coarctation of the Aorta (repair)
3. Pulmonary Artery Band (to control increased pulmonary flow)
4. Palliative Shunt (to increase pulmonary flow)
   Blalock-Taussig (left subclavian to left pulmonary artery)
   Potts' Procedure (rarely used—descending aorta to left pulmonary artery)

RIGHT THORACOTOMY

1. Palliative Shunt (to increase pulmonary flow)
   Blalock-Taussig (right subclavian to right pulmonary artery)
   Waterston-Cooley (ascending aorta to right pulmonary artery)
   Glenn (superior vena cava to right pulmonary artery)
2. Creation of an Atrial Septal Defect in Complete Transposition of the Great Vessels (Blalock-Hanlon procedure)
3. Occasionally used for repair of atrial septal defect (ASD)

MEDIAN STERNOTOMY

Complete repair of defects in:
1. The septum (VSD, ASD, endocardial cushion defects)
2. The semilunar valves (aortic stenosis, pulmonic stenosis)
3. The ventricular septum plus the pulmonary valve (tetralogy); other complex lesions
4. Complete transposition of the great arteries (Mustard or Senning or Jatene procedures)
5. Tricuspid atresia (Fontan procedure)
6. Palliation of certain congenital defects (e.g., palliative "central" pulmonary artery to aortic shunts)

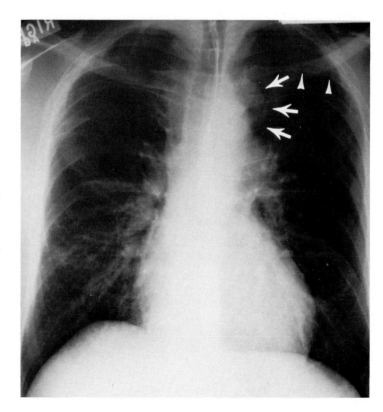

Figure 1–12. A patient with a left thoracotomy and a subclavian artery to pulmonary artery anastomosis (Blalock-Taussig shunt). Subtle rib notching is present along the left fourth (4) rib (arrowheads) and a density above the aortic knob (arrows) represents the "turned down" left subclavian artery.

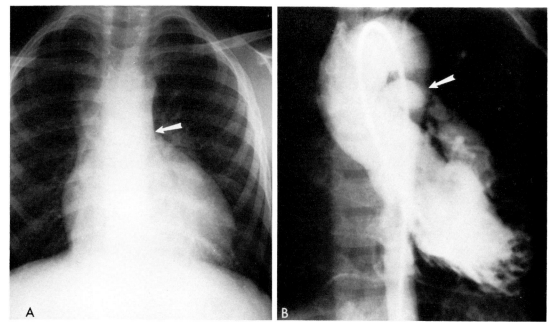

Figure 1–13. A, Posteroanterior chest radiograph in a patient who has had Potts' procedure for palliation of complex cyanotic heart disease. Note the bulge along the proximal thoracic aorta (arrow) and the prominent left pulmonary artery. B, The left ventriculogram shows the anastomosis between the descending aorta and left pulmonary artery (arrow).

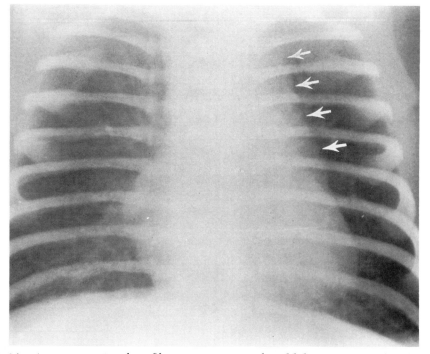

Figure 1–14. Anteroposterior chest film in a neonate with mild dyspnea. Note that the great vessel region is difficult to evaluate because of the presence of thymic tissue (arrows).

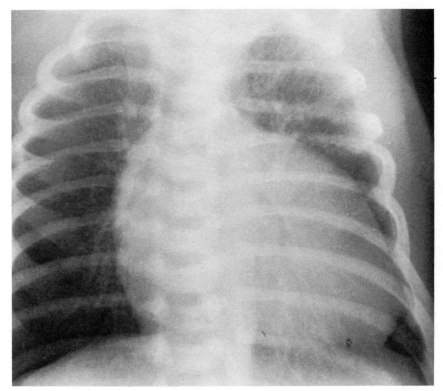

Figure 1–15. An infant with cyanotic congenital heart disease in whom the mediastinum and the great vessel region can be readily analyzed. This is due to the lack of significant thymic tissue in this stressed infant. The mediastinum is relatively narrow, there is a left aortic arch, and the pulmonary artery segment is not apparent. Note the diminished pulmonary vascularity and the prominent right atrium. This patient had pulmonary atresia with an intact ventricular septum.

Great Vessel Region

Assessment of the size and location of the aortic arch and the presence and size of the pulmonary trunk should be made early in the approach to the chest film. Again, much like clues obtained from analysis of the thoracic and abdominal regions, this area can be quite helpful in establishing a differential diagnosis. In certain specific situations, it may be highly accurate in predicting the specific cardiac lesions (for example, total anomalous pulmonary venous return to the vertical vein).

Aorta

The anterior mediastinum of the healthy neonate and the healthy child up to age six years contains variable amounts of thymic tissue. Although this suggests that the child is not stressed from a possible cardiac con-

dition, it makes analysis of the great vessel region difficult in this age group (Fig. 1–14). Fortunately, in the sick infant or young child, in whom this information is most important, reduction of thymic tissue due to stress makes assessment of this region possible (Fig. 1–15). The lateral border of the ascending aorta should not be visible on the frontal chest film of a child or adolescent. Prominence of this structure may appear as a bulge along the right upper portion of the cardiovascular silhouette (Fig. 1–16). An indirect indication of ascending aortic dilatation is deviation of the superior vena cava to the right. The left anterior oblique view is perhaps the most sensitive way to detect prominence of the ascending aorta. The presence of a dilated ascending aorta should raise the suspicion of lesions that involve pressure overload of the left ventricle (for example, systemic hypertension, aortic stenosis, and aortic coarctation).

The normal left aortic knob extends

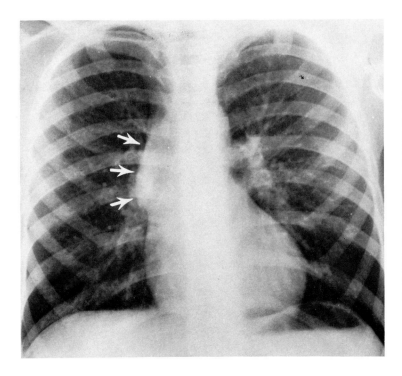

Figure 1–16. This posteroanterior chest radiograph in a ten-year-old boy shows normal vascularity and heart size. However, there is significant prominence of the ascending aorta (arrows). In this age group, this finding is suspicious for pressure overload problems involving the left ventricle (for example, systemic hypertension, aortic stenosis, and coarctation of the aorta). At cardiac catheterization this patient had significant aortic stenosis and a bicuspid aortic valve.

slightly leftward beyond the lateral wall of the descending aorta (Fig. 1–17). The side of the aortic arch is defined by the course of the transverse aorta with respect to the trachea. Even in the presence of thymic tissue, it is usually possible to ascertain the side of the arch by indirect means. First, one may appreciate an impression on the left lateral wall of the trachea (Fig. 1–18*A* and *B*) or note that it bends to the right (left arch) or left (right arch). Second, the density of the descending aorta is usually visible along the

Figure 1–17. The normal aortic knob (arrows) extends slightly leftward beyond the lateral wall of the descending aorta and should be clearly seen in most children beyond the age of five years.

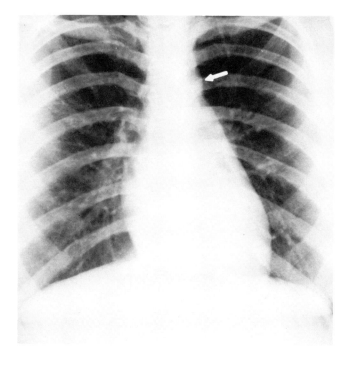

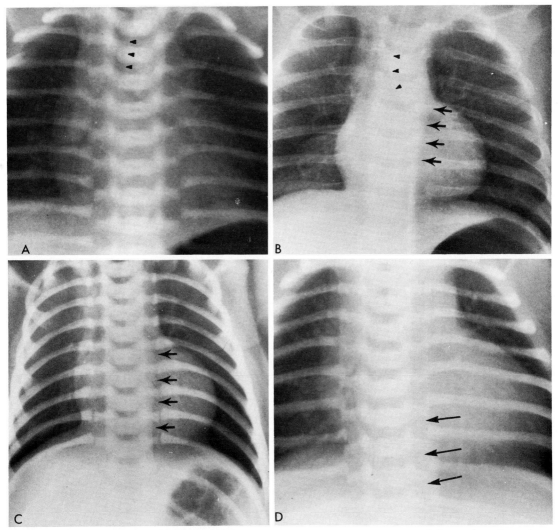

Figure 1–18. The side of the aorta may be determined by an examination of the trachea. In patients *A* and *B*, the trachea deviates to the right of the midline (arrowheads), and in patient *B* there appears to be a discrete indentation on the lower margin of the trachea at the takeoff of the left mainstem bronchus. (Note the endotracheal tube.) An additional indirect method of determining the side of the aortic arch is illustrated in patients *B* and *C*, whose chest films show the density of the descending aorta in the left paraspinous region (arrows). In the neonate one may occasionally have to use the subtle finding of increased density (whiteness) over the pedicles and paraspinous region to suggest the side of the aortic arch. This is illustrated in the patient shown in *D* (arrows).

lower left paraspinous region (Fig. 1–18*B* and *C*). Another subtle aid may be an increase in density over the left or right thoracic vertebral pedicles (Fig. 1–18*D*) even though a distinct line cannot be appreciated.

With a right aortic arch, the transverse aorta courses to the right of the trachea. There are four ways to recognize this important anomaly on the frontal film: (1) the lower tracheal indentation is on the right and the trachea is deviated to the left (Figs. 1–19 and 1–20); (2) the upper superior vena cava is deviated to the right (Figs. 1–19 and 1–20); (3) the slightly higher aortic knob is viewed on the right (Fig. 1–19); and (4) there is no aortic knob on the left (Figs. 1–20 and 1–21). The presence of barium in the esophagus may add additional direct information regarding the side of the arch (Fig.

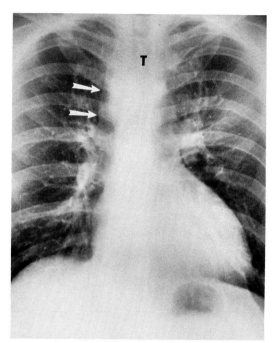

Figure 1-19. A right aortic arch is present in this patient and indicated by an impression on the right lower tracheal margin and deviation of the trachea (T) to the left. Note, in addition, that the superior vena cava density is prominent along the right upper heart margin (arrows).

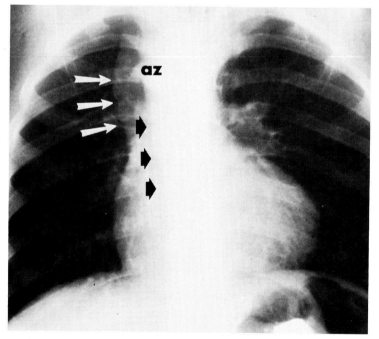

Figure 1-20. In this patient with a right aortic arch, barium in the esophagus is superimposed on the trachea. One can see that the superior vena cava and azygous vein (AZ) are deviated to the right (upper arrows). In addition, there is no evidence of the "normal"aortic knob on the left. The descending thoracic aorta is clearly seen in the right paraspinous region (lower arrows). This patient had tetralogy of Fallot.

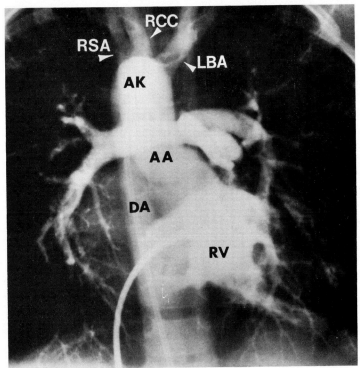

Figure 1-21. Right ventriculogram (RV) obtained in a patient with classic tetralogy of Fallot and a mirror image right aortic arch. The ascending aorta (AA), aortic knob (AK), and descending aorta (DA) are clearly delineated. This angiographic appearance should be correlated with the chest film findings previously described for a right aortic arch (Figs. 1–19 and 1–20). The order of great vessel branching with the mirror image right aortic arch is (1) the left brachiocephalic artery (LBA), (2) the right common carotid artery (RCC), and (3) the right subclavian artery (RSA).

1-22). One may also use the presence of the descending thoracic aortic density to define the side of the arch (Figs. 1–20 and 1–21), although in some cases of right aortic arch the descending aorta may descend on the left. These cases are usually associated with severe varieties of tetralogy of Fallot.

There are two common types of right aortic arch. Type I is the so-called "mirror image" right aortic arch. The order of branches is therefore the mirror image of the left aortic arch. These are: first, the left brachiocephalic artery; second, the right common carotid artery; and third, the right subclavian artery (Fig. 1–21). Since no vessels cross the mediastinum posterior to the esophagus, the Type I right aortic arch is defined by using the right arch criteria outlined above (Fig. 1–22A) coupled with a lateral barium swallow that shows no esophageal indentation posteriorly (Fig. 1–22B). This type of right aortic arch is frequently associated with congenital heart disease (an incidence of approximately 95 per cent), especially the following lesions (incidence of right aortic arch is given in parenthesis):

1. Tetralogy of Fallot (~25 per cent): note that a higher incidence of right arch exists in the more severe forms of this condition (~50 per cent).
2. Truncus arteriosus (30 to 40 per cent).
3. Transposition of the great vessels with pulmonary stenosis (5 to 10 per cent)
4. Tricuspid atresia (5 per cent)
5. Ventricular septal defect (2 per cent)

The Type II right aortic arch is associated with an aberrant origin of the left subclavian artery from the proximal descending thoracic aorta in a retroesophageal position (Fig. 1–23). This type of arch is easily recognizable using the aforementioned signs of right arch on the frontal film (Fig. 1–24A) in addition to a lateral barium swallow that demonstrates a posterior impression of variable size on the upper thoracic esophagus

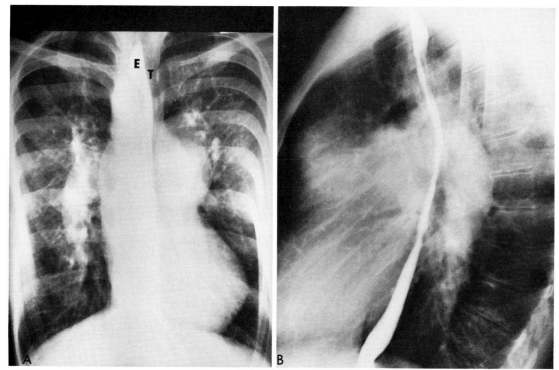

Figure 1–22. Posteroanterior *(A)* and lateral *(B)* chest radiographs in a patient with truncus arteriosus and Eisenmenger physiology. The right aortic arch causes an impression on the upper portion of the barium-filled esophagus (E) and deviates the trachea (T) to the left. On the lateral view, the esophagus shows no posterior indentation in the region of the aortic arch. This indicates that a type 1, or mirror image, right aortic arch exists. This type of right aortic arch is invariably associated with congenital heart disease.

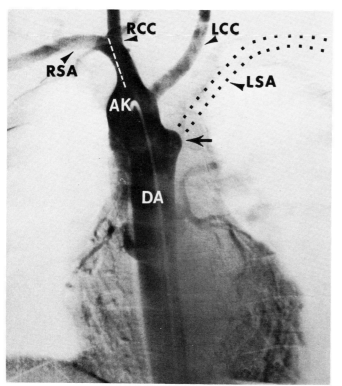

Figure 1–23. A variation of the type 2 right aortic arch. This subtraction ascending thoracic arteriogram shows the aortic knob (AK) on the right and the descending aorta (DA) in the right paraspinous region. Note the diverticular outpouching on the lateral wall of the proximal descending thoracic aorta (arrow). In the type 2 right aortic arch, this diverticulum normally gives rise to the aberrant left subclavian artery (indicated by dotted lines — LSA). In this patient the arterial segment was atretic. Note the additional great vessel branches in this patient: the left common carotid artery (LCC), the right common carotid artery (RCC), and the right subclavian artery (RSA). In other words, in this patient there are four separate great vessel origins.

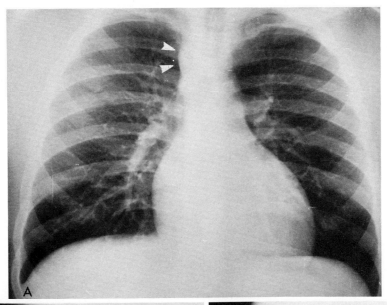

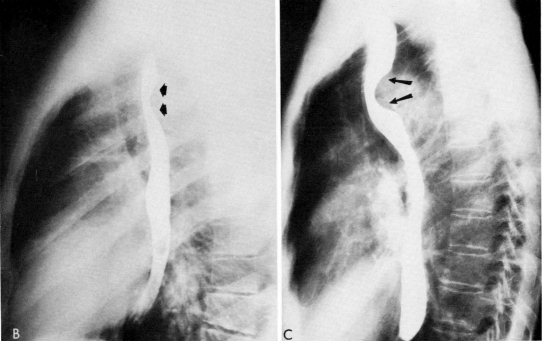

Figure 1–24. Posteroanterior (A) and lateral (B) chest radiographs in an asymptomatic male who was told he had a "mediastinal mass" after a routine physical examination and chest x-ray. Note that the trachea is deviated slightly to the left, that the aortic knob is seen on the right (arrows), and that no aortic knob is present on the left. Barium swallow demonstrates a mild anterior defect on the posterior wall of the upper barium-filled esophagus (arrows). This indicates that a type 2 right aortic arch exists. The small retroesophageal impression suggests that the ductus is on the right in this patient. Lateral chest film (C) in an elderly individual with mild dysphagia. A right aortic arch was present on the frontal film and a large extrinsic mass impresses on the upper barium-filled esophagus (arrows). The width of this impression suggests that the remnant ductal tissue relates to the left subclavian artery. In this age group the type 2 right aortic arch is not uncommonly associated with dysphagia.

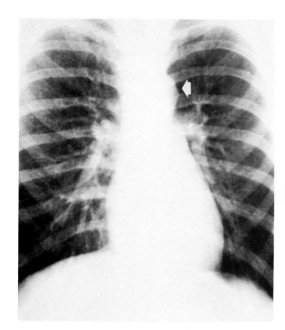

Figure 1–25. An abnormally prominent aortic knob (arrow) is seen in this patient who has an otherwise normal chest film. This twelve-year-old patient had rheumatic aortic regurgitation and mitral regurgitation.

Figure 1–26. The absence of a well-formed aortic knob (?) should raise the suspicion of coarctation of the aorta. Note that although the descending aorta is seen in this individual (lower arrow) the region of the aortic knob is not clearly defined. There is no evidence of rib notching, but at cardiac catheterization the patient had a significant aortic coarctation.

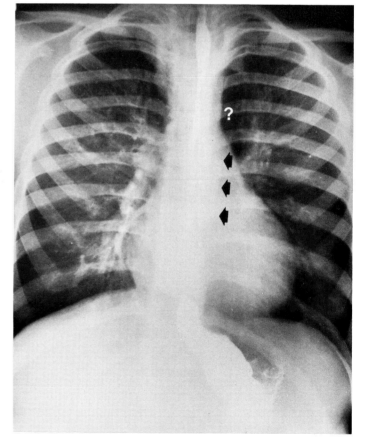

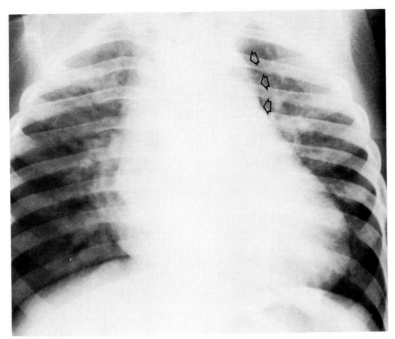

Figure 1–27. Extreme prominence of the aortic knob may also be a significant radiographic clue. In this patient with shunt vascularity, the aortic knob extends beyond the pulmonary trunk (arrows). This should suggest that the left-to-right shunt involves the aorta. This patient had a large patent ductus arteriosus.

(Fig. 1–24*B* and *C*). The ductus arteriosus is usually on the left with Type II right arch. This then forms a vascular ring (right arch → aberrant left subclavian artery → left ductus arteriosus → pulmonary artery) that is usually loose. Rarely, the ring can be tight and cause upper airway obstruction. When the ductus is on the right there is a smaller retroesophageal impression owing to the directly arising anomalous left subclavian artery (Fig. 1–24*B*). A wide retroesophageal impression is present when the ductus is on the left owing to the dilated confluence of remnant ductal tissue and left subclavian artery (Fig. 1–24*C*). Both varieties of Type II arch have a low association with congenital heart disease and the association is higher when the ductus is on the right.[5]

The junction of the transverse and descending aorta — the "aortic knob" — is visible but not prominent in childhood (Fig. 1–17). What constitutes prominence varies with individual observers. However, deviation of the knob beyond the density of the descending aorta is considered prominent by many cardiac radiologists (Fig. 1–25). The aortic knob, like the ascending aorta, can be a clue to lesions that lead to pressure

or volume overload of the left ventricle (especially aortic regurgitation). In addition, abnormalities of this region may provide the first radiographic clue to the diagnosis of coarctation of the aorta (Fig. 1–26) or a patent ductus arteriosus (Fig. 1–27).

The descending thoracic aorta "hugs" the spine in childhood (Fig. 1–28). Tortuous or overt prominence in this region is suggestive of aortic regurgitation or other lesions associated with a wide pulse pressure (Fig. 1–29). Presumably, the tortuosity is secondary to the wide pulse pressure that produces hypermobility and dilatation of the descending aorta.

Pulmonary Trunk

Once thymic tissue recedes in later childhood, the pulmonary trunk should be visible along the left upper heart border. Absence of the density may be associated with decreased flow (tetralogy of Fallot, Fig. 1–30*A*), altered position of the pulmonary trunk (complete transposition, Fig. 1–30*B*), or the "left ventricular configuration" associated with left ventricular pressure or volume overload states (Fig. 1–30*C*). The state

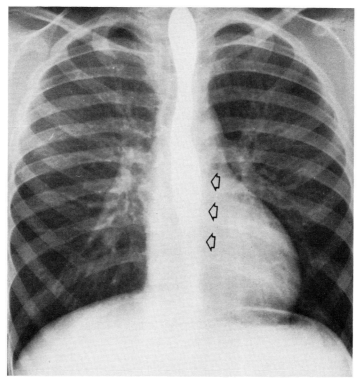

Figure 1–28. The descending thoracic aorta should "hug" the paraspinous region, even in the older child (arrows). When the descending thoracic aorta is prominent or tortuous, lesions associated with a wide pulse pressure should be considered. Aortic regurgitation is the most commonly associated lesion.

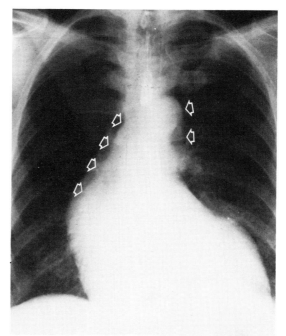

Figure 1–29. Note in this patient that the ascending aorta, aortic knob, and descending aorta (arrows) are all prominent. The pulmonary vascularity is normal and the left ventricle is enlarged. This 16-year-old male had Marfan's syndrome, cystic medial necrosis of the ascending aorta, and significant aortic regurgitation.

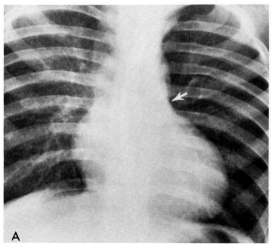

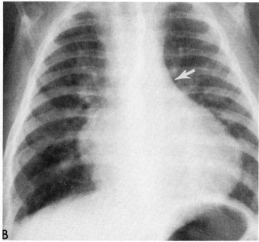

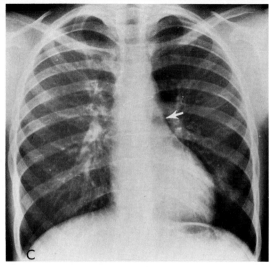

Figure 1–30. Three children in whom the pulmonary trunk is inapparent on the chest radiograph. The patient in A has tetralogy of Fallot, the patient in B has transposition of the great vessels, and the patient in C has hypertrophic subaortic stenosis (previous left ventricular myotomy). The clinical presentation of cyanosis in the first two patients, along with the presence of diminished vascularity in A and increased vascularity in B suggests the diagnosis. The patient in C was acyanotic and has normal vascularity.

of the pulmonary vascularity in the above three situations will be different in each case: diminished in tetralogy (Fig. 1–30A); increased (shunt) in complete transposition (Fig. 1–30B); and increased (pulmonary venous hypertension) or normal in left ventricular stress states (Fig. 1–30C). Therefore, the finding of an inapparent pulmonary trunk has little meaning by itself, but must be related to the clinical data (the presence or absence of cyanosis) and the appearance of the pulmonary vascularity.

Likewise, a prominent pulmonary trunk may be found in association with left to right shunts (Fig. 1–31A); left heart inflow lesions (Fig. 1–31B); high pulmonary resistance states (Eisenmenger's physiology) (Fig. 1–31C); pulmonary valve stenosis (Fig. 1–31D); or pulmonary hypertension from any cause. Therefore, for this finding to have meaning it must be related to the clinical situation and the pulmonary vascularity. The vascularity will be increased of the shunt type in moderate or large left to right shunts (Fig. 1–31A); show changes of pulmonary venous hypertension and congestion with left heart inflow lesions (Fig. 1–31B); show a high pulmonary resistance pattern in Eisenmenger states; and be normal in mild to moderate pulmonary valve stenosis (Fig. 1–31D). The pulmonary trunk is often apparent in normal teenagers (see Fig. 1–33) and this should be considered normal in this age group.

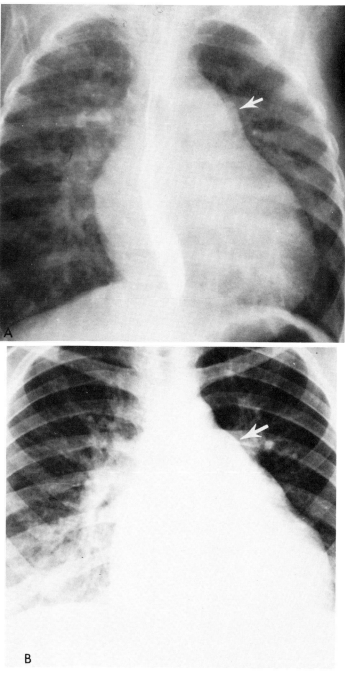

Figure 1–31. Four patients with a dilated pulmonary trunk (arrows). The patient in *A* has a large left-to-right shunt (VSD); the patient in *B* has severe rheumatic mitral regurgitation; the patient in *C* has systemic pulmonary artery pressure from a long-standing shunt (Eisenmenger's physiology); and the patient in *D* has pulmonary valve stenosis. Note that all four patients have different vascular patterns: *A,* shunt vascularity; *B,* pulmonary venous hypertension; *C,* high resistance pulmonary vascular pattern; and *D,* normal vascularity.

Illustration continued on opposite page

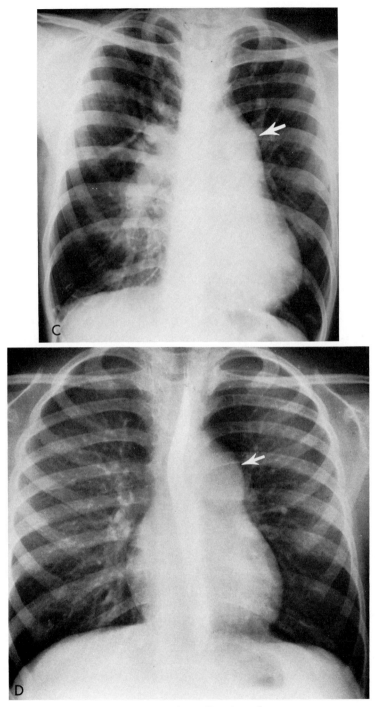

Figure 1–31. Continued

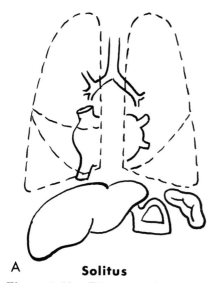
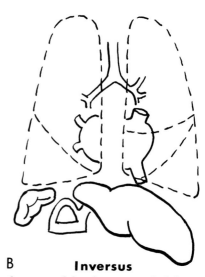

A   **Solitus**   B   **Inversus**

Figure 1–32. Diagrammatic representation of the anatomic features of the thoracic and abdominal viscera in the various body configurations. The patient with the anatomy in situs solitus is illustrated in *A;* situs inversus in *B;* the polysplenia syndrome in *C;* and the asplenia syndrome in *D.* The lungs are indicated with dashed lines, while organs that vary in position are indicated with dotted lines. (Modified from Stanger, et al.[8])

Illustration continued on opposite page

DETERMINATION OF SITUS

In approaching a case of suspected heart disease, especially complex congenital heart disease, it is important early in the analysis of diagnostic data to determine the position of the atria and viscera. The Latin translation of position is "situs," and the term visceroatrial situs has been used to describe this determination.[6] The importance of establishing the visceroatrial situs rests on the fact that cardiac ventricles, great arteries, lungs, and abdominal viscera can undergo positional and morphologic changes that render their classification into right- and left-sided structures impossible. This situation is frequently associated with congenital heart disease, often of a complex nature.

Several abdominal viscera have unique characteristics of morphology and position: the liver has two lobes (the right larger than the left) and both it and the gallbladder are located in the right upper quadrant; the solitary spleen is situated in the left upper quadrant with the stomach just medial to it; the junction of the duodenum and jejunum is in the left upper quadrant, while the ileocecal region is in the right lower quadrant. The lungs and mainstem bronchi are unique as well. The right lung has three lobes, separated by a minor and a major fissure. The left lung has two lobes, separat-

ed by a major fissure. The tracheobronchial tree has an eparterial bronchus on the right (a superiorly coursing bronchus above the right pulmonary artery), and a hyparterial bronchus on the left (a branchless bronchus that courses beneath the left pulmonary artery).

The bellwether cardiac chambers that determine right and left sidedness (and usually predict the position of the spleen and other noncardiac viscera) are the morphologic right atrium and the morphologic left atrium. These structures have their unique angiographic features (see Chapter 4). Normally, the inferior vena cava connects to the morphologic right atrium, and the right atrial appendage has a characteristic shape. Variability of superior vena caval connection makes this an unreliable indicator of atrial morphology. The left atrium can be identified only by its characteristically shaped appendage, since pulmonary venous drainage may be quite variable. The atrial morphology is independent of the position of the cardiac apex and ventricular relationships. These normal relationships are diagrammed in Figure 1–32A.

In individuals with cardiac structures and viscera in their usual positions, the term *situs* (position, situation) *solitus* (usual) is used. These individuals have normal cardiac morphology and position, and the spleen and noncardiac viscera likewise have their

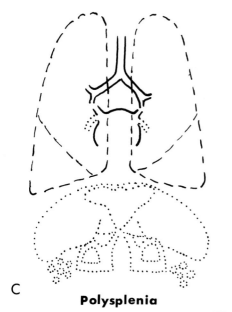

C **Polysplenia**

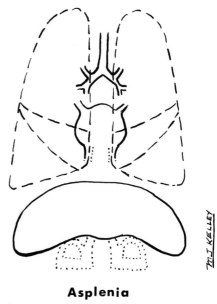

D **Asplenia**

Figure 1–32. Continued

usual morphology and position (Fig. 1–32A). In these normal individuals the right lung is trilobed (and receives the eparterial bronchus); the left lung is bilobed; and the liver, spleen, and stomach are in their ex-

pected locations (Fig. 1–33). The mirror image of this arrangement also rarely exists and is termed *situs inversus* (or mirror image visceroatrial situs). In this situation, the anatomic left atrium is on the right; the

Figure 1–33. Posteroanterior chest radiograph in a normal 17-year-old male. The minor fissure is faintly visualized in the right mid lung field (vertical arrows). The eparterial bronchus is seen emanating from the mainstem bronchus (curved arrow), and the left mainstem bronchus has its characteristic nonbranching pattern as it courses through the mediastinum (oblique arrows). The aortic knob, cardiac apex, and stomach (S) are in their expected locations.

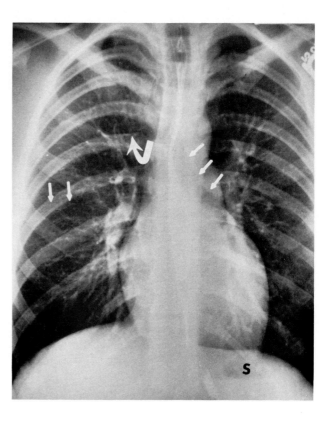

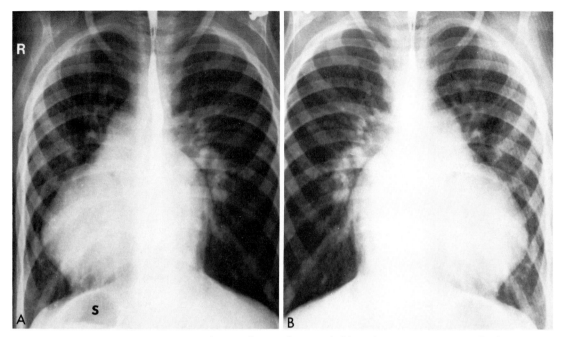

Figure 1–34. *A*, Posteroanterior chest radiograph in a child with situs inversus and a large atrial septal defect. The aortic arch, cardiac apex, and stomach (S) are all on the right (R). *B*, In individuals with situs inversus the standard chest radiograph can be reversed for easier interpretation.

anatomic right atrium is on the left; the trilobed lung and the eparterial bronchus are on the left; and the bilobed lung is on the right (Fig. 1–32*B*). Usually, the abdominal viscera will be reversed as well (situs inversus totalis). The incidence of cardiac anomalies with situs inversus is almost twice that of situs solitus.[6] The chest film in these individuals may be reversed and viewed in the usual fashion (Fig. 1–34).

The major portion of the heart and the cardiac apex in most individuals with situs solitus is on the left (Fig. 1–33). However, since the cardiac apex is independent of atrial position, it can occasionally be found in the midline *(mesocardia)* (Fig. 1–35) or rarely on the right *(dextrocardia* or right apex) (Fig. 1–36). The incidence of congenital heart disease is high in the latter case.[6] As expected, the mirror image situation exists in individuals with situs inversus. Usually the cardiac apex is on the right, but rarely it can be in the midline *(mesocardia)* or on the left *(levocardia* or left apex). These terms (mesocardia, and so on) indicate cardiac *position* only and give no information about cardiac morphology or body situs.

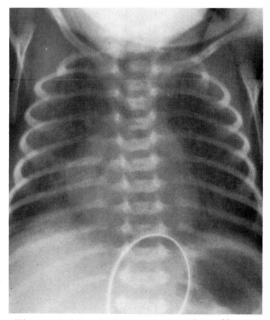

Figure 1–35. Anteroposterior chest film in a neonate with moderate respiratory distress. There is mild pulmonary parenchymal disease present. The cardiac silhouette is in a midline position (mesocardia). No cardiac murmurs or cardiac pathology was suspected.

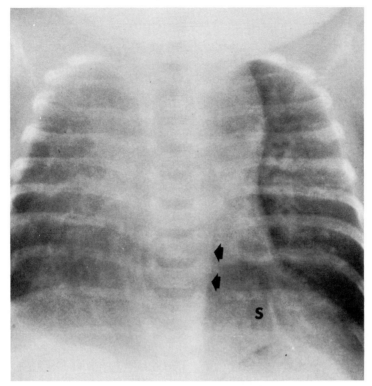

Figure 1–36. Anteroposterior chest film in a neonate with tachypnea and mild hypoxemia. Because of the severe lung disease on the right, the cardiac apex cannot be clearly defined, but no cardiac apex is present on the left. The descending aorta (arrows) and the stomach (S) are present on the left. At angiography, a right-sided cardiac apex was present. The patient had complex congenital heart disease and was classified as having situs solitus with dextrocardia.

Rarely, there are individuals whose visceroatrial situs defies classification into either situs solitus or situs inversus. In these cases, there is loss of the normal organ relationships and morphology, resulting in a loss of the usual right- and left-sided uniqueness described previously. In these individuals the positions of the viscera as well as their morphologic characteristics are indeterminate or ambiguous. The term *situs ambiguus* has been used to describe this situation.[7] Cases of situs ambiguus are invariably associated with splenic malformations—either absence of the spleen (asplenia syndrome) or multiple spleens (polysplenia syndrome). The key cardiac structures, the atria, would be expected to participate in this attempt by the body to obliterate sidedness. In fact, in many cases of situs ambiguus, there is a common atrial chamber that receives both systemic and pulmonary venous connections.

The tendency in the *polysplenia syndrome* is for the body to become bilaterally *left sided*. This is reflected by the presence of two bilobed lungs (no minor fissure) connected to two hyparterial bronchi (Fig. 1–32C). There may be hepatic symmetry and there are multiple small spleens usually situated along the greater curvature of the variably located stomach (Fig. 1–32C). A common feature of this syndrome is interruption of the hepatic segment of the inferior vena cava. Venous drainage from the abdomen occurs through the azygous system (azygous continuation of the inferior vena cava) to a right- or left-sided superior vena cava. When congenital heart disease is associated with the polysplenia syndrome, the lesions tend to be left-to-right shunts. An autopsy study has documented the variety of lesions that occur in the polysplenia syndrome (Table 1–4).[8]

The tendency in the *asplenia syndrome* is

TABLE 1–4. Cardiovascular Anomalies Associated with Splenic Syndromes°

POLYSPLENIA (17 Cases)		ASPLENIA (19 Cases)	
Atrial Septal Defect (2°)	10	Endocardial Cushion Defects	19
Interrupted Inferior Vena Cava	8	Pulmonary Atresia or Stenosis	17
Patent Ductus Arteriosus	7	Transposition (d or l)	14
Endocardial Cushion Defects	6	Double Outlet Right Ventricle	4
Ventricular Septal Defects	6		
Double Outlet Right Ventricle	5		
Aortic or Subaortic Stenosis	3		
Others	4		

°Modified from Stanger.[8]

for the body to become bilaterally *right sided.* Besides two right lungs, there are often two right atrial appendages, two superior venae cavae, and an inferior vena cava that may connect to the common atrium on the right, in the midline, or on the left[6] (Fig. 1–32D). In addition, the relationship between the abdominal aorta and inferior vena cava is frequently lost.[9] Other attempts at total right sidedness are reflected in the presence of hepatic symmetry; midline or absent gallbladder; and, of course, absence of the spleen. Malrotation of the small and large bowel is commonly associated. This syndrome invariably presents in infants with severe cyanotic congenital heart disease characterized by endocardial cushion defects, transposition complexes, and pulmonary stenosis or atresia (Table 1–4).[8] Because of the last lesion, the chest film usually demonstrates decreased vascularity.

In most infants, children, and adolescents with heart disease, the cardiac structures and viscera are in their usual position. The chest radiograph contributes valuable information and should enable the determination of situs in most individuals. Situs solitus (and, therefore, morphologically and positionally normal atria and spleen) is assumed when the cardiac apex and stomach are on the left (Fig. 1–37). When this situation does not pertain, there is a *cardiac malposition* (that is, the cardiac apex and/or stomach is other than left sided). One must then further analyze the chest film (including the upper abdomen) for the radiographic indicators of visceroatrial situs.

One of the most reliable indicators of visceroatrial situs is the tracheobronchial tree.[7] When this cannot be clearly visualized on a chest radiograph in which situs is a question, an overpenetrated (Fig. 1–38) or Bucky chest film should be obtained. One is seeking the location of the eparterial bronchus in this analysis, since it has been determined that the position of this bronchus indicates the position of the right atrium beneath it. As indicated previously, the eparterial bronchus arises superiorly as the first branch of the right mainstem bronchus and courses above the right pulmonary artery. In addition, the origin of the right mainstem bronchus is usually at a greater obtuse angle than the left. The left mainstem bronchus has no eparterial bronchus and originates at a lesser obtuse angle from the trachea. The left pulmonary artery courses over it from anterior to posterior.

When the chest film indicates that the morphologic right bronchus is on the right and the morphologic left bronchus is on the left (Fig. 1–37), then normal atria are present and situs solitus exists. When the morphologic right bronchus is on the left and the morphologic left bronchus is on the right, mirror image atria are present and situs inversus exists (Fig. 1–34A). The presence of a minor fissure should also be sought as a verification of the side of the eparterial bronchus, since in situs solitus it exists only in the trilobed right lung. Finally, the position of the stomach and liver density should be checked. In situs inversus, the stomach bubble should be on the right and the major liver density on the left (Fig. 1–34A). Hepatic symmetry (Fig. 1–40A) is present in approximately 50 per cent of cases with situs ambiguus so that a normal liver density does not exclude a splenic abnormality.[6] Generally, situs am-

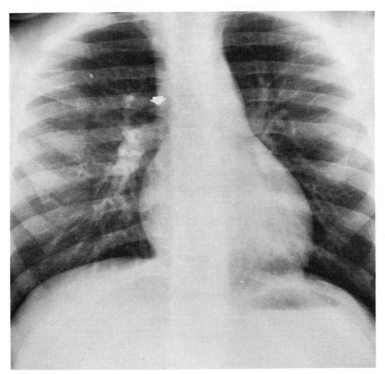

Figure 1–37. Posteroanterior chest radiograph in a six-year-old female with an infiltrate in the left lower lobe. The cardiac apex and stomach are on the left, presumptive information indicating situs solitus. The eparterial bronchus can be vaguely seen as the first branch of the right mainstem bronchus (arrow). The left mainstem bronchus has no eparterial bronchus and arises from the trachea at a lesser obtuse angle.

biguus should be suspected when the stomach and apex are not both on the left or both on the right (Fig. 1–40B). One should then seek out the eparterial bronchus.

Suspicion of the *polysplenia syndrome* should arise when the tracheobronchial tree shows two hyparterial bronchi (bilateral left sidedness) (Figs. 1–38A and 1–39A) and the absence of a minor fissure on the right. Enlargement of the azygos vein (Figs. 1–38A and 1–39A) is frequently present owing to increased flow through this system consequent to the interrupted hepatic segment of the inferior vena cava (Figs. 1–38D and E and 1–39C). The lateral chest film in normal individuals usually demonstrates the density of the inferior vena cava (Fig. 1–38C). In patients with interrupted hepatic segments of the inferior vena cava, this density may be absent (Fig. 1–38B). However, the presence of hepatic veins entering the atrium in patients with an interrupted inferior vena cava may simulate the normal inferior vena cava density (Fig. 1–39B), and, therefore, this sign should be interpreted with caution.[10] As mentioned previously, polysplenia syndrome presents in childhood with acyanotic forms of congenital heart disease. In fact, the syndrome may exist with no significant cardiac abnormalities at all.[8] A summary of the clinical and radiographic features of the polysplenia syndrome is given in Table 1–5.

The *asplenia syndrome* should be suspected when the tracheobronchial tree demonstrates two eparterial bronchi (bilateral right sidedness) (Fig. 1–40B). Two minor fissures (two trilobed lungs) should also be sought for verification (Fig. 1–40B). As mentioned previously, these cases present in infancy with severe cyanosis and diminished vascularity on the chest x-ray (Fig. 1–40) and have complex intracardiac anomalies (Table 1–4). A summary of the clinical and radiographic features of this syndrome is given in Table 1–5.

Text continued on page 49

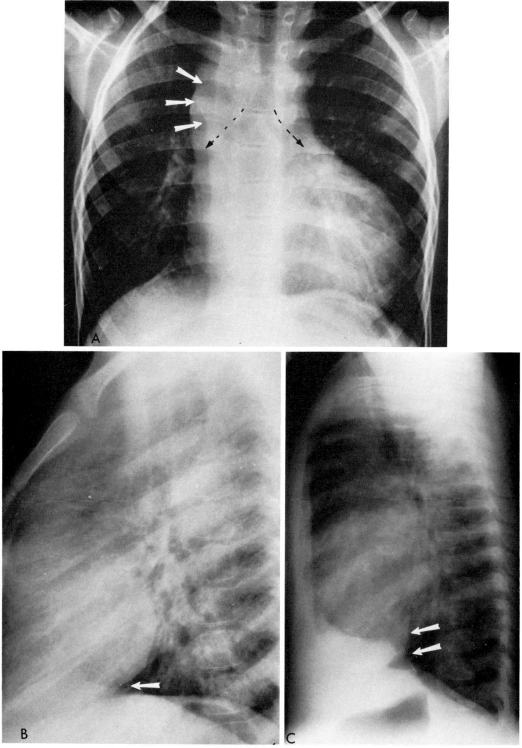

Figure 1–38. Polysplenia syndrome. On the posteroanterior chest radiograph (A) in this acyanotic patient, there is a symmetrical tracheobronchial tree with two hyparterial bronchi (arrows) indicating bilateral left sidedness. In addition, the azygous vein is enlarged (white arrows) secondary to interruption of the hepatic segment of the inferior vena cava and azygous continuation. The lateral chest radiograph (B) shows absence of the normal inferior vena caval density in the posteroinferior cardiac margin (arrow). A normal lateral chest film is shown in C for comparison. Note the inferior vena caval density (arrows). Absence of the IVC density, however, is not invariably diagnostic of interruption of the IVC (see Fig. 1–39).

Illustration continued on opposite page

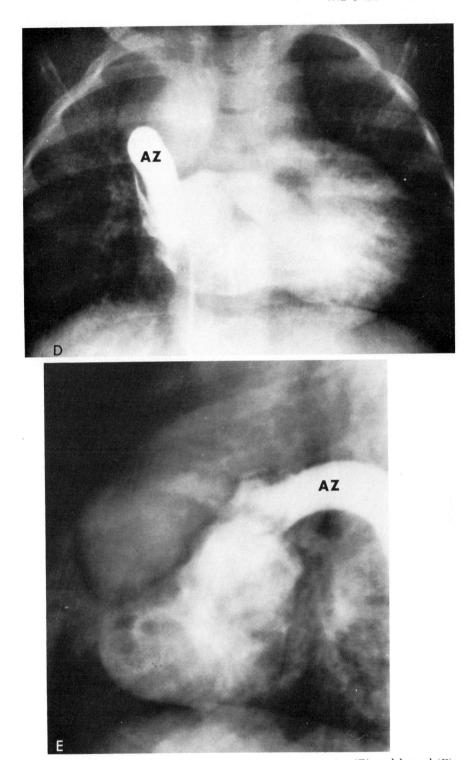

Figure 1–38 Continued. An azygous venogram in anteroposterior (D) and lateral (E) projections demonstrates that venous return from the abdomen occurs through the dilated azygous vein (AZ).

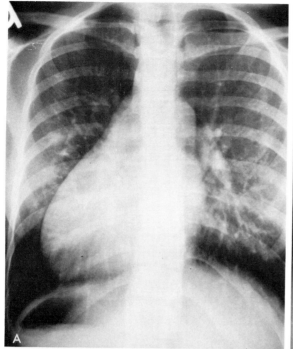

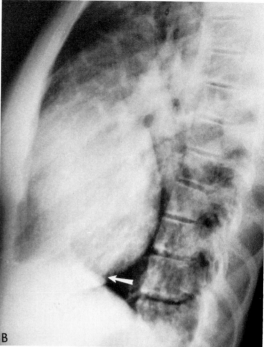

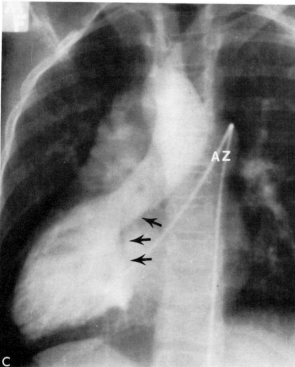

Figure 1–39. Posteroanterior (*A*) and lateral (*B*) chest radiographs in a patient with polysplenia syndrome. The cardiac apex and stomach are on the right and the tracheobronchial tree is symmetrical with bilateral hyparterial bronchi. No minor fissure is present and there is shunt vascularity. Note prominence of the left peritracheal region. The lateral film shows a "normal" density in the region usually occupied by the inferior vena cava. Catheter passage and angiocardiogram performed in the anteroposterior projection (*C*) indicate that there is azygous continuation of the inferior vena cava through a dilated azygous (AZ) vein (accounting for the density on the posteroanterior chest radiograph in the left peritracheal region). Although the left ventricle is located to the right, the angiographic appearance is typical for an endocardial cushion defect, with the so-called "gooseneck" deformity (arrows). Multiple spleens were noted on the liver-spleen scan.

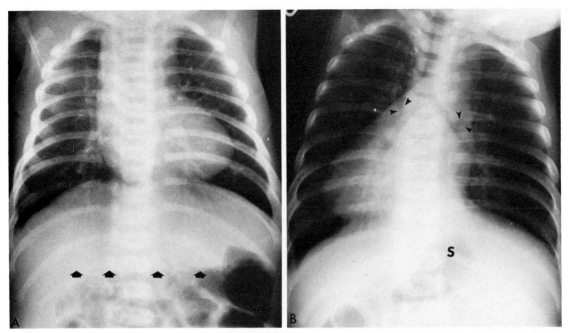

Figure 1–40. Asplenia syndrome. Anteroposterior chest radiographs in two cyanotic infants demonstrating radiographic features of the asplenia syndrome. In *A*, there is hepatic symmetry (arrows), diminished pulmonary vascularity, and an upturned cardiac apex. The stomach bubble (not clearly defined on this film) was located in the midline. In *B*, the stomach is in the midline, the tracheobronchial tree is symmetrical with bilateral eparterial bronchi (arrowheads), and there are bilateral minor fissures (poorly seen on this reproduction). The pulmonary vascularity is mildly reduced and the cardiac apex is on the right. Both patients had complex congenital heart disease characterized by endocardial cushion deformities, transposition of the great vessels, and pulmonary stenosis.

TABLE 1–5. Clinical and Radiographic Features of the Splenic Syndromes*

	POLYSPLENIA	ASPLENIA
Symptoms	Cyanosis (~20%) CHF (~80%)	Cyanosis (~95%) CHF (~5%)
Laboratory findings Heinz or Howell-Jolly bodies (blood smear) Biliary atresia	 Negative Positive	 Positive Negative
Abdomen	± Horizontal liver Stomach not midline Malrotation of bowel	Horizontal liver Stomach midline Malrotation of bowel
Lungs	Absent minor fissure Bilateral left bronchi	Bilateral minor fissures Bilateral right bronchi
Pulmonary vascularity	Usually increased	Usually decreased
SVC	Frequently bilateral	Usually bilateral
Interrupted IVC	50%	Negative
Liver/spleen scan	Multiple spleens	Absent spleen/symmetrical liver

*Modified from Stanger.[8]
CHF = congestive heart failure
IVC = inferior vena cava
SVC = superior vena cava

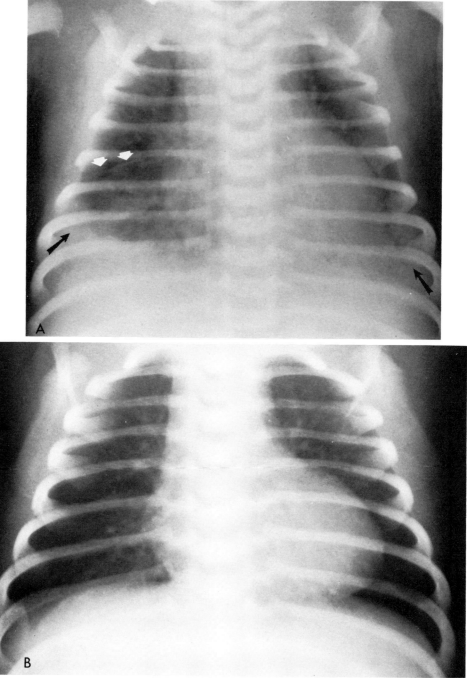

Figure 1–41. Anteroposterior chest radiograph in a patient with transient tachypnea of the newborn ("wet lung" syndrome). In A, the patient was moderately symptomatic. Note the presence of ill-defined vascular markings and bilateral pleural effusions (arrows). The minor fissure is thickened (white arrows). In a chest radiograph taken two days later (B), the lung markings have essentially returned to normal and the pleural effusions have cleared.

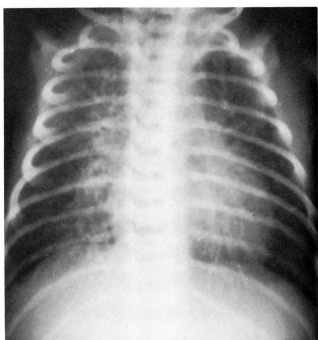

Figure 1–42. Chest radiograph in a neonate with severe respiratory distress and cyanosis. Lung markings are increased and there are bilateral interstitial infiltrates. Kerley B lines were seen on the original radiograph. These findings are indistinguishable from obstructed varieties of pulmonary venous return and other severe obstructions to left heart inflow. This infant died shortly after birth and was found to have congenital pulmonary lymphangiectasia.

LUNG PARENCHYMA

Approximately two-thirds of all cases of congenital heart disease present in the newborn period.[11] In the neonate with suspected congenital heart disease, primary lung disease presents the major differential diagnostic problem. Most pulmonary conditions that create a clinical dilemma can be diagnosed accurately by using the chest film alone. Some of these may alter or obscure the pulmonary vasculature. For these reasons, it is important to assess the lung parenchyma prior to evaluating the pulmonary vasculature in patients with suspected heart disease. It is not the purpose of this section to discuss neonatal pulmonary disease in detail, but to point out areas of possible confusion.

Certain neonatal pulmonary diseases result in an apparent increase in the pulmonary vascularity. Transient tachypnea of the newborn or the "wet lung" syndrome in its mild to moderate form may be associated with interstitial changes secondary to engorged perivascular lymphatics. These changes occur in the lower lobes and/or perihilar region and may simulate the radiographic pattern of pulmonary venous hypertension (congestion) associated with various congenital heart lesions that obstruct left

heart inflow or outflow (Fig. 1–41A). Generally, there will be progressive clearing of these interstitial infiltrates by 72 hours (Fig. 1–41B). The typical clinical picture in these acyanotic infants is tachypnea followed by dyspnea that ceases in 48 to 72 hours. Another entity, congenital pulmonary lymphangiectasia, may show a pattern in the lungs that is indistinguishable from forms of congenital heart disease associated with severe pulmonary venous obstruction (for example, total anomalous pulmonary venous connection below the diaphragm). The chest film findings in this rare condition are increased vascularity, fine reticular infiltrates, and Kerley B lines (Fig. 1–42). Clinically, these patients show severe respiratory distress and cyanosis and die soon after birth. Total anomalous pulmonary venous return below the diaphragm, a surgically correctable lesion, may have an identical radiographic picture and, if untreated, a similar clinical course.

Several conditions may result in extensive infiltrates in the lungs that obscure the pulmonary vascularity. In the chest film of the premature child with immature lungs and respiratory distress syndrome (RDS), the vascularity may be impossible to evaluate (Fig. 1–43). However, it is important to try. In the less severe forms of RDS it may

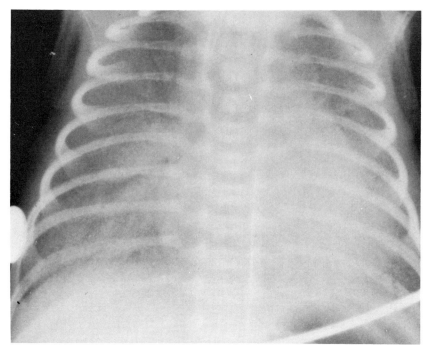

Figure 1–43. Anteroposterior radiograph in a neonate with severe respiratory distress and hypoxemia. The classic radiographic findings of respiratory distress syndrome are present. There is diffuse granular appearance in both lung fields, air bronchograms are present, and there is normal heart size. Difficulty in interpreting pulmonary vascularity in such a film is obvious.

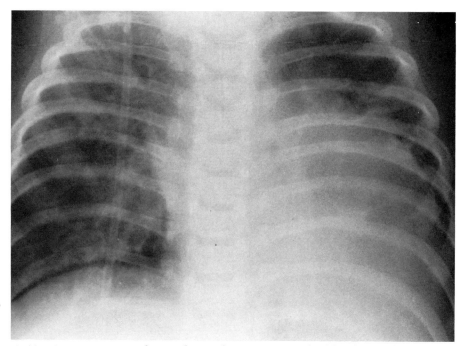

Figure 1–44. Anteroposterior chest radiograph in a two-month-old infant with chronic pulmonary disease and central nervous system problems (note the ventriculoperitoneal line overlying the right lung). There are coarse bilateral infiltrates in both lungs. Cardiomegaly in this patient was thought to be due to right heart hypertension secondary to long-standing pulmonary disease. In this case of bronchopulmonary dysplasia, an assessment of pulmonary vascularity would be impossible.

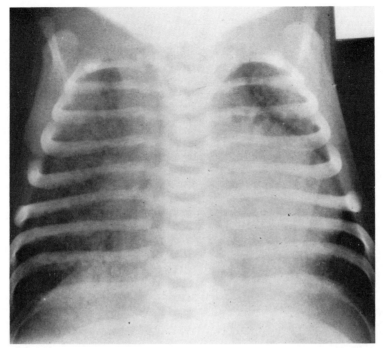

Figure 1–45. Bilateral alveolar infiltrates are noted in this infant with meconium aspiration. The chest is slightly hyperaerated so that the cardiomegaly present appears to be real. Pulmonary vascularity is obscured.

be possible to detect increased vascularity. It has been shown that there is a good correlation between increased vascularity and cardiomegaly in those infants in whom RDS is complicated by a patent ductus arteriosus (see Chapter 6).[12]

In the spectrum of diseases termed bronchopulmonary dysplasia or Mikity-Wilson syndrome, the bilateral coarse or reticular interstitial infiltrates usually obscure the pulmonary vascularity (Fig. 1–44). This is also true of the bilateral alveolar infiltrates associated with meconium aspiration (Fig. 1–45), neonatal pneumonia or pulmonary hemorrhage.

Pulmonary vascularity may be increased in symptomatic infants of diabetic mothers (Fig. 1–46A); in those with transient hypoglycemia or polycythemia (Fig. 1–46B); and in infants with erythroblastosis fetalis. Lung infiltrates (usually alveolar) often accompany these conditions. With proper therapy the increased vascularity and heart size in these infants should return to normal (Fig. 1–46C and D). If not, underlying heart disease should be suspected.

Several surgically correctable respiratory conditions may be associated with respira-

tory distress and/or cyanosis and may thus mimic heart disease. They can generally be diagnosed using the chest film and other radiographic techniques. These lesions include tracheoesophageal fistula, esophageal atresia, tension pneumothorax, diaphragmatic hernia, lobar emphysema, cystic adenomatoid malformation, mediastinal masses, and upper airway obstruction. Neonates with tracheoesophageal fistula and esophageal atresia have a high incidence of congenital anomalies and frequently have associated congenital cardiac lesions (ventricular septal defect, patent ductus arteriosus).

The lung parenchyma should also be assessed in older children with congenital heart disease. The child with an undetected left-to-right shunt commonly presents for the first time with pneumonia (Fig. 1–47). This may be indistinguishable from pulmonary edema. Children with large left-to-right shunts often have a "hyperaerated" chest with flattened hemidiaphragms, a bowed sternum, and an increased retrosternal air space (Fig. 1–48). There are several possible explanations for this picture: (1) there is increased lung volume secondary to

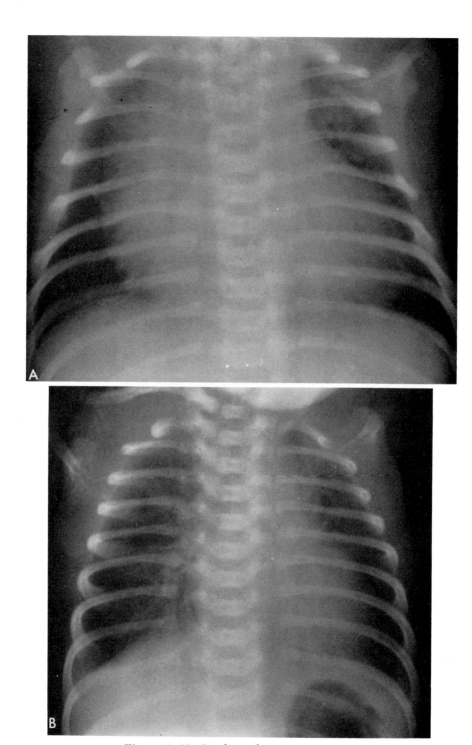

Figure 1–46. See legend on opposite page

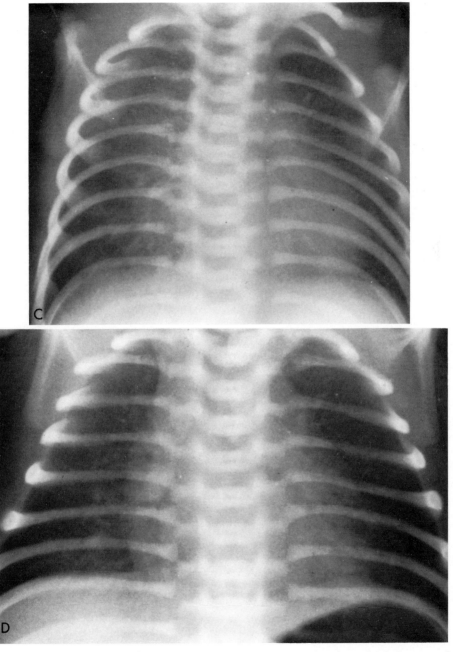

Figure 1–46. Anteroposterior chest radiographs in a symptomatic infant of a diabetic mother (A); a neonate with transient polycythemia (B); and a newborn with erythroblastosis fetalis (C). Follow-up radiograph obtained in the patient shown in (D) demonstrates clearing of the lung fields.

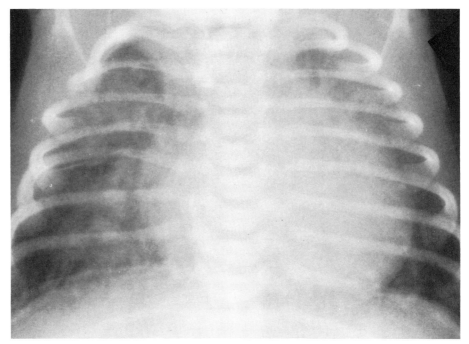

Figure 1–47. Chest radiograph in an infant with fever and tachypnea. There is right upper lobe infiltrate. Subsequent clinical examination of the child indicated the presence of a large left-to-right shunt.

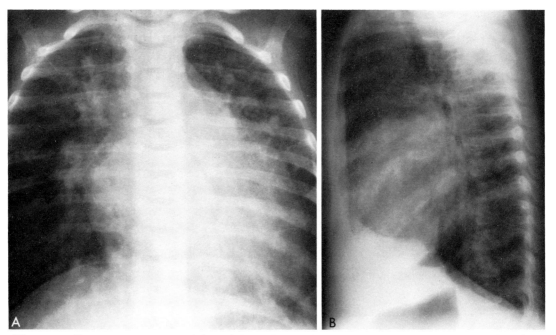

Figure 1–48. Anteroposterior (A) and lateral (B) chest radiographs in a child with a large left-to-right shunt (reflected in the pulmonary vascularity). There is also significant hyperaeration with flattening of the hemidiaphragms, a bowed sternum and increase in the retrosternal airspace.

the increase in blood flow to the lungs; (2) the presence of interstitial edema causes increased airway resistance; (3) the large arteries and veins associated with the shunt cause increased airway resistance; and (4) there is upper airway obstruction. The fourth factor should be considered especially in individuals with Down's syndrome who may have chronic upper airway obstruction.

PULMONARY VASCULARITY

General Considerations

The chest film makes perhaps its greatest contribution to the assessment of children with suspected heart disease in allowing one to evaluate the state of pulmonary vascularity. If this information, obtained from a technically adequate radiograph, is coupled with certain clinical information regarding the presence or absence of cyanosis, it provides a useful physiologic framework for considering certain differential diagnostic possibilities. A more specific diagnosis can then be made utilizing anatomic clues present on the radiograph (cardiac configuration and chamber size; presence or absence of great vessel dilatation) and anatomic and functional information provided by M-mode and two dimensional echocardiography.

The importance of interpreting technically adequate films when assessing vascularity cannot be overemphasized. The most common problems are underexposed films or those taken in expiration. Both standard posteroanterior and lateral films add unique information and each should be used. Although oblique films (especially the left anterior oblique) taken as part of a cardiac series may add confirmatory information regarding the size of vessels at the lung bases, they are primarily complementary. Generally, if the posteroanterior and lateral films show normal vascularity, the oblique views are unlikely to change this impression.

Interpretation of pulmonary vasculature admittedly involves subjective comparisons — comparisons of vessel size with volume of lung, with the age and size of the patient, and with the expected "normal" vascular appearance based on one's own accumulated experience. Hopefully, this experience is based on correlating one's own "calls" as to vascular appearance with known hemodynamic measurements. There is really no way to absolutely quantitate pulmonary blood flow on the plain chest film, and as expected there are significant intra- and inter-observer errors in evaluating increased and decreased vascularity.[13] Errors appear to be greater in conditions associated with underperfusion. However, most radiologists would agree that they should be able to detect increased flow (shunt vascularity) when the left-to-right shunt is associated with a pulmonary to systemic flow ratio (Qp:Qs) of 2:1 or greater. Although several studies have correlated radiographic signs of pulmonary venous hypertension with hemodynamic measurements in adults with chronic cardiac disease, few studies of this nature are available in infants and children.[14] In fact, infants with congestive failure may manifest different patterns on their chest radiographs than older children and adults.[14]

The presence and size of the pulmonary trunk should be assessed before analyzing the pulmonary vascularity. Taken by itself, a prominent or inapparent pulmonary trunk has little meaning. When used in conjunction with the clinical history and accurate assessment of pulmonary vascularity, however, it can add valuable information. For example, a *prominent* pulmonary trunk in an acyanotic individual with normal vascularity suggests pulmonary valve stenosis. The combination of a cyanotic child with an *inapparent* pulmonary trunk and shunt vascularity suggests the diagnosis of complete transposition or truncus arteriosus. If the vascularity is diminished in the latter situation, the diagnosis of tetralogy of Fallot is most likely.

Among individuals with suspected heart disease, changes occur in the pulmonary vasculature that are reflected on the chest radiograph. Three basic patterns can be seen: (1) normal pulmonary vasculature; (2) prominent pulmonary vasculature; and (3) decreased pulmonary vasculature.

Normal Pulmonary Vascularity

Although this vascular pattern is present in normal individuals, it may also be seen in association with significant hemodynamic lesions. These include obstructive lesions

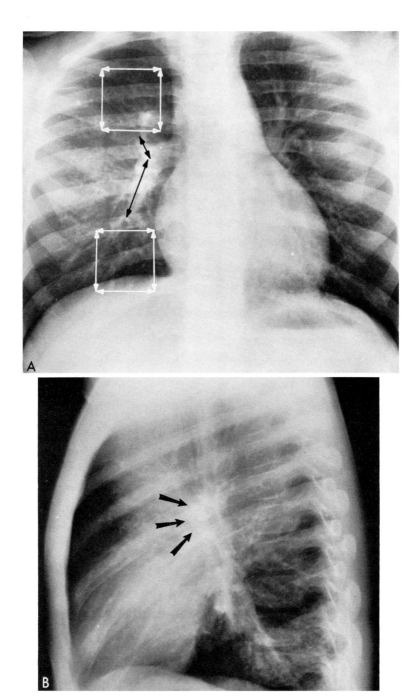

Figure 1–49. Posteroanterior and lateral chest radiographs in a child with no cardiac lesions. Normal pulmonary vascularity is present on the frontal (A) and lateral (B) films. The "hilar angle" formed by the right upper lobe pulmonary vein and the right descending pulmonary artery is indicated on the frontal film (arrows). Note that the ratio of vessel size in the lower vs. the upper lobes is approximately 2:1. The areas demarcated by boxes are those frequently used to assess vessel size. On the lateral view, the right main pulmonary artery density is indicated (arrows).

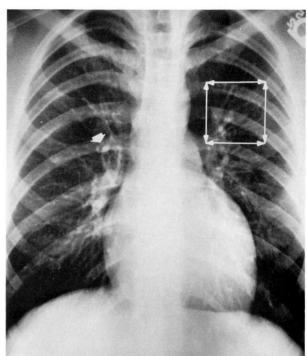

Figure 1–50. Posteroanterior chest radiograph in a normal teenager demonstrates that pulmonary vessels can be seen through the cardiac silhouette in the left lung. These should be compared in size with vessels in the upper lung fields in the square indicated (arrows). Note additionally the presence of similar size bronchus and artery seen on end in the right perihilar region (arrow).

involving the left heart (aortic stenosis, coarctation), and right heart (pulmonary valve stenosis), and myocardial disease (myocardiopathy, myocarditis). In addition, individuals with small left-to-right shunts (Qp:Qs < 2:1) or "balanced" lesions (ventricular septal defect with pulmonary valve stenosis) may have normal vascularity. The normal pulmonary trunk should be apparent as a straight or somewhat concave density along the left upper heart border just below the density formed by the transverse and descending aortic junction or aortic knob (Fig. 1–49). Its location should not be confused with that of the left atrial appendage (a more inferior convexity located just beneath the left mainstem bronchus), which is not usually present on a normal chest film.

The structures that contribute most to the densities in the hilar regions include the distal portions of the right and left main pulmonary arteries. The pulmonary trunk overlies part of the left main pulmonary artery on the frontal film. In healthy children under six years of age, thymic tissue may obscure both of these structures on the frontal film and the lateral view becomes the only method of evaluating their size. Using the lateral film, one should be able to evaluate the size of the right main pulmona-

ry artery as a *round* density and occasionally the left main pulmonary artery as a *curved* density crossing over the left mainstem bronchus (Fig. 1–49*B*). The variability of appearance of these arteries on the lateral film is due to the fact that they take origin from the pulmonary trunk at different angles — the right arising at almost 90° and the left at about 10° — as essentially a direct posterior continuation of the pulmonary trunk. Additional contribution is made to the hilar densities by the upper lobe pulmonary veins. On the frontal film, the right upper lobe vein often forms a discrete angle with the proximal portion of the right descending pulmonary artery—the so-called "hilar angle" (Figs. 1–49*A* and 1–50).

Generally, when one speaks of the pulmonary vasculature as normal, increased, or decreased, one is assessing three things: (1) the size and distinctness of the hilar vessels; (2) the size and distinctness of extrahilar pulmonary vessels; and (3) the distribution of the extrahilar pulmonary vessels. In normal upright individuals, the extrahilar vessels taper uniformly from the hila to the periphery and the vessels coursing to and from the lower lobes are larger than those supplying and draining the upper lobes (Figs. 1–49*A* and 1–50). The ratio of vessel size in the lower versus upper lobes is approximately 2:1. Although a point is often made of distinguishing pulmonary veins from pulmonary arteries in the assessment of extrahilar vasculature, this is more of an exercise in anatomy than physiology. For practical purposes, it is not necessary to distinguish arteries from veins, since conditions that are associated with increased pulmonary vasculature (pulmonary venous hypertension, left-to-right shunts, bronchial circulation) or diminished pulmonary vasculature (severe obstruction to pulmonary flow) are associated with increased or decreased flow to *both* pulmonary arteries and veins.

Abnormal Pulmonary Vascularity

Prominent Pulmonary Vascularity

Prominent pulmonary vascularity is divided into three basic patterns: (1) that which results from excess flow to the pulmonary vessels secondary to a systemic (left) to pulmonary (right) shunt — *shunt vascularity;* (2) that which is associated with pulmonary venous obstruction or hypertension — *pulmonary venous hypertension pattern;* and (3) that which is associated with increased lung flow through bronchial or systemic arteries arising from the aorta—*bronchial vascularity.* Two other prominent patterns (both related to left-to-right shunts) may be seen. When very large left-to-right shunts are associated with congestive failure, interstitial edema may be superimposed on the basic shunt pattern, producing the *flow-failure pattern.* This is often seen in neonates. In certain patients, the initial left-to-right shunt is associated with high pulmonary resistance and pulmonary arterial thickening, resulting in Eisenmenger's physiology and eventually a right-to-left shunt. The chest radiograph in these individuals frequently reveals a discrepancy in extrahilar and hilar vessels —*the high pulmonary resistance pattern.*

SHUNT VASCULARITY. In the presence of a moderate to large systemic (left) to pulmonary (right) shunt and as a response to increased pulmonary blood flow and pressure, the pulmonary arteries and veins dilate. The magnitude of systemic-to-pulmonary shunts varies from small to large and depends upon (1) the size of the communication between the two circuits and (2) the relative resistance to flow into the

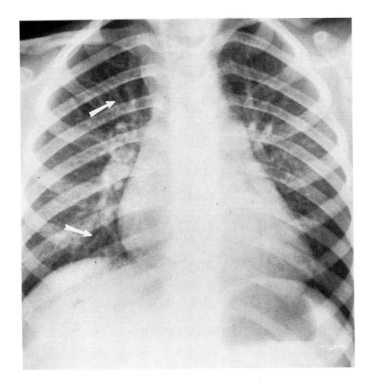

Figure 1–51. Posteroanterior chest radiograph in a patient with a 1.75:1 left-to-right shunt at the atrial level. There is uniform prominence of pulmonary vascularity both in the lower and upper lung zones as indicated by arrows. This pattern may be seen in left-to-right shunts that result in a pulmonary to systemic flow ratio of less than 2:1.

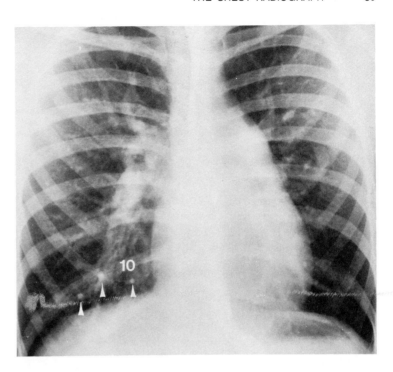

Figure 1–52. Posteroanterior chest radiograph in a 15-year-old with an atrial septal defect and a pulmonary to systemic flow ratio of 3:1. Note that there is generalized dilatation of lower and upper lobe vessels, but that the lower lobe vessels are larger. The hilar angle is well preserved and there are sharp, smooth margins to the vessels. Note the vessels on end (arrows) in the right lower lung field. It is unusual to see vessels of this size below the tenth posterior rib (10), unless pulmonary blood flow is increased.

two circuits. In patients with left-to-right shunts in which the pulmonary-systemic flow ratio is less than 2:1, the chest film may be normal or at most there will be a reduction of the normal gradient of vessel size between upper and lower lung zones (Fig. 1–51). This is due to the "recruitment" of reserve areas of the normally underperfused upper lung zones. As the magnitude of the shunt approaches 3:1 or 4:1, the increased size (from 1½ to 2 times normal) of vessels in all lung zones is appreciated (Fig. 1–52). Veins and arteries are affected equally as are both central and peripheral vessels. Sharp, smooth margins of these enlarged vessels are usually maintained unless interstitial edema is superimposed. Dilatation takes place in a rather uniform manner throughout the lungs, with the large central pulmonary arteries and veins maintaining their *distinct* outlines (Fig. 1–52). In other words, shunt vascularity is an accentuation of the normal vascular pattern. Several clues will aid in the appreciation of this pattern. First, distinct "shunt" vessels may be seen below the tenth posterior rib (Fig. 1–52). Second, in suggesting shunt vascularity, one may compare the size of an extrahilar pulmonary artery with its companion bronchus when these structures are seen on end. The most productive area to

look for this relationship is just lateral and superior to the hilar vessels (Fig. 1–53). Finally, the increased size and density of enlarged hilar vessels are often best appreciated on the lateral chest film (Fig. 1–54).

The diameter of the right descending pulmonary artery and the trachea may be measured with accuracy in children over two years of age. We have observed that 90 per cent of normal children have tracheal and right descending pulmonary artery diameters that are the same or within 2 mm of each other.[15] Furthermore, no child with a left-to-right shunt (whether small, moderate, or large) has a right descending pulmonary artery diameter *less than* the tracheal diameter (Fig. 1–55). Although accurate radiographic assessment of pulmonary vascularity is a matter of experience, this objective measurement would appear to be of value in borderline cases. The right descending pulmonary artery should be measured where it parallels the right intermediate bronchus and crosses the right upper lobe pulmonary vein. The tracheal diameter is taken just above the impression of the aortic knob (Fig. 1–55).

The size of the pulmonary trunk is not an accurate predictor of the magnitude of the shunt, since it may be large in small shunts and only moderately enlarged in large

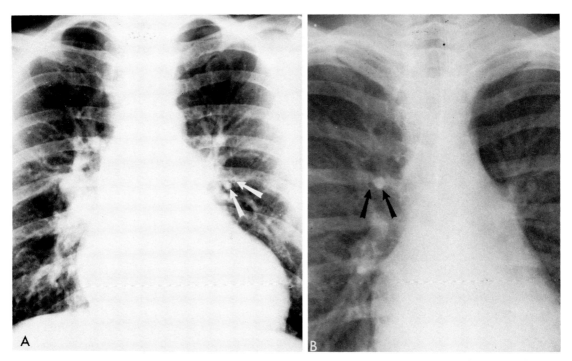

Figure 1–53. Posteroanterior chest radiographs in two patients with moderate left-to-right shunts. In *A*, the vessel seen on end with its companion bronchus in the left upper lobe is too large (arrows). In *B*, the same situation is seen in the right upper lobe (arrows). This appearance of vessel size in the upper lung fields may also be seen in patients who have redistribution of pulmonary flow secondary to pulmonary venous hypertension. Therefore, the lower lobe vessels must also be assessed for size in distinguishing redistribution from shunt vascularity. Both of these patients had moderate left-to-right shunts.

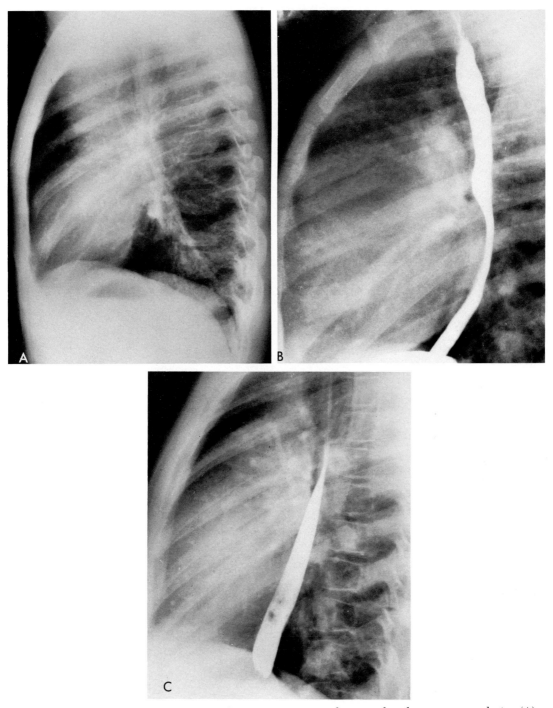

Figure 1–54. Lateral chest radiographs in a patient with normal pulmonary vascularity (A); a patient with a large ventricular septal defect (B); and a patient with a large atrial septal defect (C). Note the prominence of the hilar vessels in the two patients with left-to-right shunts. Notice also that the barium-filled esophagus demonstrates left atrial enlargement in the patient with the VSD, while the left atrium is normal in size in the patient with the ASD.

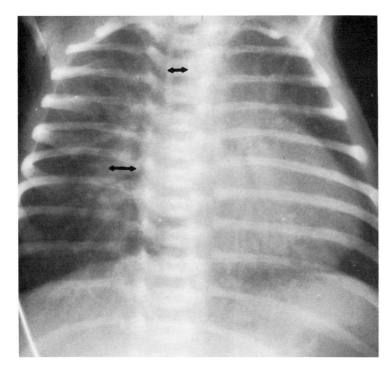

Figure 1–55. Comparison of the diameter of the right descending pulmonary artery (lower arrow) with that of the trachea (upper arrow) may be helpful in assessing pulmonary vascularity in borderline cases. In children with left-to-right shunts, the descending pulmonary artery diameter is never less than that of the trachea. This infant had a moderately sized VSD.

shunts. In addition, it varies considerably in size in normal individuals and may be dilated as an isolated finding.

In the infant whose left heart failure is secondary to a large left-to-right shunt, a flow-failure pattern will predominate, with generalized vascular engorgement being the predominant feature (Fig. 1–56).

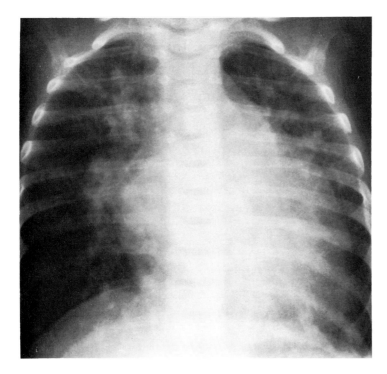

Figure 1–56. Anteroposterior chest radiograph in an infant with a large left-to-right shunt and congestive failure. Notice the ill-defined yet prominent pulmonary vascular markings. Lower lobe pulmonary vessels remain dilated in the face of a large left-to-right shunt, even though interstitial pulmonary edema makes them less distinct than in the uncomplicated left-to-right shunt.

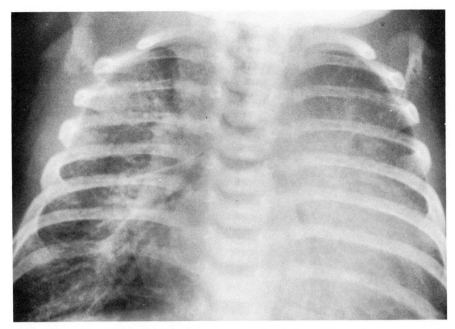

Figure 1–57. One-day-old infant with severe congestive failure. The pulmonary vascular markings are prominent; the hilar vessels are obscured by interstitial edema; and the lower lobe vessels are ill-defined. Although the cardiac silhouette is difficult to define because of the parenchymal abnormalities, cardiomegaly is present.

PULMONARY VENOUS HYPERTENSION PATTERN. The radiographic signs of elevated pulmonary venous pressure secondary to left heart failure or to lesions involving obstruction distal to the pulmonary veins manifest themselves differently in the newborn or young infant as compared with the older child. Several pulmonary conditions that may simulate the radiographic pattern of pulmonary venous hypertension have been discussed. These include infants of diabetic mothers and those with transient tachypnea of the newborn or transient hypoglycemia—all conditions that lead to volume overload of the heart. Generally these conditions present in the first day of life and show gradual improvement with therapy. The heart is normal in size or minimally enlarged.

Infants with congestive failure generally present after the first day of life. There is usually moderate to severe cardiomegaly. The cardiac silhouette often has a nonspecific, globular appearance. If lung disease is not severe, one can usually detect prominent vascularity, although pulmonary redistribution is not apparent. Bilateral perihilar edema may obscure hilar vessels and interstitial edema results in ill-defined lower lobe vessels (Fig. 1–57). The lungs may be hyperinflated. These findings reflect pulmonary venous hypertension secondary to left-sided heart failure. If secondary right heart failure ensues, hepatomegaly may be noted.

The first manifestation of pulmonary venous hypertension in the older child is seen in the extrahilar vessels. The vessels show redistribution from their usual 2:1 lower to upper lobe ratio. This may take the form of equalization of vessel size (1:1 distribution) in the face of mild elevations of pulmonary venous pressure (Fig. 1–58). As pulmonary pressure elevations become higher, a reversal of the vessel size in upper and lower lobes is noted (Fig. 1–59). The presence of interstitial edema around small lower lobe vessels that raises the resistance to flow in these vessels is theorized to cause this redistribution phenomenon.[16] The edema may not be visible radiographically until mean pulmonary capillary wedge pressures reach 20 mmHg. At this point, vessels may become ill-defined or may seem to "disappear" from the lung bases as they become silhouetted by edema fluid (Fig. 1–60). Kerley B lines indicate fluid in the perilymphatic interlobular septa of the lung bases and reflect mean pulmonary capillary

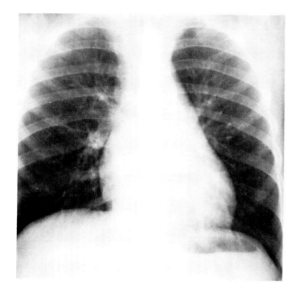

Figure 1–58. Posteroanterior chest radiograph in a three-year-old with aortic stenosis. There is a 1:1 pulmonary vascular distribution indicating mild elevation of pulmonary venous pressure.

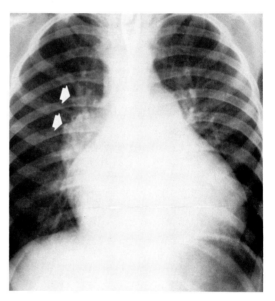

Figure 1–59. Posteroanterior chest radiograph in a 10-year-old with chronic rheumatic mitral valve disease. Obvious redistribution of pulmonary vascularity is present and there is obliteration of the normal hilar angle (arrows).

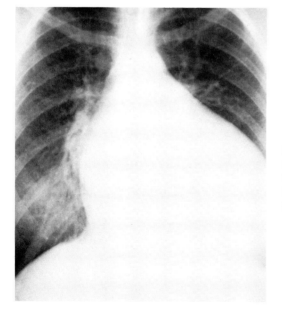

Figure 1–60. Posteroanterior chest radiograph in a child with chronic rheumatic mitral valve disease demonstrating poorly defined lower lobe vessels and pulmonary vascular redistribution. This patient had a mean pulmonary capillary wedge pressure in the mid 20 mmHg range.

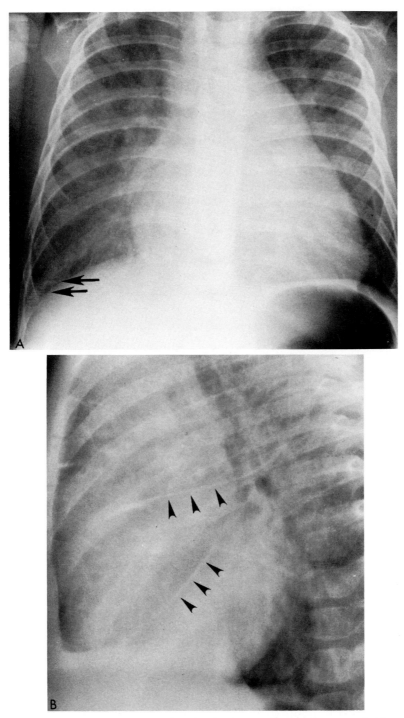

Figure 1–61. Posteroanterior (A) and lateral (B) chest radiographs in a child with significant obstruction to pulmonary venous return by a membrane in the left atrium (cor triatriatum). Kerley B lines are present on the frontal film (arrows) as thin horizontal lines in the right costophrenic region (arrows). Fluid in the fissures seen on the lateral film (arrowheads) is another manifestation of pulmonary venous hypertension.

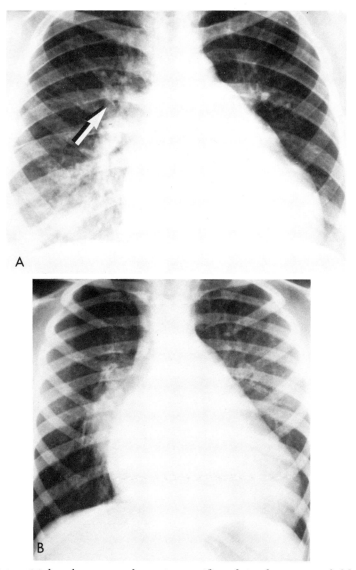

Figure 1–62. Interstitial pulmonary edema is manifested in these two children with chronic rheumatic mitral valve disease, as prominent yet ill-defined hilar vessels (A) and obliteration of the normal hilar angle (B). A thick cuff of edema fluid is seen around the upper lobe bronchi in patient A (arrow).

wedge pressures of 20 to 25 mmHg. These are best visualized in the costophrenic angles as thin horizontal lines extending to the pleural surface (Fig. 1–61). Fluid in the fissures and pleural effusion are other manifestations of moderate pulmonary venous hypertension (Fig. 1–61). Interstitial pulmonary edema will cause the hilar vessels to appear prominent yet ill-defined (Fig. 1–62A). Often there is loss of the normal hilar angle (Fig. 1–62B). Occasionally, bronchi seen on end may reveal thick cuffs (>2

mm) of edema fluid around their periphery (Fig. 1–62A). This sign should be used with caution, since diseases that cause inflammation or fibrosis of the bronchi may thicken their wall. Overt pulmonary alveolar edema, the extreme manifestation of elevated pulmonary venous pressure, suggests marked left ventricular dysfunction or inflow obstruction. Often these fluffy densities have an evanescent quality, shifting in location and density (Fig. 1–63).

BRONCHIAL VASCULARITY. This rela-

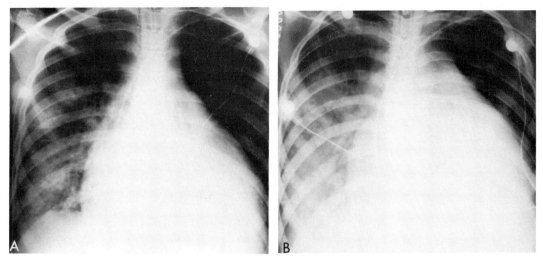

Figure 1–63. A, B, Portable chest radiographs in a ten-year-old child with acute rheumatic pancarditis. The fluffy alveolar densities vary in location and density over a two-hour period.

tively uncommon pattern occurs in cyanotic children with pulmonary atresia and right-to-left shunting (usually through a large VSD). It is really a manifestation of a severe reduction of pulmonary flow. In this situa-

tion, pulmonary blood supply is derived from systemic arteries (usually bronchials) arising from the aorta. These vessels tend to give a "prominent" vascular pattern (Fig. 1–64). However, this pattern differs from

Figure 1–64. Posteroanterior chest radiograph in a cyanotic child with "prominent" pulmonary vascularity. Further analysis reveals that well-defined pulmonary arteries are lacking, that the pulmonary trunk density is absent, and that the lung densities are composed of fine reticular markings. Note the presence of a right aortic arch and an upturned apex in this patient with pulmonary atresia/VSD. This pulmonary vascular pattern is due to systemic ("bronchial") collaterals.

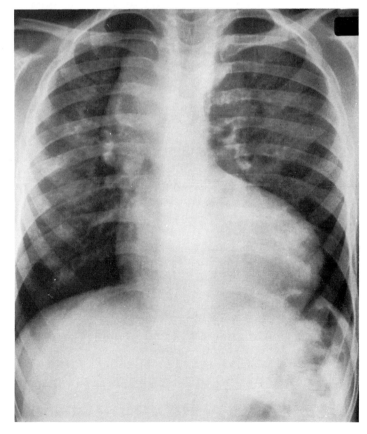

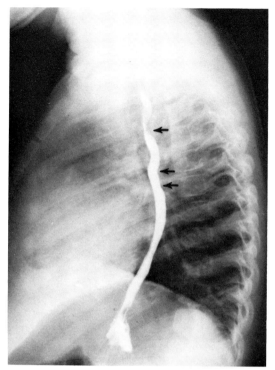

Figure 1–65. Lateral chest radiograph in a cyanotic child with pulmonary atresia/VSD. Note the poorly defined hilar region and small pulmonary branches at the lung bases. The upper broad impression on the barium-filled esophagus (single arrow) is due to an aberrant left subclavian artery. However, the smaller impressions below this (double arrows) are due to systemic (bronchial) collaterals coursing from the aorta to the lungs.

the shunt pattern in that, although the hilar regions may appear prominent, the lateral view will reveal this region to be poorly defined rather than prominent (Fig. 1–65). In the mid lung zones the branching pattern will often be unusual and present a reticulated appearance (Fig. 1–64). The peripheral lung zones contain thin, stringy vessels or no vessels at all (Fig. 1–64). The barium swallow may reveal small impressions caused by the systemic collaterals (Fig. 1–65).

HIGH PULMONARY RESISTANCE PATTERN. Early evidence of the development of increased pulmonary arterial resistance (pulmonary vascular obstructive disease) may be seen serially as a reduction in diameter of vessels 2 to 3 cm from the pleura. Reduc-

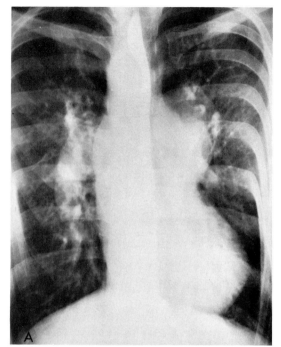

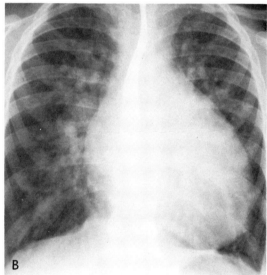

Figure 1–66. Two patients with Eisenmenger's physiology. The patient in *A* had a truncus arteriosus. Note the huge central pulmonary arteries, rapid tapering of vessels in the mid lung fields, and the absence of vessels in the outer third of the lung fields. Incidentally, note the right aortic arch. The patient in *B* has a chest radiograph that should be interpreted as a large left-to-right shunt. A VSD was present, but predominant shunting was right to left and pulmonary artery pressure and pulmonary vascular resistance were markedly elevated.

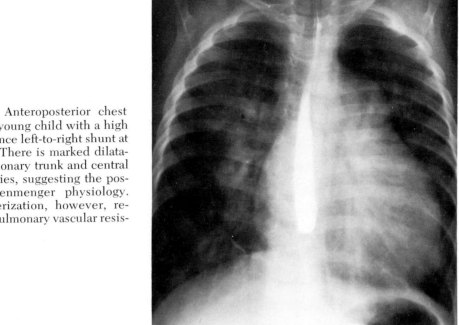

Figure 1–67. Anteroposterior chest radiograph in a young child with a high flow, low resistance left-to-right shunt at the atrial level. There is marked dilatation of the pulmonary trunk and central pulmonary arteries, suggesting the possibility of Eisenmenger physiology. Cardiac catheterization, however, revealed normal pulmonary vascular resistance.

tion in caliber of segmental and lobar arteries followed by increasing dilatation of the central pulmonary arteries may be seen subsequently.

Individuals who develop pulmonary arterial changes and elevated peripheral pulmonary resistance secondary to left-to-right shunts (Eisenmenger's physiology) may have a variety of pulmonary vascular patterns. Although the classic findings are those of a large pulmonary trunk and hilar pulmonary arteries with discrepantly small second and third order pulmonary arteries (Fig. 1–66A), the film may also look like a typical large left-to-right shunt (Fig. 1–66B) or even appear relatively normal. In addition, older children with high flow, low resistant shunts may present with vascular patterns similar to those with Eisenmenger's physiology (Fig. 1–67).

Decreased Pulmonary Vascularity

Reduction of pulmonary blood flow results from severe obstruction to right heart outflow. This is reflected on the chest film as a general reduction in the size of intrapulmonary arteries and veins. Generally,

the pulmonary trunk in these cases is inapparent or small (Figs. 1–68A, 1–69A). The hilar regions are reduced in size and decreased in density. This is best appreciated on the lateral view (Figs. 1–68B, 1–69B). The extrahilar vessels are thin and stringy (Fig. 1–68A and C). The chest of a child with diminished vascularity will appear hyperlucent even though the radiographic technique is adequate as judged by thoracic disc space visualization (Fig. 1–68A). When the obstruction is mild the vascularity may appear relatively normal.

CARDIOVASCULAR SILHOUETTE

The Newborn

In the initial radiographic evaluation of the neonate with suspected heart disease, a frontal and lateral film will usually suffice for the assessment of lung parenchyma, pulmonary vascularity, and heart size. Oblique films of the chest with barium in the esophagus are rarely of value in this age group unless a vascular ring is suspected.

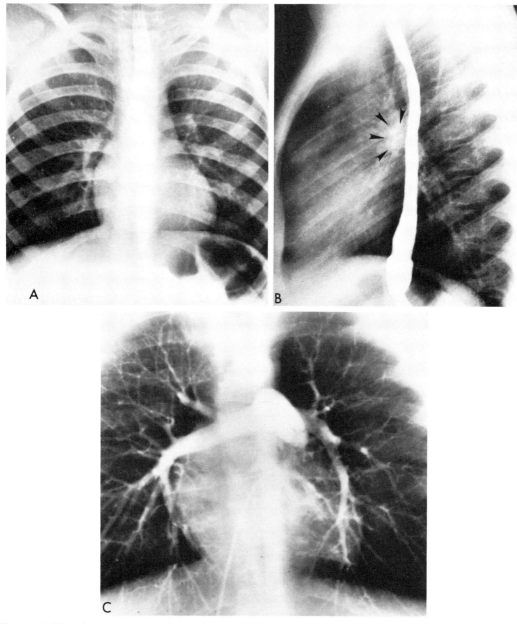

Figure 1–68. Anteroposterior *(A)* and lateral *(B)* chest radiographs with barium in the esophagus obtained in a cyanotic child. The right hilar pulmonary vessels are small, while vessels in the mid and outer lung fields are thin and stringy. The lateral view reveals that the hilar vessels are reduced in size (arrowheads). The right ventriculogram *(C)* obtained in this patient with tetralogy of Fallot shows diffuse reduction in pulmonary arterial caliber suspected on the chest film.

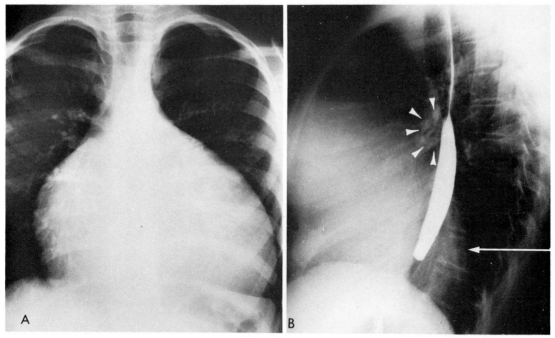

Figure 1–69. Posteroanterior (A) and lateral (B) chest radiographs in a cyanotic patient with Ebstein's anomaly of the tricuspid valve. Because of the massive heart size, it is difficult to appreciate the small size of the pulmonary vessels on the frontal film, although they are reduced in size as visualized through the cardiac silhouette. The lateral view shows a small hilar density (arrowheads) with small vessels emanating from this region. Note the massive right heart dilatation in the retrosternal area and the posterior projecting, dilated right atrium (arrow).

Profound changes in the cardiovascular system occur after birth and these may influence the appearance of the pulmonary vascularity and heart size on the newborn chest film. After the first breath, a fall in pulmonary vascular resistance occurs, while there is vasoconstriction of the ductus arteriosus. Subsequent increase in arterial oxygen tension and decrease in carbon dioxide tension lead to decrease in pulmonary arterial tone and increase in muscular tone in the ductus. However, bidirectional shunting through the ductus is common in the first hour after birth and may persist for up to six hours.[17] Left-to-right shunting through the ductus may occur up to 12 hours depending on the relative rates of change in resistance of the systemic and pulmonary circuits. Bidirectional shunting through the foramen ovale may also persist for several hours in the neonate.[18] These factors tend to produce a normal "increase" in pulmonary vascularity in the first 12 hours. There follows a gradual decrease in vascularity until a basal state is reached at about 24 hours.

Decreased blood flow through the right heart, secondary to clamping the umbilical cord, causes a decrease in cardiac size in the first 12 hours. This and the cessation of ductal and foraminal shunting at 12 to 24 hours contribute to a generalized decrease in cardiac size during this time period. Stabilization of the heart size after 72 hours is the rule.[19]

Dogmatic statements about cardiac size should be avoided in the neonatal period unless one is certain that a film was obtained during quiet respiration. Significant changes in heart size occur with the Valsalva (decrease) and the Müller (increase) maneuvers, both of which commonly accompany crying.[20] One study suggests that the cardiothoracic (CT) ratio of the newborn varies little with respiration.[20] Following the first 24 hours (in which the most significant hemodynamic changes have occurred), one may safely use a CT ratio of 0.57 as the upper limit of normal for a film obtained during quiet respiration.[21] Calculation of the CT ratio by two reliable methods is

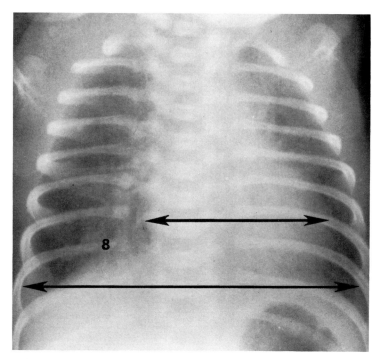

Figure 1–70. Calculation of the cardiothoracic ratio may be accomplished by comparing the maximal width of the cardiac silhouette with a thoracic dimension calculated at either the inner margins of the eight ribs or the maximal internal chest width (arrows). The normal range in the neonate is 43 to 56.5 per cent.[21]

shown in Figure 1–70. Whether the thoracic dimension is taken at the inner margin of the eighth ribs or at the maximal internal chest width, the normal CT ratio range in neonates is similar, namely 43 to 56.5 per cent.[21]

The cardiac apex in the normal newborn often has an upturned appearance (Fig. 1–71A). Although this may be a reflection of physiologic right ventricular hypertrophy, it may also be a reflection of the lordotic position assumed in most neonatal chest films. In addition, it is not unusual in the neonatal period to visualize a "ductus bump" along the lateral margin of the upper thoracic aorta (Fig. 1–71B). This finding, which represents the obliquely viewed ductus arteriosus, has no pathologic significance beyond the first few days of life.

The Cardiac Series

The conventional four views of the heart with barium in the esophagus include a posteroanterior (PA) view, a lateral view, a 60° right anterior oblique (RAO) view (all with barium), and a 45° left anterior oblique

(LAO) view (without barium) (Fig. 1–72). Modification of this to exclude the little used RAO view has proved worthwhile. This group of three films (the cardiac series) may be used in the initial evaluation of the child with suspected heart disease. The additional radiation exposure and cost involved in obtaining the LAO view are minimal and the addition of barium allows accurate evaluation of the aortic arch region and left atrium. Cardiac fluoroscopy has little use in the evaluation of children with suspected heart disease unless it is to better define suspected vascular anomalies not clearly seen on the cardiac series.

The internal and border-forming anatomy of the cardiac silhouette in the four conventional views is depicted graphically in Figure 1–72.

The Infant and Child

After the thymus regresses in the first few years of life, the border-forming cardiac and vascular structures can be readily identified (Fig. 1–73). The straight right upper border

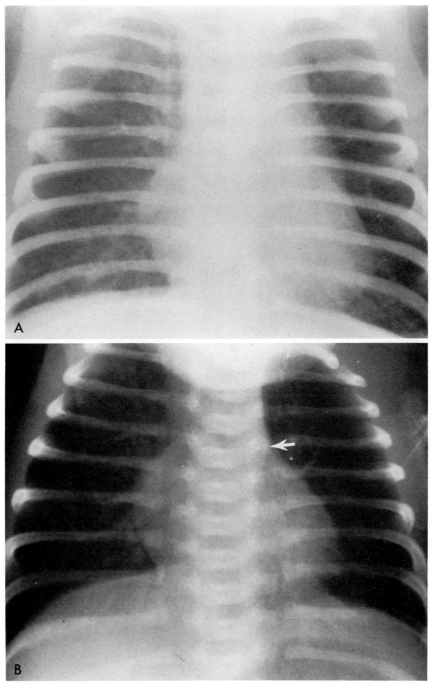

Figure 1–71. Anteroposterior chest radiographs obtained in two neonates. An upturned apex (A) is frequently found in this age group. Although this may be a reflection of physiologic right ventricular hypertrophy, it may also be secondary to the lordotic position assumed in most neonates. In (B), a slight bulge is seen in the proximal portion of the descending thoracic aorta. This is the so-called "ductus bump" and should not be viewed as a significant finding beyond the first few days of life.

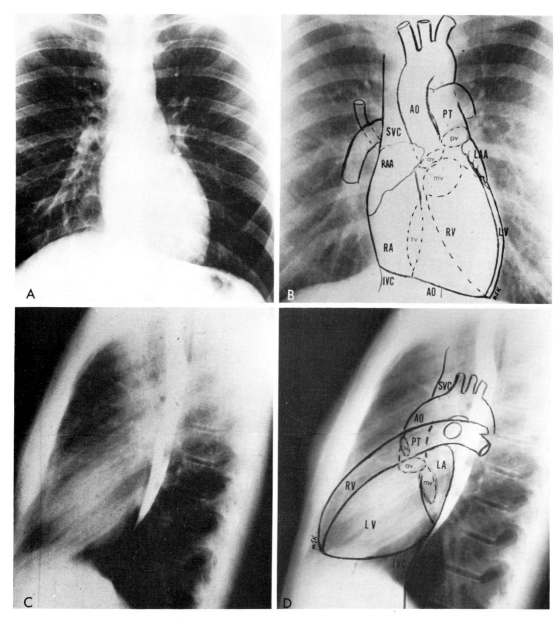

Figure 1–72. Conventional four-view cardiac series. This includes the posteroanterior view with barium *(A)*, a lateral view with barium *(C)*, a 60° right anterior oblique (RAO) view with barium *(E)*, and a 45° left anterior oblique (LAO) without barium *(G)*. The internal and border-forming cardiovascular structures in these four views are diagrammatically depicted in Figures *B, D, F,* and *H*. (AO = aorta, av = aortic valve, E = esophagus, IVC = inferior vena cava, LAA = left atrial appendage, LA = left atrium, LMB = left mainstem bronchus, LV = left ventricle, mv = mitral valve, PT = pulmonary trunk, pv = pulmonary valve, RAA = right atrial appendage, RA = right atrium, RV = right ventricle, SVC = superior vena cava, and tv = tricuspid valve).

Illustration continued on opposite page

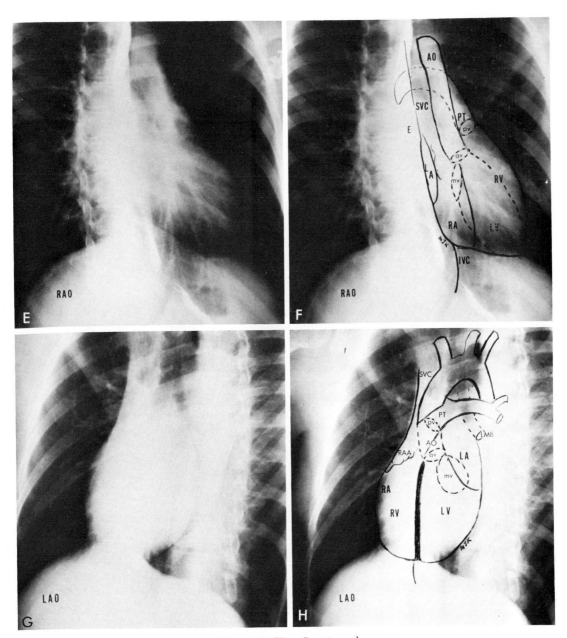

Figure 1–72. Continued

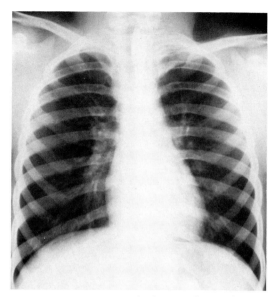

Figure 1–73. Normal chest radiograph in a five-year-old child.

of the cardiac silhouette is formed by the superior vena cava (Fig. 1–73). The lower convex bulge is formed by the right atrial appendage superiorly and the body of the right atrium inferiorly (Fig. 1–73). The left heart border is made up of three apparent convexities and one small, flat region. The convexities from superior to inferior are the junction of the transverse and descending thoracic aorta (the aortic knob); the pulmonary trunk (pulmonary artery segment); and a rim of left ventricular myocardium (Fig. 1–73). The small, flat region situated between the pulmonary trunk and left ventricle is the left atrial appendage (Fig. 1–73). This structure is usually not convex. The cardiac apex in this age group shows no evidence of the upward tilt of the neonate. Forming a continuous inferior density from the aortic knob is the linear perivertebral density of the descending thoracic aorta (Fig. 1–73). Prominence of any of the aforementioned structures should be viewed with suspicion in the infant and young child.

The Older Child and Adolescent

The cardiac silhouette in this age group may have the previously described appearance of the young child (Fig. 1–74A) or

begin to take on the appearance of the adult heart. The main feature that distinguishes the normal cardiac silhouette of the adult from that of the child is that the pulmonary trunk becomes less apparent and the apex points more inferiorly (Fig. 1–74B). The region of the pulmonary trunk may even be characterized by an overt concavity (Fig. 1–74B) and the aortic knob becomes a prominent feature of the silhouette (Fig. 1–74B). This "adult" type cardiac silhouette should be viewed with suspicion, as it may be seen in children with various left ventricular stress problems (aortic stenosis, systemic hypertension, coarctation, and so on). Prominence of the ascending aorta may serve as another clue in separating these cases from the normal.

Right Heart Structures

The right atrium and right atrial appendage form the right border of the cardiac silhouette on the frontal film and the upper third of the heart border on the LAO view (Fig. 1–72A,B,E, and F). It is difficult to diagnose isolated right atrial enlargement even using the more sensitive LAO view. In practical terms, this is not a problem, since few lesions cause isolated right atrial enlargement without additionally enlarging the right ventricle. Because of this, it is rare that separating the two structures in analysis of films will be helpful in suggesting a diagnosis. Therefore, the term right heart enlargement to include both structures will be used throughout this text.

On the frontal film, right heart enlargement is indicated by an abnormal convexity in the right atrial region and extension of the right atrium to the right and superiorly (Figs. 1–75A and C and 1–76A). There may be obliteration of the normal indentation between the pulmonary trunk and left ventricle as the enlarged right ventricle becomes border forming (Fig. 1–75C). On the lateral view, there is projection of the right heart structures (right atrial appendage and right ventricular outflow tract) higher on the sternum than is usual (Figs. 1–75B and D and 1–76B). Normally the junction of the right heart and sternum should not exceed 40 per cent of the distance between the sternal-diaphragmatic junction and the manubrial-sternal junction. This determination

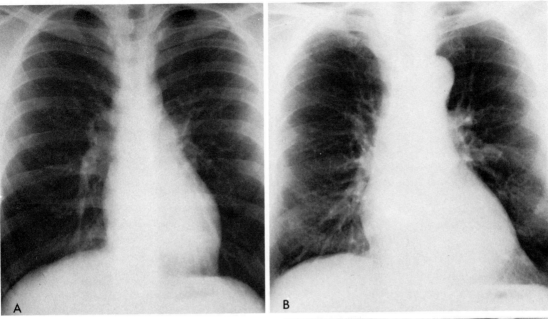

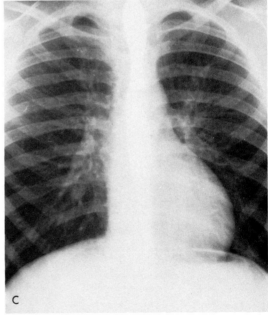

Figure 1–74. *A,* Posteroanterior chest radiograph in a 16-year-old boy. The shape of the cardiovascular silhouette is quite similar to that seen in the child depicted in Figure 1–73. *B,* Chest radiograph in a 60-year-old man showing the typical "adult" cardiovascular silhouette. The pulmonary trunk is no longer apparent, the cardiac apex points somewhat more inferiorly than that of the teenager, and the aortic knob is a prominent feature of the cardiovascular contour. *C,* This 10-year-old child has an "adult" type cardiovascular silhouette. Although this may be a normal appearance in some children of this age, one should be concerned that it is related to cardiac lesions that stress the left ventricle (for example, aortic stenosis, systemic hypertension, and aortic coarctation). The child had hypertrophic obstructive cardiomyopathy.

cannot be made when there is significant thymic tissue present or when the anteroposterior diameter of the chest is narrowed (an anteroposterior to transthoracic ratio less than 30 per cent).[22] In cases where the right heart (and especially the right atrium) becomes huge, there may be a posterior projection of the right atrium on the lateral film. This is most commonly seen in Ebstein's anomaly of the tricuspid valve

(Fig. 1–75D). The left ventricle can be affected by right heart enlargement and, when it is, it may be displaced posteriorly behind the shadow of the inferior vena cava (Fig. 1–76B). A left anterior oblique view will demonstrate that the left ventricle is being displaced by dilated right heart structures (Fig. 1–76C). Although it may be impossible in this situation to rule out left ventricular enlargement, it is important not

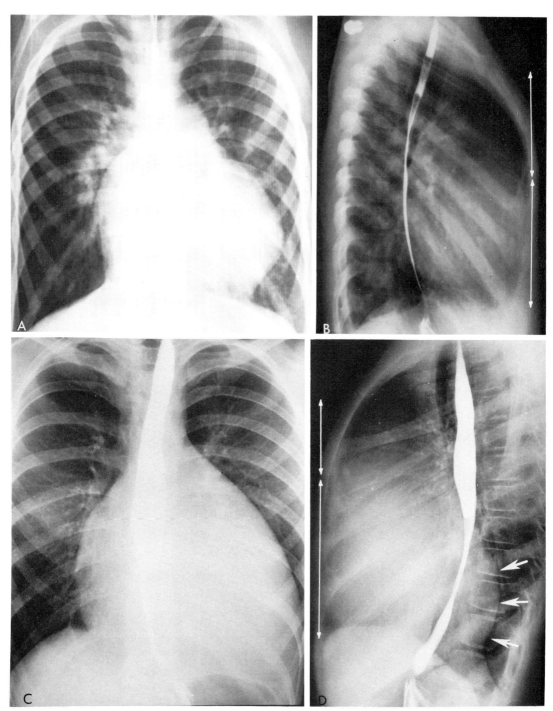

Figure 1–75. Right heart enlargement is suggested on the frontal films *A* and *C* by the prominent convexity of the right atrium and extension of the right atrial density superiorly and rightward. In *A*, the cardiac silhouette shows an upturned apex. In *C*, the normal indentation between the pulmonary trunk and left ventricle is obliterated by dilated right heart structures. On the lateral views *B* and *D*, the right heart structures project high on the sternum (arrows). When this distance exceeds 40 per cent of the distance between the manubrial-sternal junction and the sternal-diaphragmatic junction, right heart enlargement is present. Note in *D* that the dilated right atrium has projected posteriorly behind the shadow of the inferior vena cava (arrows). Note also how the pulmonary vascularity aids one in evaluating these two cases associated with right heart enlargement. In the first case, the presence of shunt vascularity and the lack of left atrial enlargement suggests an atrial septal defect, while in the second case the presence of diminished pulmonary vascularity suggests the diagnosis of Ebstein's anomaly of the tricuspid valve.

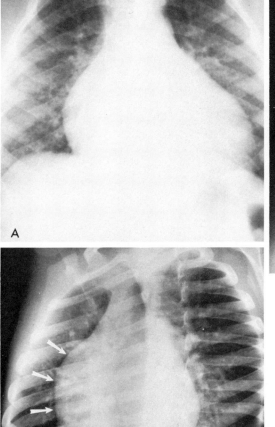

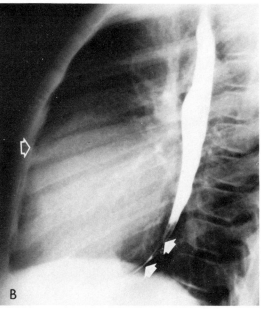

Figure 1–76. Cardiomegaly in this child noted on the posteroanterior view *(A)* is due primarily to right heart enlargement, which is best appreciated in the retrosternal area on the lateral view *(B)* (arrow). There has been displacement of the left ventricle posteriorly into the barium-filled esophagus (arrows). The presence of right heart enlargement and the posterior displacement of the left ventricle is further appreciated on the LAO projection *(C)* (arrows).

to erroneously suggest that it is enlarged on the basis of the lateral view above. It is important, therefore, to rule out right heart enlargement before suggesting that this sign of left ventricular enlargement is positive.

In conditions associated with right ventricular hypertrophy, there may be little actual enlargement of right heart structures (for example, the cardiothoracic ratio in tetralogy of Fallot is usually normal). However, these conditions often produce a change in contour of the cardiac silhouette in the form of an upturned or unusually rounded cardiac apex (Fig. 1–77A and B). The former is due to the superior displacement of the

left ventricle by the hypertrophied right ventricle. The latter is due to superimposition of the right ventricle over the usual border-forming left ventricle. The LAO view is particularly sensitive to changes in right heart size. Enlargement is indicated by varying degrees of convexity of the right heart border just below the junction with the superior vena cava (Fig. 1–76C).

Left Atrium

The normal left atrium is centrally placed within the cardiac silhouette and is not border forming in the frontal projection

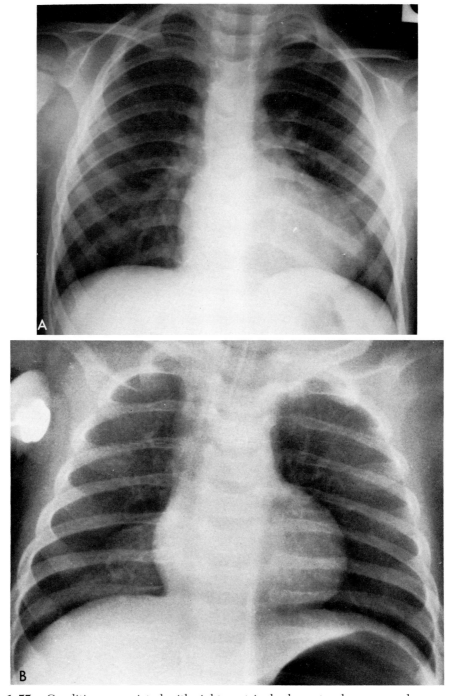

Figure 1–77. Conditions associated with right ventricular hypertrophy may produce an upturned cardiac apex *(A)* or an unusually rounded cardiac apex *(B)*. The former is due to the superior displacement of the left ventricle by the hypertrophied right ventricle, while the latter is due to superior position of the right ventricle over the usual border-framing left ventricle. Both patients had tetralogy of Fallot.

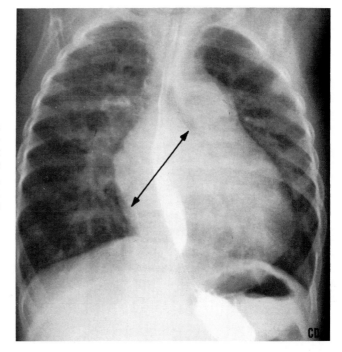

Figure 1–78. In this child with a large ventricular septal defect, the distance between the right wall of the left atrium ("double density") and the left mainstem bronchus is 5.5 cm (arrow). This is an abnormally large dimension in this one-year-old child and indicates left atrial enlargement.

(Fig. 1–72*A* and *B*). It makes up the upper half of the posterior margin of the heart on the lateral view (Fig. 1–72*C* and *D*). It is here in intimate contact with the esophagus. As mentioned, the left atrial appendage is inconspicuous between the pulmonary trunk and left ventricle. In the LAO view, the left atrium lies beneath the left mainstem bronchus (Fig. 1–72*G* and *H*). The left atrioventricular groove may also be visualized in this projection.

Left atrial enlargement is an important

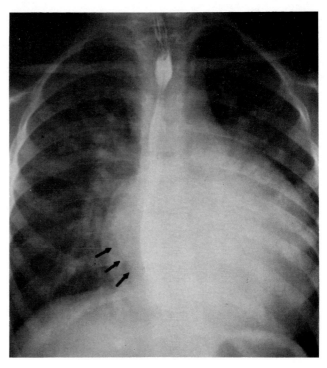

Figure 1–79. Deviation of the barium-filled esophagus to the right is due to a dilated left atrium in this child with endocardial cushion defect and significant mitral regurgitation. Note additionally the presence of double density along the right heart border (arrows).

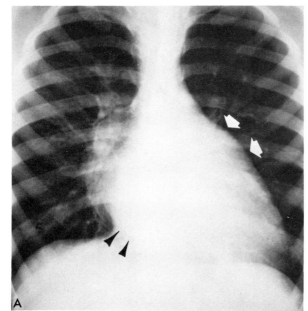

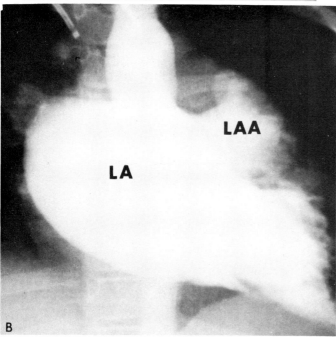

Figure 1–80. A, Dilatation of the left atrial appendage (white arrows) and an inferiorly displaced right wall of the left atrium (black arrows) is noted in this 12-year-old patient with chronic rheumatic mitral regurgitation. B, Left ventriculogram obtained in patient shown in A demonstrates massive mitral regurgitation with marked dilation of the left atrium (LA) and left atrial appendage (LAA).

finding in helping to distinguish specific lesions within various hemodynamic categories. In the frontal projection, the following are signs of left atrial enlargement: (1) increased distance (>3.5 cm in infants, >4.5 cm in children) between the right wall of the left atrium (the "double density") and the left mainstem bronchus (Fig. 1–78); (2) deviation of the barium-filled esophagus to the right (Fig. 1–79); and (3) prominence of the left atrial appendage (Fig. 1–80). The upper limits of normal for the left atrial dimension (double density to left mainstem bronchus measurement) has been determined in adults.[23] A left atrial dimension of 7 cm or 7.5 cm is considered abnormal in adult females and males, respectively. It should be noted that the double density

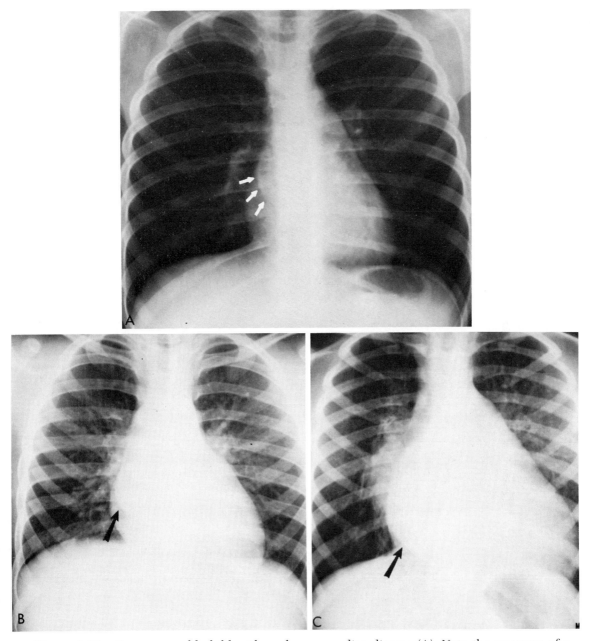

Figure 1–81. Seven-year-old child with no known cardiac disease *(A).* Note the presence of a "double density" along the right upper cardiac margin (arrows). This represents mediastinal reflection on the pulmonary veins and may be seen in normal children. However, when the double density is more inferiorly displaced *(B)* (arrow) or horizontal in position *(C)* (arrow), it should be considered an abnormal finding indicating significant left atrial enlargement. The two patients in *(B)* and *(C)* had chronic rheumatic mitral valve disease.

may be seen in normal children (Fig. 1–81*A*). In this situation, it represents a confluence of pulmonary veins, mediastinal pleura, and pericardium. An inferior and horizontal appearance to the double density, however, should usually be viewed as ab-

normal (Fig. 1–81*B* and *C*). It is rare to see left atrial appendage enlargement (even when there are other signs of left atrial enlargement) unless rheumatic mitral valve disease is present.[24] Elevation of the left mainstem bronchus on the frontal view is

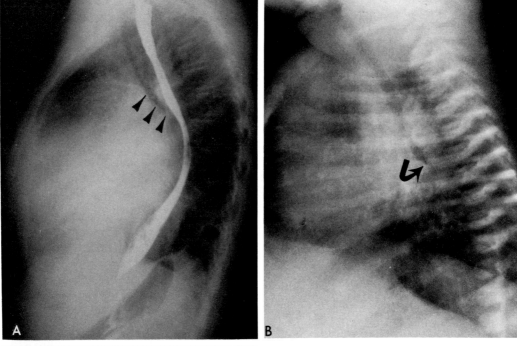

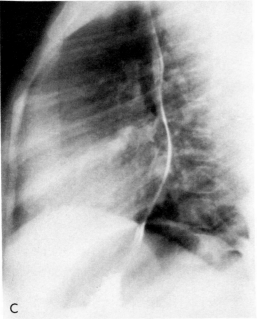

Figure 1–82. A, Posterior deviation and elevation of the left mainstem bronchus (arrows) is noted in the patient with chronic rheumatic mitral valve disease. The finding is confirmed with the barium swallow showing significant left atrial enlargement. B, In this infant, posterior deviation and elevation of the left mainstem bronchus is noted (arrows). In addition, there is a discrete bulge in the region of the left atrium. This child had a large ventricular septal defect. C, True left atrial enlargement should involve both an anterior impression on the barium column as well as posterior deviation of the esophagus.

difficult to assess in children and is therefore an unreliable indicator of left atrial size.

In the lateral view, left atrial enlargement may be detected when there is posterior deviation and elevation of the left mainstem bronchus and/or a discrete bulge in the region of the left atrium (Fig. 1–82A). This may be a useful sign in infants in whom a barium swallow is rarely obtained (Fig. 1–82B). A more accurate assessment of left atrial size is made with barium in the esophagus. True left atrial enlargement should involve both an anterior impression on the barium column and posterior deviation of the esophagus (Fig. 1–82A and C). Pseudo left atrial enlargement may be encountered

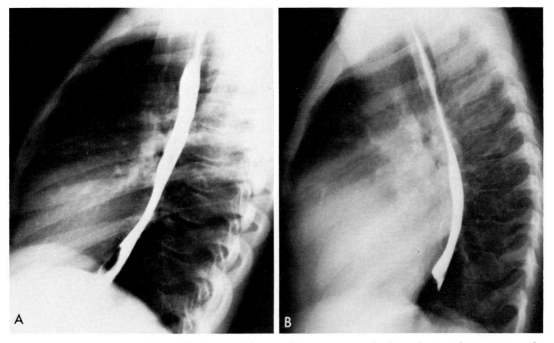

Figure 1–83. Pseudo left atrial enlargement may be encountered when the esophagus is overdistended with barium, as in this case *(A)*, or in the face of right heart enlargement, which may push the left atrium into the esophagus *(B)*.

when the esophagus is overly distended with barium (Fig. 1–83A); in some normal persons when the right heart is in atrial diastole (ventricular systole); and in some cases of right heart enlargement, in which the left atrium is pushed into the esophagus (Fig. 1–83B). In the latter case, there is rarely a discrete anterior impression on the

Figure 1–84. One can estimate left atrial size by drawing a line from the anterior wall of the pulmonary artery parallel to the lower third of the esophagus. This line passes through the mitral valve, and the dimension between the mitral valve and posterior wall of the left atrium (left atrial size) can readily be obtained. The values obtained with this measurement are similar to those obtained using M-mode echocardiography.

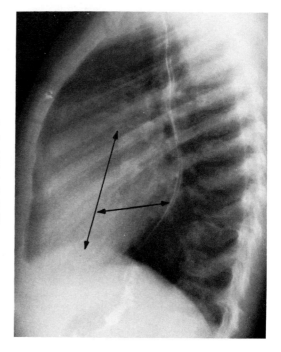

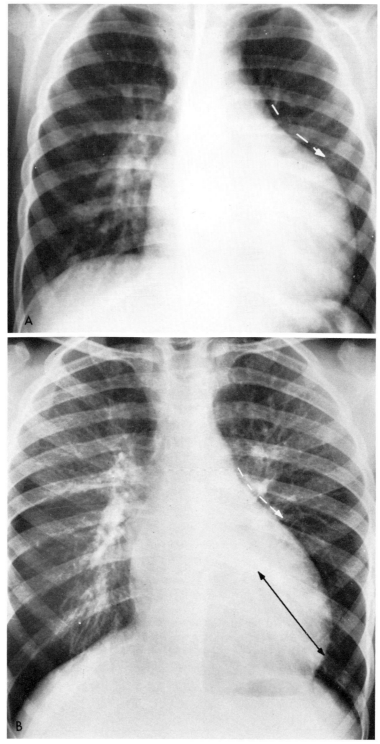

Figure 1–85. *A*, Left ventricular enlargement. Posteroanterior chest radiograph in a patient with a large ventricular septal defect. Note that the cardiac apex is inferiorly displaced and projects below the left hemidiaphragm. *B*, In this patient with hypertrophic obstructive cardiomyopathy, the vector of the left ventricular apex is inferiorly displaced (arrow). In both patients the concave left mid heart border is indicated (dotted arrows).

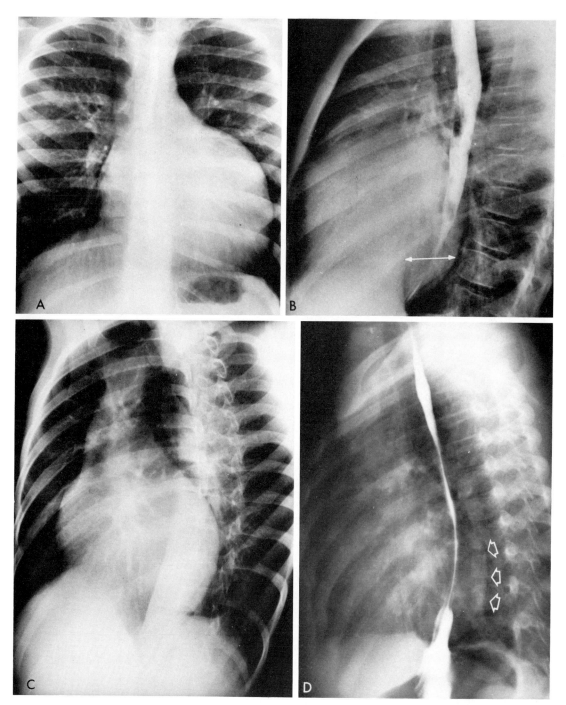

Figure 1–86. *A,* Posteroanterior chest radiograph in a patient with hypertrophic obstructive cardiomyopathy. There is massive left ventricular enlargement. *B,* On the lateral film, the left ventricle is posteriorly displaced from the inferior vena caval density by 4 cm (arrow). *C,* There is no evidence of right heart enlargement on the LAO view of this patient. Note that the left ventricle projects well beyond the spine in this projection. *D,* Marked right atrial dilatation in this patient with an atrial septal defect simulates left ventricular enlargement. Usually the left ventricle will cause posterior deviation of the barium-filled esophagus, whereas the right atrium will not.

barium column (Fig. 1–83B). If one can clearly define the right pulmonary artery on the lateral film, one can actually measure the left atrial dimension in a plane that is similar to that obtained with M-mode echocardiography.[25] One drops a "plumb line" from the anterior margin of the right pulmonary artery, parallel to the lower third of the esophagus. This line normally passes through the mitral valve (Fig. 1–84). A line drawn from the anterior margin of the left atrium, just above the mitral valve, to the posterior wall of the left atrium (as demarcated by the esophagus) gives the left atrial dimension. In infants and children, the normal range for this left atrial dimension is 2 to 3 cm. Caution should be used that a correctly positioned lateral view is obtained for this measurement.

Left Ventricle

The apex of the normal left ventricle is usually slightly lower than that of the right ventricle and rests on the left hemidiaphragm. It is posterior and to the left of the right ventricle and forms the rim of the left heart border in the normal individual. In the lateral view it makes up the lower half of the posterior border of the cardiac silhouette (Fig. 1–72C and D).

Left ventricular enlargement due to dilatation or combined dilatation/hypertrophy states produces a change in the vector of the heart in that the apex points downward, often projecting below the left hemidiaphragm (Fig. 1–85A and B). An additional helpful clue to the presence of left ventricular enlargement is the shape assumed by the heart. An overt concavity to the left mid heart border in the region normally occupied by the pulmonary trunk often exists. This combination of the prominent left heart border and mid left heart concavity has been termed the "left ventricular configuration."[26] The significance of this finding can be determined only after analysis of the pulmonary vascularity and great vessel region coupled with a knowledge of the patient's age. In children and adolescents, a left ventricular configuration with normal vascularity and prominent ascending aorta suggests aortic stenosis, systemic hypertension, or other left ventricular stress problems (Fig. 1–85B). In young adults, this configuration has less significance and may be normal. In older adults, the left ventricular configuration is the rule rather than the exception. The importance of interpreting the pulmonary vascularity prior to assigning the left ventricular configuration to a left ventricular stress lesion is pointed out by the fact that patients with tetralogy of Fallot (and diminished vascularity) may have a "left ventricular configuration" (see Fig. 1–77A). In this situation the cardiac contour is really due to right ventricular hypertrophy and a hypoplastic pulmonary trunk.

The lateral view may suggest left ventricular enlargement when the posterior edge of the heart projects more than 2 cm beyond a line drawn from the left hemidiaphragm 2 cm up the inferior vena cava (Fig. 1–86B).[27] This sign should be interpreted with caution, however. As pointed out previously, right heart enlargement can push the left ventricle posteriorly and thus this should be ruled out before left ventricular size is assessed. This is most easily accomplished by obtaining a left anterior oblique view (Fig. 1–86C). In a 45° LAO projection, the edge of the left ventricle should not project more than halfway over the spine. Left ventricular enlargement should be suspected when it does (Fig. 1–86C). A poor inspiratory effort or improperly positioned lateral film may also give false positive or negative results. Occasionally, the right atrium will be dilated to a sufficient degree to produce a posterior "pseudo left ventricular" density (Fig. 1–86D). The barium-filled esophagus will not be deviated posteriorly by a dilated right atrium (Fig. 1–86D).

REFERENCES

1. Luke, M. J., McDonnel, E. J.: Congenital heart disease and scoliosis. J. Pediatr 73:725, 1968.
2. Greenwood, R. D., Rosenthal, A., Parisi, L., Fyler, D. C., Nadas, A. S.: Extracardiac abnormalities in infants with congenital heart disease. Pediatrics 55:485, 1975.
3. White, R. I., Jordan, C. E., Fisher, K. C., Lampton, N. L., Neil, C. A., Dorst, J. P.: Skeletal changes associated with adolescent congenital heart disease. Am J Roent 116:531, 1972.
4. Fellows, K. E., Jr., Rosenthal, A.: Extracardiac roentgenographic abnormalities in cyanotic congenital heart disease. Am. J Roent 114:371, 1972.
5. Stewart, J. R., Kincaid, O. W., Edwards, J. E.: An Atlas of Vascular Rings and Related Malforma-

tions of the Aortic Arch System. Springfield, Charles C Thomas, 1964.

6. Elliott, L. P.: An angiocardiographic and plain film approach to complex congenital heart disease: Classification and simplified nomenclature. Current Problems in Cardiology III, #3, 1978.

7. Van Mierop, L. H. S., Eisen, S., Schiebler, G. L.: The radiographic appearance of the tracheo-bronchial tree as an indicator of visceral situs. Am J Cardiol 26:432, 1970.

8. Stanger, P., Rudolph, A. M., Edwards, J. E.: Cardiac malpositions: An overview based on the study of sixty-five necropsy specimens. Circulation 56:159, 1977.

9. Elliott, L. P., Cramer, G. C., Amplatz, K.: The anomalous relationships of the inferior vena cava and abdominal aorta as a specific sign of asplenia. Radiology 87:841, 1966.

10. O'Reilly, R. J., Grollman, J. H.: The lateral chest film as an unreliable indicator of azygous continuation of the inferior vena cava. Circulation 53:891, 1976.

11. Lambert, E. C., Canent, R. V., Hohn, A. R.: Congenital cardiac anomalies in the newborn: A review of conditions causing death or severe distress in the first month of life. Pediatrics 37:343, 1966.

12. Higgins, C. B., Rausch, J., Friedman, W. F., Hirshlaugh, M. J., Kirkpatrick, S. E., Goergen, T. G., Reinke, R. T.: Patent ductus arteriosus in preterm infants with idiopathic respiratory distress syndrome. Radiographic and echocardiographic evaluation. Radiology 124:189–195, 1977.

13. Arnois, D. C., Silverman, F. N., Turner, M. E.: Radiographic evaluation of pulmonary vasculature in children with congenital cardiovascular disease. Radiology 72:689–698, 1959.

14. Simon M.: The pulmonary vasculature in congenital heart disease. Radiol Clin North Am 6:303, 1968.

15. Kelley, M. J.: Personal observations of 1000 chest films in infants and children.

16. West, J. B., Dollery, C. T., Heard, B. E.: Increased pulmonary vascular resistance in the dependent zone of the isolated dog lung caused by perivascular edema. Circ Res 17:206, 1965.

17. Avery, M. E.: The Lung and its Disorders in the Newborn Infants, 3rd ed. W. B. Saunders Co., Philadelphia, 1974.

18. Rowe, R. D., Freedom, R. M., Mehrizi, A., and Bloom, K. R.: The Neonate with Congenital Heart Disease, 2nd ed. W. B. Saunders Co., Philadelphia, 1981.

19. Kjellberg, S. R., Rudhe, R., Zetterstrom, R.: Heart volume variations in the neonatal period. Acta Radiol 42:173, 1954.

20. Burnard, E. D., James, L. S.: The cardiac silhouette in newborn infants: A cinematographic study of the normal ranges, Pediatrics 28:545, 1961.

21. Edwards, D. K., Higgins, C. B., Gilpin, E. A.: The cardiothoracic ratio in newborn infants. Abstract #202, RSNA, Nov 1980, p. 16.

22. Twigg, H. L., deLeon, A. C., Perloff, J. K., Majid, M.: The straight back syndrome: Radiographic manifestations. Radiology 88:274–277, 1967.

23. Higgins, C. B., Reinke, R. T., Jones, N. E., Broderick, T.: Left atrial dimension on the frontal thoracic radiograph: a method for assessing left atrial enlargement. Am J Roent 130 (2):251–255, 1978.

24. Kelley, M. J., Elliott, L. P., Shulman, S. T., Ayoub, E. M., Victorica, B. E., Gessner, I. H.: The significance of the left atrial appendage in rheumatic heart disease Circulation 54:146, 1976.

25. Westcott, J. L., Ferguson, D.: The right pulmonary artery–left atrial axis line. A method for measuring left atrial size on lateral chest radiographs. Radiology 118(2):265–74, 1976.

26. Elliott, L. P., Schiebler, G. L.: X-Ray Diagnosis of Congenital Cardiac Disease. 2nd ed. Springfield, Charles C Thomas, 1979.

27. Eyler, W. R., Wayne, D. L., Rhodenbaugh, J. E.: The importance of the lateral view in the evaluation of left ventricular enlargement in rheumatic heart disease. Radiology 73:56, 1959.

Chapter 2

THE ECHOCARDIOGRAPHIC EXAMINATION

Echocardiography provides anatomic information using a technique that is both nonionizing and noninvasive, while at the same time is unique and complementary to the other diagnostic tests employed in the diagnosis of congenital heart disease. M-mode echocardiography is restricted to a unidimensional, linear view of anatomy, permitting measurement of chamber dimensions or valve motion as a function of time. From it some inferences can be made concerning anatomic relationships in two dimensions. Because M-mode information is so sparse, the development of two-dimensional real-time cross-sectional techniques was considered a major breakthrough when it occurred. These techniques allow temporal and spatial relations to be displayed as a continuous two-dimensional representation of cardiac structures at speeds of up to 60 frames per second. The first device of this type was the linear array that provided a rectangular field of view.[1] The usefulness of this technique is restricted by a low line-to-line information density and by the large size of the multi-transducer head, which is difficult to fit within the rib spaces. The sector scanner,

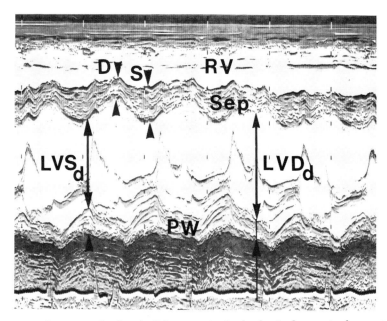

Figure 2–1. M-mode scan at the level of the ventricular body. Left ventricular posterior wall (PW), left ventricular internal cavity measurement in systole (LVS$_d$), and diastole (LVD$_d$) are demonstrated. The interventricular septum (Sep) is shown in both diastole (D) and systole (S). The right ventricular cavity (RV) is visualized in the anterior portion of the scan between the right ventricular wall and the right ventricular aspect of the interventricular septum.

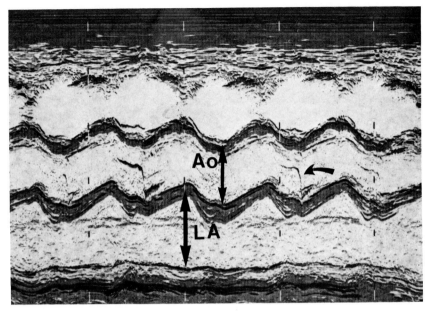

Figure 2–2. M-mode scan at the level of the aortic root. The aortic root (Ao) is visualized anterior to the left atrial cavity (LA). The aortic valve leaflets (curved arrow) are seen within the aortic root. Measurement of the left atrium and aortic root may provide indirect evidence of the left-to-right shunting at the ventricular and/or ductal level. In normals the ratio should be less than 1.2.

which may be mechanically[2] or electronically swept,[3] provides a triangular view of the heart with the apex at the skin surface and is well suited for cardiac applications because it permits unobscured access to the heart through the narrow soft tissue window between ribs. The narrowest portion of the near field is not problematic, since excellent visualization of all four cardiac chambers can be achieved by approaching the heart from either apical[4] or subxiphoidal[5] views. These views place the anatomic structures of interest in the more distant, wider aspects of the sector triangle. These two-

$$\text{Pulm STI} = \frac{PEP}{ET}$$

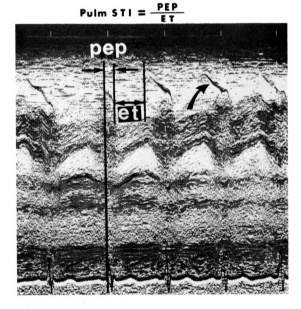

Figure 2–3. Pulmonary systolic time intervals (Pulm STI). Measurement of pulmonary valve systolic time intervals has been used to estimate pulmonary artery end-diastolic pressure and pulmonary vascular resistance. The pre-ejection period (pep)—the time between the onset of electrical systole and initial opening of the pulmonic valve (small arrows)—and the ventricular ejection time (et)—the time between the onset of valve opening to the closure of the valve — can be directly measured from the M-mode echocardiogram and simultaneous electrocardiogram.

dimensional images show excellent detail of neonatal as well as general pediatric and adult cardiac anatomy.[6] M-mode techniques still remain useful for measurement of chamber size[7] and can be used to estimate left ventricular[8, 9] and pulmonary artery[10, 11] pressures as well as the time of opening and closing of the intracardiac valves (Figs. 2–1, 2–2, 2–3).

Recent advances in technology that allow the examiner to use higher frequency transducers (for example, 5 MHz) have substantially improved image resolution and are particularly advantageous for neonatal examinations.

REAL-TIME TWO-DIMENSIONAL ECHOCARDIOGRAPHIC EXAMINATION[6]

Parasternal Examination

Long Axis View (Fig. 2–4A)

With the patient in the supine or in the left decubitus position, the transducer is placed in the third or fourth left intercostal

space over the "echocardiographic window." With the scanner oriented in the longitudinal or sagittal axis of the heart, a view is obtained providing a tomographic plane parallel to a line drawn between the right shoulder and the apex of the heart through the patient's left flank. This "long axis view" allows visualization of the left atrium, both mitral valve leaflets, the left ventricular inflow region, and the left ventricular outflow tract. The interventricular septum and the anterior leaflet of the mitral valve are seen in fibrous continuity with the aortic root. Anterior to the aortic root is the right ventricular outflow tract (infundibulum) and, anterior to the interventricular septum, a portion of the right ventricular body. The attachment of the septal leaflet of the tricuspid valve to the septum can frequently be visualized in this view.

The Right Ventricular Outflow Tract (Fig. 2–4B)

If the examiner rotates the transducer 30° clockwise from the long axis view of the left ventricle, the tomographic plane is oriented along the long axis of the right ventricular

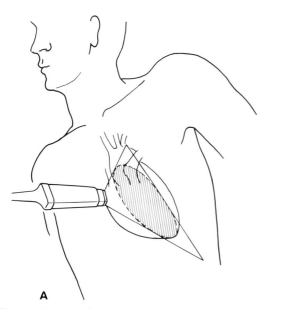

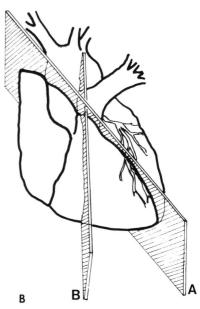

Figure 2–4. Left ventricular long axis anatomy. A, With the patient lying supine or slight left decubitus, the transducer is placed over the "echocardiographic window" in the third to fourth left intercostal space parasternally. The long axis of the sector passes through the sagittal plane of the heart, along a line between the right shoulder and the cardiac apex (see also Fig. 2–8). B, Long axis imaging from the precordium allows sectioning the heart along two-dimensional planes that permit examination of the left ventricular inflow and outflow tracts (plane A). By rotating the transducer 30° clockwise from the long axis view of the left ventricle, a plane that visualizes the right ventricular outflow tract can be obtained (plane B) (see also Fig. 2–11).

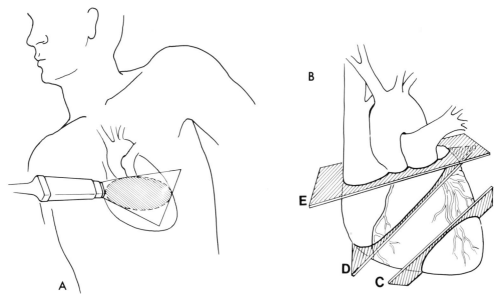

Figure 2–5. Short axis (transverse view). *A,* Further clockwise rotation by 60° creates a tomographic plane at right angles to the long axis view and provides a short axis or transverse section of the left and right ventricles. With the transducer maintained in the third to fourth intercostal space, serial cross-sectional views can be obtained from the apex through the great artery roots by gradual tilting of the transducer. *B,* With the transducer tilted toward the ventricular apex (plane C), cross-sectional views of the left ventricular apex and mitral valve papillary muscles are obtained. Further cranial orientation of the transducer (plane D) provides cross-sectional evaluation of the mitral orifice, left ventricular free wall, and right ventricular cavities. Plane E provides a cross-sectional view of the roots of the great arteries (see also Figs. 2–15 to 2–17).

outflow tract. This provides a view of the infundibulum of the right ventricle, the pulmonic valve, and the pulmonary trunk (main pulmonary artery). The point of bifurcation of the trunk into right and left pulmonary arteries can frequently be seen. This view is especially valuable in evaluating the width of the right ventricular outflow tract and the integrity of the membranous portion of the interventricular septum.

Short Axis or Transverse View (Fig. 2–5)

By rotating the transducer clockwise an additional 60°, the tomographic plane is placed at right angles to the long axis view, providing a short axis or transverse sectional view of the left ventricle and the anterior crescent-shaped right ventricle. With the transducer positioned in the third or fourth left intercostal space, serial cross-sectional views can be obtained from the apex of the heart through the origins of the great arteries by tilting the transducer from the left ventricular apex to the aortic root, in a manner similar to the standard M-mode echocardiographic "sweep." With the trans-

ducer oriented toward the ventricular apex, cross-sectional views of the left ventricular apex and papillary muscles are obtained. Further cephalad tilt of the transducer allows cross-sectional evaluation of the mitral valve leaflets and the mitral orifice, the left ventricular free wall, and the right and left ventricular cavity dimensions. The transducer may be further tilted to show a cross section of the left ventricular outflow tract and the origins of the great arteries. The normal cross-sectional view of the great arteries creates an image referred to as the "circle and sausage" (referring to the circular aorta and the "sausage-shaped" right ventricular outflow tract anterior to it). The three aortic valve cusps can usually be seen within the center of the circle. The coronary ostia are often visualized as well. The tricuspid valve is located to the right of the aortic root and the sweep of the right ventricular outflow tract to the level of the pulmonic valve lies anterior to the aorta, forming the "sausage." The normal pulmonic valve is anterior and to the left of the aorta. The main pulmonary artery can be visualized as it dives posteriorly to its bifurcation. The left atrium and a portion of the

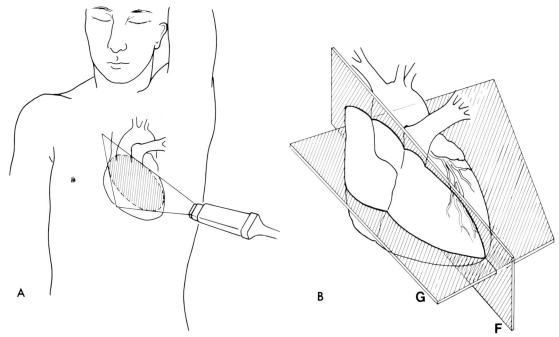

Figure 2–6. Apical imaging. *A,* With the patient in the left lateral decubitus position the transducer is placed over the apical impulse and oriented similar to a short axis view but tilted to point toward the right shoulder to create a four-chamber, or hemiaxial, view. With the transducer maintained over the apex, but rotated 90° clockwise so as to align the plane along the long axis of the ventricle, a right anterior oblique equivalent view is produced.

B, Orientation of the two-dimensional scanning planes from the apex. The right anterior oblique equivalent view arises from a long axis image of the left ventricle transecting the inferior, apical, and anterolateral left ventricular walls and the mitral valve (plane F) (see also Fig. 2–20). Plane G shows the transducer transecting the interventricular septum at right angles to the right anterior oblique equivalent view, thus generating a hemiaxial view that allows simultaneous visualization of the four cardiac chambers, intracardiac septae, and atrioventricular valves (see also Fig. 2–18).

interatrial septum are seen posterior to the aortic root.

Apical Imaging[4] (Fig. 2–6)

With the examination plane oriented in the "short axis" of the left ventricle and the patient in the left lateral decubitus position, the transducer is placed over the point of maximal impulse. This orientation creates a tomographic plane from the apex of the heart through the right shoulder, allowing imaging of the four cardiac chambers, both atrioventricular valves, the interatrial and interventricular septa, and the central fibrous body (the point of union of the septa and both atrioventricular valves). This has been referred to as the "hemiaxial equivalent" view. The left lower pulmonary vein may be seen entering the left atrial cavity, and both ventricular inflow regions can be examined simultaneously. The posterior or inflow portion of the interventricular septum is also seen in this view. In addition, the relative levels of origin of the atrioventricular valves may also be evaluated. If the transducer is rotated 90°, a long axis view of the left ventricle that is bordered by the inferior ventricular wall, apex, and anterolateral left ventricular walls is obtained with simultaneous visualization of the left atrium and left ventricular inflow and outflow regions. This has been called the "right anterior oblique equivalent" view.

Subxiphoid (Subcostal) Imaging[5] (Fig. 2–7)

From a subxiphoid position in the upper abdomen, with the transducer elevated by 45° from the anterior abdominal wall and placed to the right of the midline along the long axis of the body, the inferior vena cava

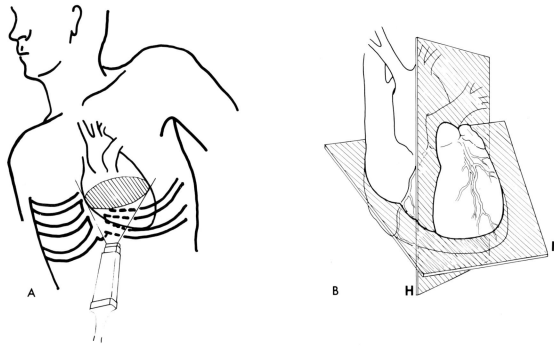

Figure 2–7. Subxiphoid views. *A,* With the transducer in the subxiphoid region oriented along the long axis of the body, the inferior vena cava may be followed to its insertion in the right atrial cavity (see Fig. 2–21). With 90° clockwise rotation of the transducer, the coronal view of the heart is obtained. Tilting the transducer 45° to the abdominal wall will visualize the heart in a four chamber configuration, allowing examination of the interatrial and interventricular septa and both ventricular inflow tracts (see Fig. 2–22). With the transducer tilt decreased to 35 to 40°, the left ventricular outflow tract and aortic valve are visualized (see Fig. 2–24). Further decrease in the elevation of the transducer angle to 30° provides visualization of the anterior right ventricular outflow tract, pulmonary valve, and main pulmonary artery (see Fig. 2–25). *B,* Subxiphoid imaging. In the long axis, plane H allows imaging of the inferior vena cava and the right ventricular inflow and outflow tract. The four-chamber view is illustrated by plane I, allowing evaluation of both ventricular inflow tracts and intracardiac septae.

is visualized and may be followed to its insertion in the right atrium. Ninety degrees of clockwise rotation of the transducer provides a four-chamber, or coronal, view of the heart. Both atrial chambers are visualized with the ultrasound beam striking the interatrial septum perpendicularly, providing a view of the entire septum. Both ventricular inflow tracts and the crest of the interventricular septum are visualized. With the transducer in the subxiphoid position and oriented along the same axis, the elevation of the transducer may be decreased to 35 to 40° in order to visualize the left ventricular outflow tract and aortic root. Further decrease of the transducer elevation angle to 30° from the abdominal wall, provides a view of the anterior right ventricular outflow tract, pulmonic valve, and main pulmonary artery.

SEQUENTIAL APPROACH TO CONGENITAL HEART DISEASE

By integrating the information obtained from the physical examination, the plain chest radiograph, and the electrocardiogram with that obtained from the echocardiogram, it is possible to deductively analyze complex congenital cardiac anomalies.[12] From the information obtained on physical examination, the patient with congenital heart disease may be classified as either cyanotic or acyanotic.

The chest film provides valuable information concerning the position of the heart within the thorax and the situs of the patient (See Chapter 1). Over- or underperfusion of the lungs is determined by an assessment of the pulmonary vascular markings. A reasonable differential diagnosis can usually be

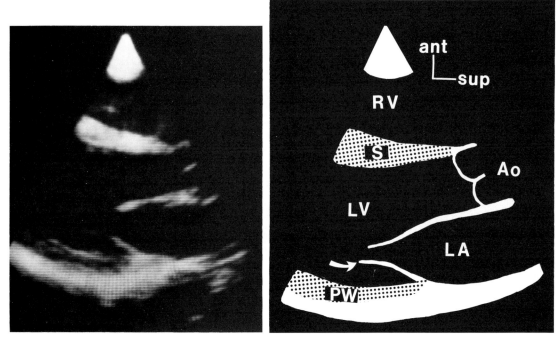

Figure 2-8. Normal anatomy—long axis view of the left ventricle. A 60° sector of the left ventricular long axis. The right ventricular outflow (RV) is seen in the upper portion of the sector, anterior to the interventricular septum (S). The mitral valve (curved arrow) separates the left atrium (LA) from the left ventricle (LV). Mitral-aortic and septal-aortic fibrous continuity are demonstrated. The epi- and endocardial surfaces of the left ventricular posterior wall (PW) are also well defined.

achieved at this point (this will be dealt with in subsequent chapters). The atrial situs is further delineated by using the two-dimensional echocardiogram to locate the inferior vena cava in the long axis subxiphoidal view. The inferior vena cava is then traced to its insertion into the right atrium, which is further identified by the location of the eustachian valve. This also identifies the rare patient with bilateral inferior venae cavae or the patient with ambiguous abdominal situs and absent inferior vena cava. Based on the chest film and echocardiographic findings, patients are then classified into those with situs solitus (S), situs inversus (I), and situs ambiguus (A).

Using two-dimensional echocardiographic imaging techniques, it is possible to evaluate the trabecular pattern of the ventricular chambers and the interventricular septum and to provide information concerning the direction of ventricular looping (an event that took place during embryonic development of the heart). It is possible to determine whether the coarsely trabeculated right ventricle has looped to the right

(dextro or d-loop) in the usual fashion or to the left (levo or l-loop). Further information concerning the ventricular loop may be obtained by locating the position of the mitral valve, which is identified in most cases by its direct fibrous continuity with a great artery, and the position of the ventricular conal tissue. The great arteries may be individually identified in the long axis view by determining which of the two vessels dives posteriorly and bifurcates, and is thus the pulmonary artery. In the short axis view, the origin of the coronary arteries identifies the aortic root. Moreover, in the short axis view of the great arteries of the normal person, one sees the circular aortic cross section and anterior crescent-shaped sweep of the right ventricular outflow tract joining the pulmonary trunk. In transposition or malposition complexes, the ascending aorta is located anterior to or alongside the pulmonary trunk and both great arteries are visualized as circles. The labeling of the spatial relationships between the arteries is determined by the right-left orientation of the arteries (anterior rightward aorta, "D"; anterior leftward aorta, "L"; directly an-

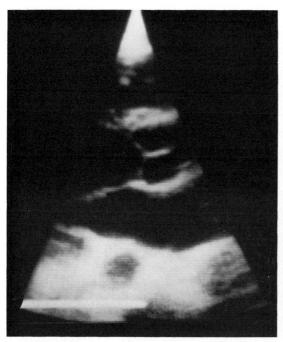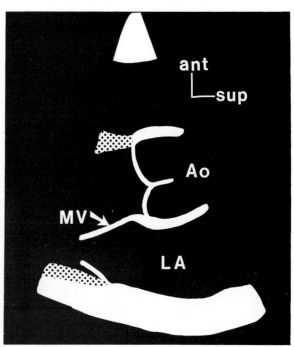

Figure 2–9. Normal anatomy — long axis of the left ventricle. A 45° sector oriented higher in the left ventricular outflow tract allows detailed examination of the ascending aorta and mitral valve leaflets (MV). The aortic valve leaflets (Ao) are seen within the aortic root. The left atrium (LA) lies posterior to the aortic root. In this view, the LA/Ao ratio may be measured.

teroposterior orientation, "A"). In these patients, the intracardiac anatomy can be classified noninvasively according to the segmental approach that has been suggested by Van Praagh:[12]

Situs — solitus (S), inversus (I), or ambiguus (A)

Ventricular Loop — right (D) or left (L)

Aortic Position — anterior rightward (D), anterior leftward (L), directly anteroposterior (A)

NORMAL TWO-DIMENSIONAL ECHOCARDIOGRAPHIC ANATOMY

The *long axis view* (Fig. 2–8) provides information about the normal anatomy of the left ventricle. The mitral valve is characterized by its direct continuity with the posterior great vessel (aorta). Mitral-aortic and septal-aortic fibrous continuity can easily be demonstrated. In addition, one can determine the relationship between the aortic root and the right ventricular outflow tract and between the left atrium and aortic root. Coarse trabeculation in the anterior aspect of the interventricular septum marks the position of the morphologic right ventricle. In normal individuals, this ventricle has looped to the right and is anterior and to the right of the left ventricular cavity. With further cephalad orientation of the transducer in the long axis (Fig. 2–9), the ascending aorta is identified as a vessel that arches to the left and gives rise to the vessels to the head and extremities. This view is useful for identification of the size and shape of the ascending aorta and the left atrium posterior to the aortic root. With orientation of the transducer in the long axis and angulation toward the right side of the sternum, the right ventricular inflow tract is seen (Fig. 2–10). Using this view, the right atrium may be measured and the integrity of the tricuspid valve evaluated.

Rotation of the transducer 30° clockwise from the long axis view gives a long axis view of the right ventricular outflow tract (Fig. 2–11) and demonstrates the infundibular region of the right ventricle. The pulmonic valve is seen, separating the conal region of the right ventricle from the pulmo-

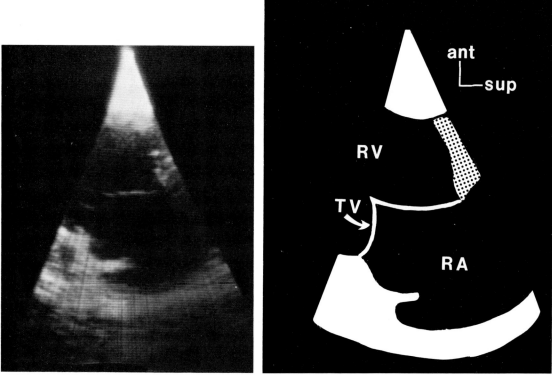

Figure 2-10. Normal anatomy — long axis of the right ventricular inflow tract. This view is obtained by angulating the transducer off the long axis of the left ventricle toward the right flank of the patient and orienting the scan plane beneath the sternum. The tricuspid valve (TV) is seen between the right atrial cavity (RA) and right ventricular cavity (RV). This view is especially useful for evaluating the integrity of the tricuspid valve leaflets and for estimating the size of the right atrial cavity.

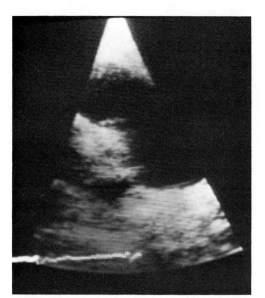
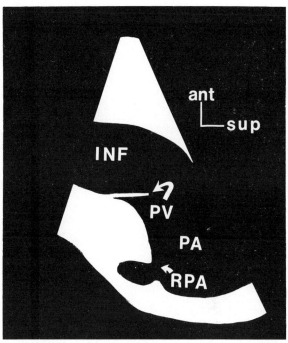

Figure 2–11. Normal anatomy — long axis of the right ventricular outflow tract. The transducer can be rotated 30° clockwise from the left ventricular outflow tract view to obtain visualization of the right ventricular outflow tract. The infundibular region of the right ventricle (INF) is seen below the level of the pulmonary valve (PV). In this image, only the posterior leaflet of the pulmonic valve is seen. The main pulmonary artery (PA) dives posteriorly above the level of the valve and the take-off of the right pulmonary artery (RPA) can be defined.

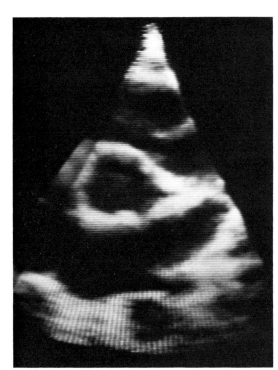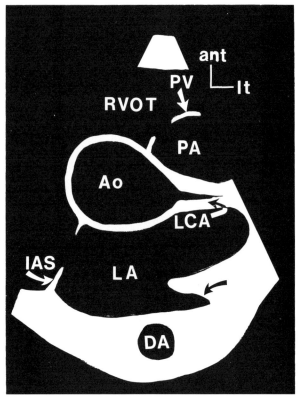

Figure 2–12. Normal anatomy — short axis (or transverse) view of the great arterial roots. In the short axis view of the great arterial roots, the aorta (Ao) appears as a circular cross section with the anterior sausage-shaped right ventricular outflow tract (RVOT) sweeping to the pulmonary artery (PA). The pulmonic valve (PV) is anterior to and to the left of the aortic root. The left coronary artery (LCA) can be seen arising from the aortic root. The left atrium (LA) is posterior to the aortic root. The left lower pulmonary vein (black curved arrow) is seen entering the left atrial cavity. The interatrial septum is posterior to the aortic root (IAS). The descending aorta (DA) can be seen posterior to the left atrium (LA).

nary trunk, which can be followed as it dives posteriorly to its bifurcation. The long axis view of the heart, therefore, may be used (1) to evaluate the patency of both the left and right ventricular inflow and outflow tracts and (2) to identify the integrity of the semilunar and atrioventricular valve leaflets.

With further clockwise rotation of the transducer the *short axis view* is obtained. This view, which is at right angles to the long axis view, allows the spatial interrelationship of the great arteries to be evaluated (Fig. 2–12). The normal pulmonic valve is found anterior, superior, and to the left of the aortic valve. In this short axis view, the left atrium lies posterior to the aortic root, and the origin of the left main coronary artery from the left coronary cusp can be visualized. It is often possible to identify the entry of the left lower pulmonary vein

into the cavity of the left atrium in this view. The morphology of the aortic valve cusps (Fig. 2–13) and their opening pattern (Fig. 2–14) can be evaluated, allowing secure identification of aortic valve malformations, such as the bicuspid aortic valve. This view may also be used in measuring the aortic valve annulus when cardiac surgery for valve replacement is considered. With slight cephalad orientation in the short axis view from the aortic root, the pulmonary trunk may be followed to its bifurcation (Fig. 2–15). Direct visualization of the bifurcation and the proximal portions of the right and left pulmonary artery branches is usually possible. Apical orientation of the transducer in the short axis permits examination of the left ventricular cavity posterior and to the left of the crescentic, anterior right ventricular cavity. The mitral valve is seen within the normal circular cross section of

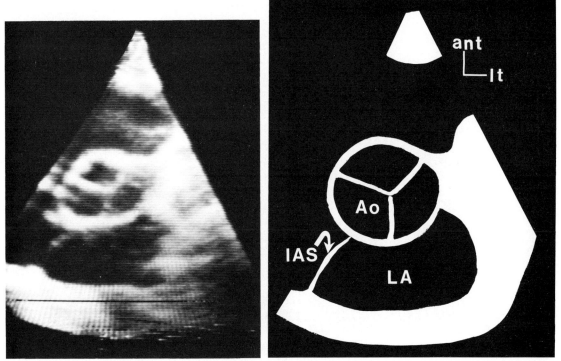

Figure 2–13. Normal anatomy — short axis view of aorta. The three-cusped aortic valve can be visualized within the cross section of the aortic root (Ao) at end-diastole. The interatrial septum (IAS) lies posterior to the aortic root and forms one border of the left atrium (LA).

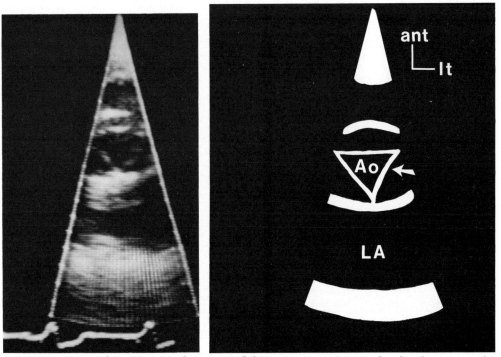

Figure 2–14. Normal anatomy — short axis of the aortic root. In systole, the three aortic leaflets open in a triangular fashion (arrow) and verify the three-leafed arrangement of the valve. (Ao = aortic root; LA = left atrium).

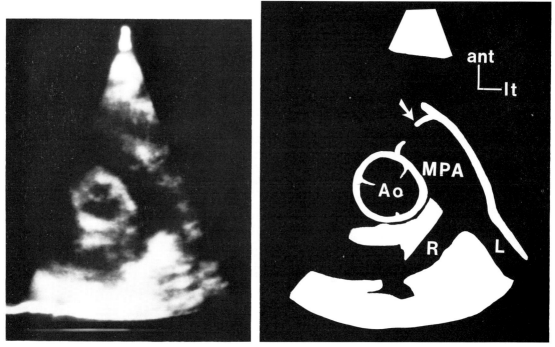

Figure 2–15. Normal anatomy — pulmonary artery in short axis. Slight cranial direction of the transducer in the short axis plane permits identification of the bifurcation of the main pulmonary artery (MPA) into its right and left components (R) (L). The right pulmonary artery can be seen posterior to the aortic root (Ao).

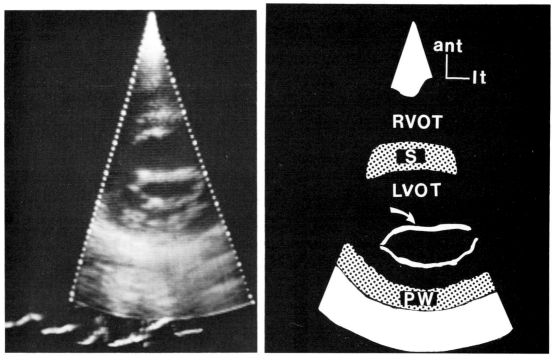

Figure 2–16. Normal anatomy — short axis of the ventricular cavities. Short axis view at the mid portion of the ventricles showing the circular cross section of the left ventricular cavity at the level of the mitral valve. The interventricular septum (S) can be seen between the crescent-shaped anterior right ventricular outflow tract (RVOT) and the circular left ventricular outflow tract (LVOT). The mitral valve (curved arrow) is seen in the open position within the left ventricular cavity. The thickness of the left ventricular posterior wall (PW) can be measured in this view.

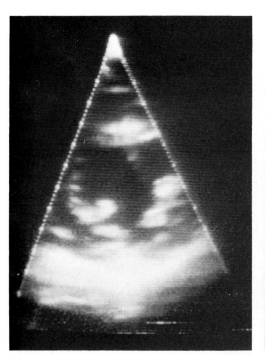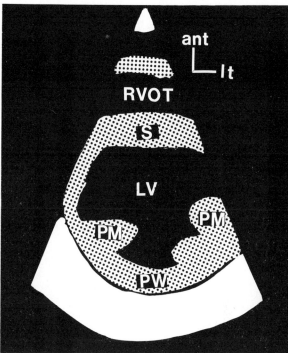

Figure 2-17. Normal anatomy — short axis of the ventricles toward apex. Short axis view of the ventricular apex shows the circular cross section of the left ventricle (LV) and the two papillary muscles (PM) in their normal medial and lateral positions along the posterior wall (PW). The septum (S) lies below the right ventricular outflow tract (RVOT).

the left ventricular cavity (Fig. 2–16). This "en-face" view of the mitral valve throughout the cardiac cycle allows measurement of the mitral valve orifice directly from the two-dimensional image.[13] With further tilting of the transducer toward the apex in the short axis, the anteromedial and posterolateral papillary muscles of the mitral valve are identified (Fig. 2–17).

With the patient in the left decubitus position and the transducer placed over the apical impulse, the *hemiaxial or four chamber view*[4] is obtained (Fig. 2–18). This allows one to evaluate the four cardiac chambers simultaneously. The inflow portion of the interventricular septum, the inflow regions of both ventricles, and the insertion of the atrioventricular valves can all be examined. A portion of the interatrial septum primum may also be visualized between the atrial cavities and the left lower pulmonary vein entry into the left atrium. With slight posterior angulation, the coronary sinus may also be evaluated (Fig. 2–19).

With rotation of the apical transducer into the long axis of the heart, the left ventricular inflow and outflow tract may be identified from the *"right anterior oblique equivalent view"*[4] (Fig. 2–20). This also allows measurement of the size of the left atrial cavity. The apical views, therefore, are useful for (1) evaluating the positions of the atrioventricular valves and the inflow portions of both ventricles, and (2) evaluating the inflow portion of the interventricular septum and the interatrial septum primum. The right anterior oblique equivalent view is useful for allowing measurement of the left ventricle and left atrium as well as for evaluating the patency of the left ventricular inflow and outflow regions.

In the *subxiphoidal view*, the visceroatrial situs can be evaluated by identifying the inferior vena cava as it traverses the liver and enters the right atrium (Fig. 2–21). The four chamber (coronal) view from the subxiphoid position (Fig. 2–22) permits the interatrial septum to be identified and examined in detail.[5,14] Because this view is perpendicular to the plane of the interatrial

Text continued on page 110

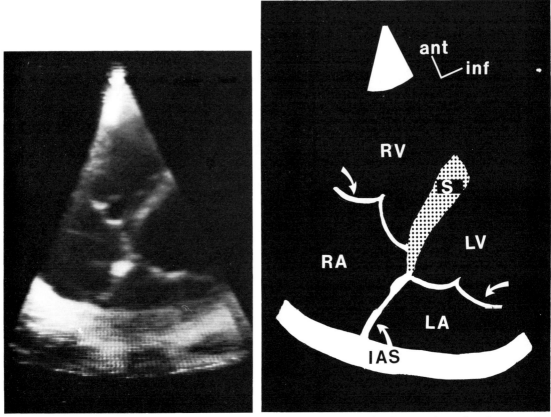

Figure 2–18. Normal anatomy — apical or four-chamber view. The four cardiac chambers can be viewed in the hemiaxial equivalent or apical four-chamber view. The interventricular septum (S) is seen between the right (RV) and left (LV) ventricular cavities. The atrioventricular valves (curved arrows) separate the right (RA) and left (LA) atria from their respective ventricles. Note that the insertion of the tricuspid valve is somewhat more apical than the insertion of the mitral valve. The interatrial septum (IAS) lies between the atrial cavities.

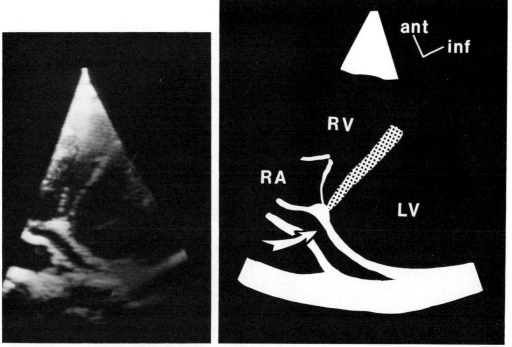

Figure 2–19. Normal anatomy — coronary sinus view from apex. With slight clockwise rotation from the apical four-chamber view, the left (LV) and right (RV) ventricles are displayed and the coronary sinus (arrow) may be seen entering the right atrial cavity (RA).

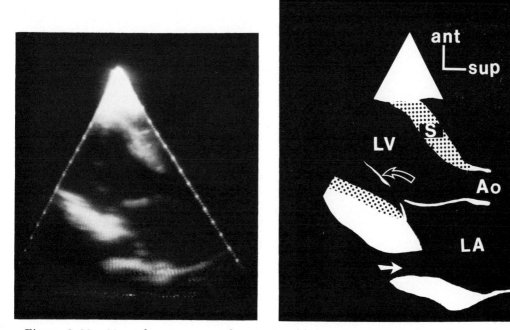

Figure 2–20. Normal anatomy — right anterior oblique view. With the transducer at the apex and oriented along the long axis of the ventricle, the right anterior oblique equivalent view can be created. This allows visualization of the septum (S), left ventricular cavity, and the ventricular inflow and outflow tracts. The left atrium (LA) and its inflow into the left ventricle (LV) are well seen. (Ao = aorta; solid arrow = pulmonary vein; open arrow = chordae tendineae).

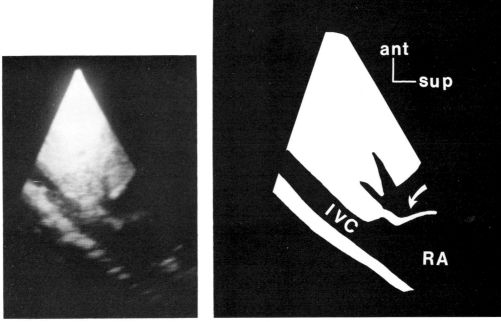

Figure 2–21. Normal anatomy — subxiphoidal long axis view of inferior vena cava. The inferior vena cava (IVC) can be seen entering the right atrium (RA). The eustachian valve (arrow) is seen at the junction of IVC entry into RA.

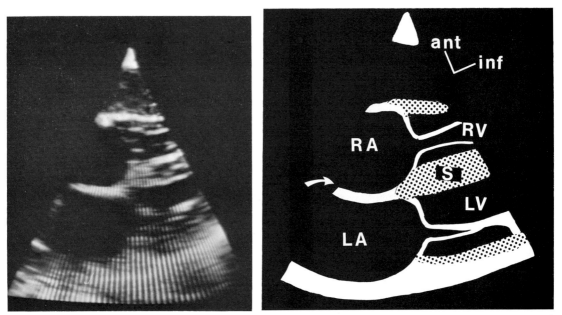

Figure 2–22. Normal anatomy—subxiphoidal view of ventricular inflow tract. The interatrial septum (arrow) is most clearly defined in this view because the scan plane is oriented perpendicularly to the plane of the septum. The septum separates the atria (LA and RA). The inflow portion of the ventricular septum (S) is identified in this view. The right and left ventricular inflow tracts (RV and LV) are also displayed.

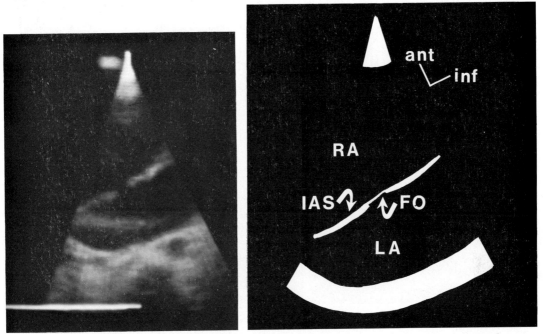

Figure 2-23. Normal anatomy—subxiphoidal view of interatrial septum. The interatrial septum (IAS) can be examined best from the subxiphoid short axis view. This view allows identification of the foramen ovale (FO), as well as the right (RA) and left (LA) atrium.

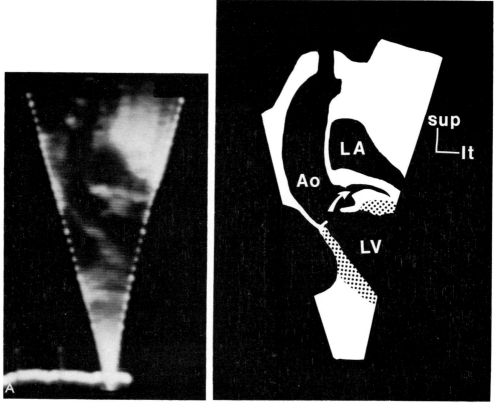

Figure 2–24.   A, Normal subxiphoidal view—left ventricular outflow tract. Subxiphoid view showing the ascending aorta (Ao) and the left ventricle (LV). The origin and proximal portion of the left
main coronary artery (arrow) is seen to arise from the coronary sinus above the aortic valve leaflets. The
left atrium (LA) lies lateral to the aortic arch. (Note that this image has been electronically inverted.)

Illustration continued on opposite page

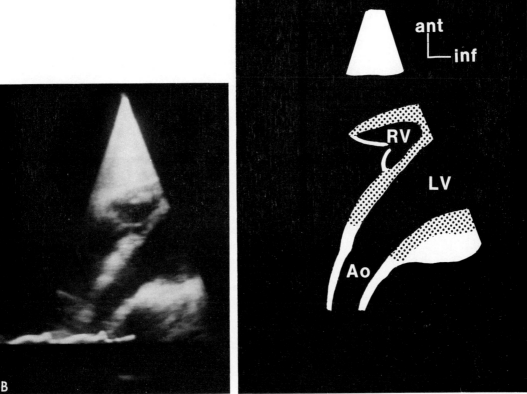

Figure 2–24 Continued. B, Normal anatomy—short axis subxiphoidal view of the left ventricular outflow tract. With the transducer elevated 35° from lower abdominal wall in the short axis, the subxiphoidal view of the left ventricular outflow tract is seen. In this view, the left ventricle (LV) is seen leading to the aorta (Ao). This view is especially useful in the evaluation of possible left ventricular outflow tract obstructions. A truncated portion of the right ventricle (RV) is present in the anterior portion of this plane.

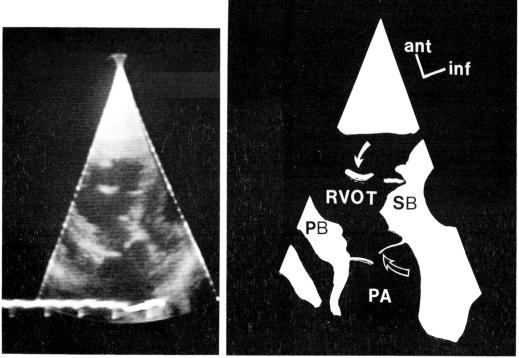

Figure 2–25. A, Normal anatomy — short axis subxiphoidal view of the right ventricular outflow tract. With a further decrease in elevation of the transducer to 30° from the abdominal wall the right ventricular outflow tract (RVOT) is seen in an upside-down fashion from the subxiphoid view. The septal and parietal limbs of the crista are well visualized. (SB = septal band; PB = parietal band of the crista). The pulmonic valve is well seen (dark arrow) and the main pulmonary artery (PA) is visualized to the level of the bifurcation. The papillary muscle of the conus is frequently visualized in this view (white arrow).

septum, the integrity of the atrial septum secundum and patency of the foramen ovale can usually be determined (Fig. 2–23). The inflow region of both ventricular cavities is also evaluated and, by decreasing the elevation of the transducer from the abdominal wall, the left ventricular outflow tract can be traced to the level of the ascending aorta (Fig. 2–24) and aortic arch (Fig. 2–24A). With further decrease in the elevation of the transducer, toward the abdominal wall, the right ventricular outflow is seen coursing anterior to the left ventricular outflow tract (Fig. 2–25). The relationship between the outflow tracts and the great arteries may, therefore, be completely evaluated from this view.[14] The subxiphoid view has great utility for the evaluation of visceroatrial situs as well as for evaluation of the integrity of the interatrial septum, interventricular septum, atrioventricular valves, and ventricular outflow tracts and great arteries.

In summary, the combination of precordial, apical, and subxiphoidal echocardiographic imaging allows complete evaluation of the internal anatomy and structural relationships of the cardiac chambers and great vessels.

REFERENCES

1. Bom, N., Lancee, C. T., Van Zwieten, G., et al.: Multiscan echocardiography. Circulation 48:1066, 1973.
2. Griffith, J. M., Henry, W. L.: A sector scanner for real-time two-dimensional echocardiography. Circulation 49:1147, 1974.
3. Von Ramm, O. T., Thurstone, F.: Cardiac imaging using a phased array ultrasound system. Circulation 53:258, 1976.
4. Silverman, N. H., Schiller, N. B.: Apex echocardiography: A two-dimensional technique for evaluating congenital heart disease. Circulation 57:503, 1978.
5. Lange, L. W., Sahn, D. J., Allen, H. D., Goldberg,

S. J.: Subxiphoid cross-sectional echocardiography in infants and children with congenital heart disease. Circulation 59:513, 1979.

6. Tajik, A. J., Seward, J. B., Hagler, D. J., Mair, D. D., Lie, J. T.: Two-dimensional real-time ultrasonic imaging of the heart and great vessels: Technique, image orientation, structure identification and validation. Mayo Clin Proc 53:271, 1978.

7. Roge, C. L., Silverman, N. H., Hart, P. A., Ray, R. M.: Cardiac structure growth pattern determined by echocardiography. Circulation 57:285, 1978.

8. Bennett, D. H., Evans, D. W., Raj, M. V.: Echocardiographic left ventricular dimensions in pressure and volume overload. Br Heart J 37:971, 1975.

9. Gewitz, M. H., Werner, J. C., Kleinman, C. S., Hellenbrand, W. E., Talner, N. S.: Role of echocardiography in aortic stenosis: Pre- and post-operative studies. Am J Cardiol 43:67, 1979.

10. Hirschfeld, S., Meyer, R., Schwartz, D. C., Korfhagen, J., Kaplan, S.: The echocardiographic assessment of pulmonary artery pressure and pulmonary vascular resistance. Circulation 52:642, 1975.

11. Hirschfeld, S., Meyer, R., Schwartz, D. C., Korfhagen, J., Kaplan, S.: Measurement of right and left ventricle systolic time intervals by echocardiography. Circulation 51:304, 1975.

12. Solinger, R., Elbl, R., Minhas, K.: Deductive echocardiographic analysis in infants with congenital heart disease. Circulation 50:1072, 1974.

13. Henry, W. L., Griffith, J. M., Michaelis, L. L., McIntosh, C. L., Morrow, A. G., Epstein, S. E.: Measurement of mitral orifice area in patients with mitral valve disease by real-time two-dimensional echocardiography. Circulation 51:827, 1975.

14. Bierman, F. Z., Williams, R. G.: Prospective diagnosis of a d-transposition of the great arteries in neonates by subxiphoid, two-dimensional echocardiography. Circulation 60:1496, 1979.

Chapter 3

NUCLEAR MEDICINE PROCEDURES

by Harvey J. Berger, M.D.,

*Assistant Professor of Diagnostic Radiology
and Medicine; Director of Cardiovascular Imaging,
Yale University School of Medicine*

Alexander Gottschalk, M.D.,

*Professor of Diagnostic Radiology;
Vice-Chairman, Department of Diagnostic Radiology,
Yale University School of Medicine*

Barry L. Zaret, M.D.,

*Associate Professor of Medicine and Diagnostic
Radiology; Chief, Section of Cardiology,
Yale University School of Medicine*

INTRODUCTION

The use of radioactive tracers to evaluate heart disease in children dates to 1948 when Prinzmetal and associates initially described the characteristics of the first-pass radiocardiogram in three patients with congenital cardiac lesions.[1] They used a Geiger-Müller counter as a radiation detector and iodine-131 sodium iodide as the radiotracer. Since then, there have been major advances in available radiopharmaceuticals, instrumentation, and computer systems. Development of high resolution stationary detector systems, such as the gamma scintillation camera, coupled to dedicated computers and microprocessors has made possible dynamic quantitative imaging of the heart, both in children and in adults.

The application of nuclear medicine techniques to the study of congenital heart disease has focused primarily on the use of first-pass radionuclide angiocardiography for detection, localization, and quantification of intracardiac shunts and shunts between the great vessels. In addition, the first transit study can be used to determine

From the Nuclear Medicine Section, Department of Diagnostic Radiology, and the Cardiology Section, Department of Internal Medicine, Yale University School of Medicine, New Haven, Connecticut 06510. Supported in part by NHLBI Grant RO 1 HL 21690. Dr. Berger is an Established Investigator of the American Heart Association.

left and right ventricular ejection fractions, as well as regional wall motion. Recently, gated equilibrium cardiac blood pool imaging and thallium-201 myocardial perfusion imaging have been utilized in children with congenital and acquired heart disease. These radionuclide techniques are not traumatic to the patient, carry no known physical risks, and deliver an acceptably low whole body radiation burden. Because only tracer amounts of radionuclides are injected, these agents do not result in altered physiologic states, such as is encountered when iodinated contrast agents are employed.

At the onset, it is important to stress that radionuclide methods should be used in conjunction with the chest radiograph and echocardiogram. Radionuclide assessment of biventricular performance and cardiac flow patterns provides data directly complementary to the cross-sectional echocardiographic examination and can be used to help focus the echocardiographic study, if it is performed first. In addition, radionuclide assessment of the degree of left-to-right shunting can be quantified. Nevertheless, in most clinical situations, patients still require cardiac catheterization and angiography for precise anatomic definition of all congenital lesions and for measurement of intracardiac and vascular pressures and oxygen saturations, and subsequent calculation of vascular resistances and valve areas. Following cardiac catheterization and corrective surgery, radionuclide studies can be utilized to follow the patient's cardiac status, imposing minimal discomfort or risk to the patient.

In this chapter, the major radionuclide techniques applicable to the study of children with cardiac disease will be described. These include first-pass radionuclide angiocardiography, gated equilibrium cardiac blood pool imaging, and thallium-201 myocardial perfusion imaging. In addition, pulmonary perfusion imaging and liver/spleen scanning, which have occasional applications in children with heart disease, will be discussed briefly. Following description of each method, selected clinical applications and potential future directions will be reviewed. Emphasis will be placed upon application in children but, when appropriate, discussion of uses in adults with congenital heart disease will also be included.

FIRST-PASS RADIONUCLIDE ANGIOCARDIOGRAPHY

General Description

Radionuclide angiocardiography provides both qualitative and quantitative data in patients with congenital heart disease.[2-6] This technique involves serial imaging of the first transit of the radionuclide bolus through the central circulation with a gamma scintillation camera (Fig. 3–1). Each study requires injection of a separate radionuclide bolus. The volume of injectate must be small. The brief period of data acquisition (usually less than 30 seconds at a resting heart rate) makes this approach especially suitable for children, even severely ill neonates. Anatomic and morphologic data are obtained with the scintillation camera and a video playback system. Quantitative analysis requires a dedicated computer system that allows definition of regions of interest and generation of high frequency time-activity curves from these regions. Gamma cameras and computers are now fully portable and can be brought directly to the patient's bedside, facilitating study of critically ill patients in the pediatric or newborn intensive care unit.

Radiopharmaceuticals

Any of the technetium-99m radiotracers, except macroaggregated albumin or microspheres, can be used for a first transit study. In children, technetium-99m pertechnetate is usually employed in a dose of approximately 200 μCi/kg body weight, but a minimal dose of 2 to 3 mCi is always used, even in neonates.[2] In adults, a total dose of 15 to 25 mCi is used. The radionuclide employed must be of high specific activity so that its volume is less than 0.5 ml. In children, prior to radionuclide administration, sodium perchlorate (intravenous) or potassium perchlorate (oral) should be given in a dose of 3 to 6 mg/kg body weight. Perchlorate blocks the uptake of technetium-99m pertechnetate by the choroid plexus, thyroid, and gastrointestinal tract, and thereby promotes excretion of the radionuclide in the urine. In addition, this lowers the overall radiation burden (Table 3–1). If serial studies are required, the initial study can be

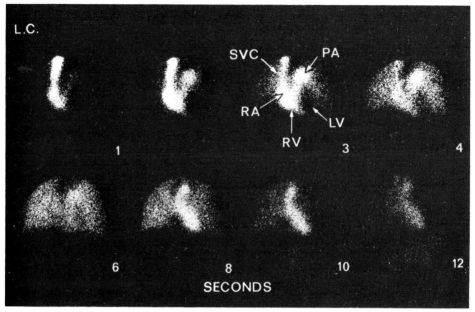

Figure 3–1. Normal first-pass radionuclide angiocardiogram obtained on a single crystal scintillation camera in the anterior position. The time after appearance of radioactivity at the superior vena cava is designated in seconds. Each of the images in the upper row represents one-second accumulations, while each of the images in the lower row represents two-second accumulations. Note the distinct right and left heart phases. By 12 seconds, most of the activity has left the central circulation. SVC = superior vena cava. RA = right atrium. RV = right ventricle. PA = pulmonary artery. LV = left ventricle. (Reproduced with permission from Treves, Maltz, and Adelstein.[4])

TABLE 3–1. Common Radiopharmaceuticals Used in Pediatric Cardiopulmonary Studies

RADIONUCLIDE	USES	ADMINISTERED DOSE (mCi)*	CRITICAL ORGAN	WHOLEBODY RADIATION DOSE (rads)†
99mTc-pertechnetate	First-pass radionuclide angiocardiography	2–25	Colon (after perchlorate blockade)	0.07–0.33
99mTc-red blood cells	First-pass radionuclide angiocardiography Multiple-gated blood pool imaging	2–25	Spleen	0.14–0.50
99mTc-human serum albumin	First-pass radionuclide angiocardiography Multiple-gated blood pool imaging	2–25	Blood	0.12–0.38
99mTc-macroaggregated albumin	Pulmonary perfusion imaging	0.2– 4.0	Lung	0.01–0.60
Thallium-201	Myocardial perfusion imaging	0.25– 2.0	Kidney	0.25–0.36

*Range from minimal to maximal doses.
†Range from a one-year-old to an adult expressed per imaging dose.
99mTc = technetium-99m
From Kereiakis, J., et al.: Radiopharmaceutical dosimetry in pediatrics. Semin Nucl Med 2:316, 1972.

performed with either technetium-99m DTPA (diethylenetriaminepentaacetic acid) or sulfur colloid. DTPA is used for renal scanning and is cleared from the blood pool by glomerular filtration, while sulfur colloid is used for liver/spleen scanning and is cleared by the reticuloendothelial system. Both radionuclides result in lower residual background levels in the blood pool than does technetium-99m pertechnetate.[6]

Alternatively, first-pass radionuclide angiocardiography can be combined with subsequent equilibrium cardiac blood pool imaging by using either technetium-99m labeled human serum albumin or labeled autologous red blood cells. In the latter case, approximately 0.05 mg/kg of unlabeled stannous pyrophosphate is injected 15 to 20 minutes prior to injection of technetium-99m pertechnetate, providing in vivo labeling of the patient's own red blood cells. In the adult, 3 mg of stannous pyrophosphate are administered.[7]

Radionuclide Injection

Generally, sedation is not required, even in young children. Depending upon the patient's size and age, either a 23 or 21 gauge butterfly needle or an 18 or 19 gauge 1½ inch polyethylene catheter is used for injection of the radionuclide dose. The largest possible size should be employed. The medial right antecubital vein is the preferable injection site, but in some cases an external jugular vein may be employed. It is important to emphasize that careful *bolus administration* is essential to ensure the validity of derived quantitative data. Meticulous care is needed in order to obtain reliable results, and the injection site should be chosen with this in mind.[3, 6] An intravenous infusion is established to ensure patency of the injection site. To facilitate bolus injection, the catheter or butterfly needle is attached to an extension tube and a three-way stopcock. After the tube is filled with normal saline, the radioactive bolus is introduced into the tube with small air interfaces before and after the radionuclide material. (The air is omitted if there is a possibility of a right-to-left shunt.) The flush syringe is connected directly to the tubing so that the bolus is introduced directly by the flush. The radionuclide then is injected as a bolus using a normal saline flush of 1 to 20 ml depending upon the patient's body size. Care should be taken to ensure that the injection is made when the child is not crying or breathing irregularly, as these may cause fragmentation of the bolus or may directly affect the patient's cardiac status by altering sympathetic tone. If the bolus injection is fragmented or prolonged, the study should be repeated. The bolus dose should have a duration of less than two seconds as estimated from a computer-derived time-activity curve from a region of interest over the superior vena cava.

Instrumentation and Data Acquisition

Studies may be performed using either a conventional single crystal scintillation camera or the computerized multicrystal camera. Most pediatric cases have been carried out with the single crystal camera. For evaluation of intracardiac shunts and delineation of cardiac flow patterns, the single crystal camera is clearly preferable. The major advantages of the single crystal camera are its high intrinsic resolution and mobile capability, which are particularly valuable in clinical assessment in the newborn special care unit or intensive care unit. A limiting factor of conventional single crystal cameras, however, is the relatively *low maximal count rate* of raw data. These systems have linear response rates up to approximately 60,000 to 80,000 counts/sec, above which dead time losses and data distortion occur. These factors are most critical when high frequency studies needed for evaluation of ejection fraction and wall motion are performed.[6] These studies, especially in adolescents and adults, are best performed on the multicrystal scintillation camera, which has a greater count rate capacity (up to approximately 450,000 counts/sec) without data distortion.

Depending upon the diagnostic information sought, data may be collected in several ways. For qualitative assessment in patients with congenital heart disease, data are acquired at two to three frames/sec using a

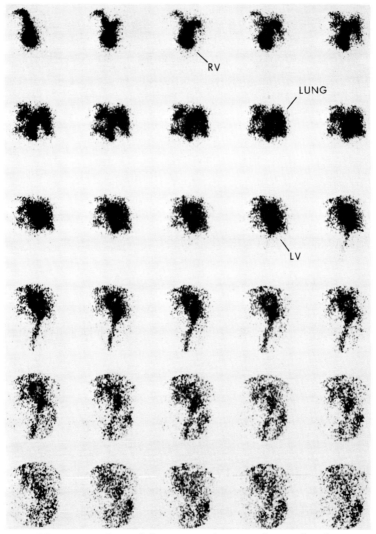

Figure 3–2. Normal first-pass radionuclide angiocardiogram obtained in the anterior position. This study is displayed at three frames per second. Note the distinct right and left heart phases. Activity clears from the lungs quickly. In the fourth row, activity is clearly demonstrated in the descending aorta. In the lower two rows, there is activity in the systemic circulation. RV = right ventricle. LV = left ventricle.

multiformat display to record the serial analog images (Fig. 3–2). The same data should be collected simultaneously on a computer in frame mode. If necessary, the study can be replayed from the computer at a slower rate, or individual frames can be combined and scrutinized carefully. For evaluation of ventricular performance, such as ejection fraction, data need to be acquired at 20 to 40 frames/sec depending upon the patient's heart rate. Choice of the appropriate framing interval is particularly important in infants who frequently manifest significant resting tachycardia.

Most commonly, studies are performed with a low energy, high sensitivity parallel hole collimator. For evaluation of neonates or small children, converging collimators may be useful, because they provide magnification of the image and augmented sensitivity. In general, studies should be recorded on at least a 64×64 computer matrix. Visual analysis may be performed from an interpolated 128×128 matrix. Studies are obtained in the anterior position with the chest centered in the field of view. This provides the best separation of the heart and lung and is the most reproducible.

Depending upon the results of the anterior position study, it may occasionally be necessary to repeat the study in the left anterior oblique position, which provides maximal separation of the right and left ventricles.

Qualitative Analysis

The first step in analysis of the first-pass radionuclide angiocardiogram involves visual evaluation of the series of images.[2, 8-10] The morphology of the cardiac blood pool and of the great vessels is viewed to determine the overall flow pattern. The normal first-pass radionuclide angiocardiogram shows the radionuclide bolus as it passes sequentially through the central circulation. There is both temporal and anatomic segregation of radioactivity within individual cardiac structures (Figs. 3–1 and 3–2). Initially, the absolute and relative chamber sizes should be evaluated. Gross structural abnormalities often can be detected from visual assessment of the flow patterns, which are similar to those that would be encountered on a contrast angiogram. For example, in obstruction of the superior vena cava, there is interruption of the normal flow pattern into the right heart, occasionally associated with collateral thoracic circulation. Post-stenotic dilatation of the pulmonary artery or of the aorta can be detected. In right-to-left shunts, there will be early appearance of radionuclide in the left side of the heart and the aorta concomitant with visualization of the lungs. At times, the level of the right-to-left shunt can be determined. For example, in Ebstein's anomaly, the tracer may flow from the right atrium to the left atrium, instead of the normal temporal sequence. In right-to-left shunting at the ventricular level, such as in tetralogy of Fallot, the radionuclide flows directly from the right ventricle to the left ventricle, with minimal lung activity. In left-to-right shunting, the radionuclide angiocardiogram classically demonstrates persistently high levels of activity in the lungs and/or the right ventricle owing to early recirculation (Figs. 3–3 and 3–4). In large shunts, it may be possible to demonstrate dilution of the radioactive bolus with unlabeled shunted blood as it reaches the level of the shunt, as well as extremely poor visualization of the left ventricle and the aorta. Persistent pulmonary activity and poor visualization of the left heart on a first transit study are virtually diagnostic of a left-to-right shunt. The persistence of pulmonary activity is all the more striking when one considers that pulmonary blood flow and thus pulmonary transit are augmented in left-to-right shunts. It is important to stress that *poor bolus injection*, congestive heart failure, or tricuspid or pulmonic regurgitation can mimic the appearance of a left-to-right shunt. These variables should be considered when evaluating the results of the study.

Additional qualitative information can be obtained with the use of relatively simple computer techniques. Regions of interest are placed over specific cardiopulmonary structures, and time-activity curves are generated from each region of interest.[4, 11] The configurations of the curves are helpful in determining if a shunt is present and, if so, in determining its anatomic location (Figs. 3–5 and 3–6). Particular attention should be directed to the pulmonary time-activity curve. Normally, this curve has a sharp peak as radioactivity reaches the lungs and then a sharp fall as the bolus leaves the lungs and enters the left heart. Thereafter, following disappearance of the radioactivity from the lungs, there is a second wider, but lower, peak due to normal recirculation of blood through the systemic circuit. In a left-to-right shunt, the pulmonary time-activity curve shows a characteristic early reappearance of radioactivity, which interrupts the normal monoexponential decay of radioactivity after the initial peak. The amount of early pulmonary recirculation is proportional to the shunt flow.

Although in large left-to-right shunts the early pulmonary recirculation peak will be obvious, in smaller left-to-right shunts further standardization may be required for diagnostic purposes. Evaluation of the pulmonary dilution curve can be facilitated using computer methods[11, 12] (Fig. 3–7). The time interval between the first appearance of radioactivity and the peak activity is defined as t_1. The same time interval, t_2, is measured from the peak of the pulmonary curve. Radioactive counts at times t_1 and t_2 are defined as C_1 and C_2, respectively. The ratio of counts C_2/C_1 ($\times$ 100) is used as a marker to evaluate the presence or absence of a left-to-right shunt. Several studies have

Text continued on page 122

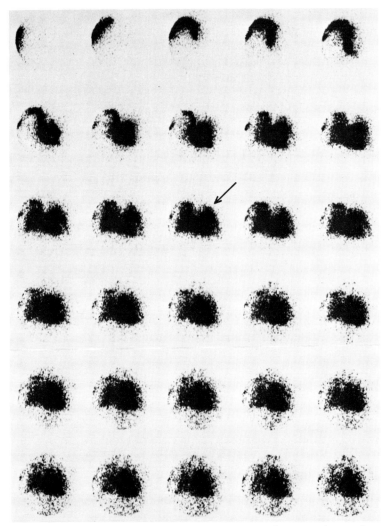

Figure 3–3. Anterior position first-pass radionuclide angiocardiogram obtained in an adult with an atrial septal defect. Note activity in the enlarged right ventricle at a time when activity is demonstrated in the lungs. In addition, there is persistent pulmonary activity, consistent with a large left-to-right shunt (arrow). By gamma variate computer analysis, the Qp:Qs ratio was 2.4:1.

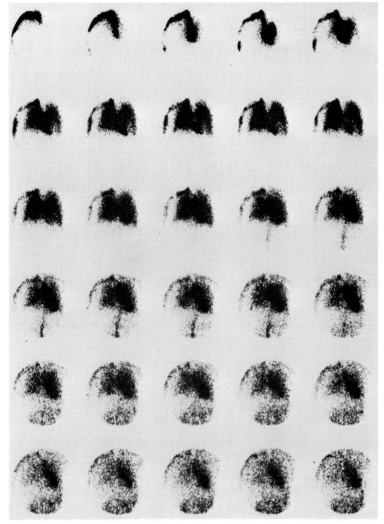

Figure 3–4. First-pass radionuclide angiocardiogram in a young adult with a small ventricular septal defect. Note the persistent pulmonary activity in the second and third rows. However, there is good visualization of the descending aorta, suggesting that the left to right shunt is relatively small. By computer analysis, the Qp:Qs ratio was 1.7:1. In the fourth and fifth rows, when there still is substantial activity in the lungs, the left ventricle is visualized. This also suggests the presence of a left-to-right shunt.

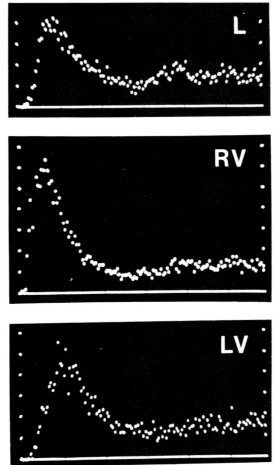

Figure 3–5. Time-activity curves obtained from the lung (L), right ventricle (RV), and left ventricle (LV) in an infant with a patent ductus arteriosus. These curves were generated with a relatively simple microprocessor system and are displayed at three frames per second. Note the delayed washout from the lung region of interest, consistent with pulmonary recirculation. In addition, there is a second smaller recirculation peak after the initial clearance of the bolus. The curves generated from the right ventricular and left ventricular regions of interest are normal. This analysis confirmed the clinical diagnosis of a patent ductus arteriosus. Following therapy with a prostaglandin synthetase inhibitor, the left-to-right-shunt closed, and the curve generated from the lung region of interest normalized.

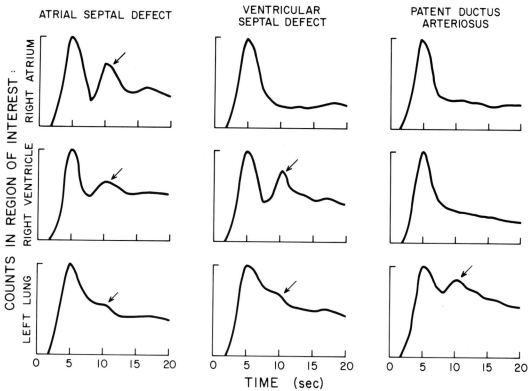

Figure 3–6. Regional time-activity curves corresponding to left-to-right shunts. These diagrammatic representations illustrate how regional time-activity curves can be used to localize the level of the left-to-right shunt. There is recirculation in the lungs for shunts at each level. However, as noted in the previous example, in a patent ductus arteriosus, there is recirculation only in the lungs, with a normal washout in the right atrium and right ventricle. In a ventricular septal defect, there is recirculation (arrows) in both the right ventricular and pulmonary regions of interest. In an atrial septal defect, there also is recirculation at the level of the right atrium. It is important to note that in the presence of multiple shunts only the most proximal shunt can be localized. (Modified with permission from Treves, Maltz, and Adelstein.[4])

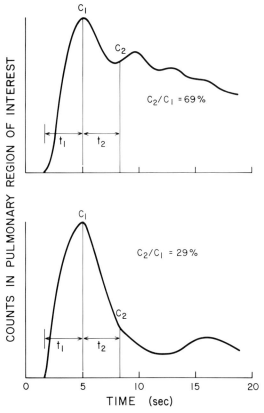

Figure 3–7. Standardized technique for analysis of the pulmonary time-activity curve in assessment of a left-to-right shunt. As described in the text, the C_2/C_1 ratio can be used to standardize analysis of the time activity curve. A normal example is shown below, with a C_2/C_1 ratio of 29 per cent. An example of a patient with a left-to-right shunt is shown above, with a C_2/C_1 ratio of 69 per cent. In the presence of pulmonary recirculation due to a left-to-right shunt, the C_2/C_1 ratio is usually greater than 35 per cent.

demonstrated that a C_2/C_1 ratio of less than 32 per cent is normal. In the presence of pulmonary recirculation due to a left-to-right shunt, the C_2/C_1 ratio is usually greater than 35 per cent. This relatively simple technique does not provide *quantitative* data on the size of the shunt, as it does not correlate well with the size of the shunt. The C_2/C_1 ratio may also be elevated in some patients with right-to-left shunts. *Careful standardization* should be performed by any laboratory employing this approach.

Further information concerning the site of a left-to-right shunt can be obtained from the composite regional time-activity curves already generated (Figs. 3–5 and 3–6). The reliability of this analysis depends upon valvular competence and the generation of noncontaminated regional curves.[4] If more than one shunt is present, only the most *proximal* shunt can be localized accurately. For example, in an atrial septal defect, there is early recirculation in the right atrium, right ventricle, and lung. However, in a ventricular septal defect recirculation occurs only in the right ventricle and the lung, and a normal right atrial time-activity curve is demonstrated. In a patient with a patent ductus arteriosus, recirculation is evident only in the lungs. Furthermore, there is greater early pulmonary recirculation in the left lung as compared with the right, because of preferential flow to the left side through the shunt.[3]

Quantitative Analysis

Quantification of the magnitude of left-to-right shunting is now possible using computerized analysis of the pulmonary time-activity curve.[13-16] Based upon the studies of Maltz and Treves,[13] a series of algorithms have been developed that allow determination of the pulmonic to systemic flow ratio (Fig. 3–8). This approach uses a gamma variate model in which the initial portion of the primary peak of the pulmonary dilution curve is used to predict the shape of the remainder of the curve, assuming no recirculation. The curve determined by the gamma variate fit is subtracted from the original raw data, and the early points in the remaining curve, as well as a new gamma variate function, are used to predict the shape of the second peak, which represents early pulmonary recirculation. From the integrated areas of these two curves, pulmonic to systemic flow ratios (Qp:Qs) in the range of 1.2 to 3.0 can be determined. Data obtained with this method correlate closely with values obtained using oximetry at the time of cardiac catheterization[13,14] (Fig. 3–9). Qp:Qs ratios greater than 3.0 produce a flattened pulmonary dilution curve that is difficult to analyze. Ratios less than 1.2 cannot be differentiated from normal. Although analysis is performed using automated computer programs, careful visual assessment of the computer-generated curves is required. Accuracy and reliability of the quantitative assessment depend upon *sig-*

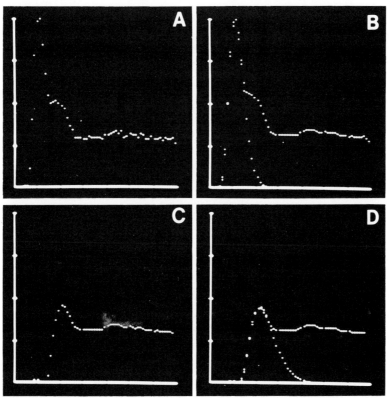

Figure 3–8. Method for determining pulmonary to systemic flow (Qp:Qs) ratio, as developed at Childrens Hospital Medical Center, Boston, Massachusetts. A smoothed pulmonary time-activity curve is shown in panel *A*. The first portion of the time-activity curve is fit to a gamma variate in panel *B*. The area in the initially fit portion shown in panel *B* is proportional to the pulmonary flow (Qp). The derived histogram then is subtracted from the original curve, resulting in another histogram that represents shunt and systemic recirculation (panel *C*). This residual histogram also is fit to a gamma variate, as shown in panel *D*. The area of this new gamma variate fit is proportional to shunted flow. The difference between the areas of the two fitted curves is proportional to systemic flow. This allows estimation of the Qp:Qs ratio. These curves are derived from the programs initially described in Maltz and Treves.[13]

Figure 3–9. Comparison of Qp:Qs ratio obtained by oximetry during cardiac catheterization and by the gamma variate analysis from first-pass radionuclide angiocardiography in 105 patients. The mean age of the patients was ten years with a range of one month to 31 years. Note the excellent correlation between these two techniques over a range of Qp:Qs ratios from 1.0 to 3.0. (Reproduced with permission from Askenazi, Ahnberg, Korngold, et al.[14])

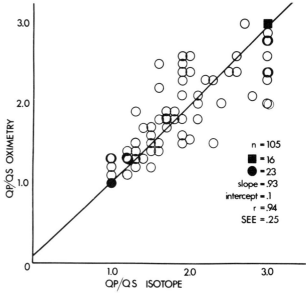

ANT

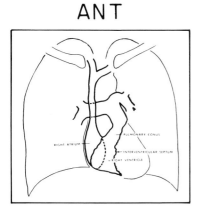

LAO

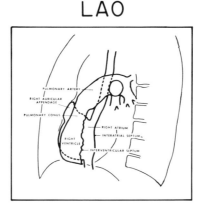

RAO

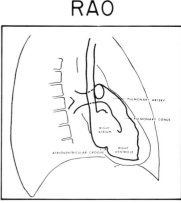

Figure 3–10. Idealized angiocardiographic outlines of the right heart structures in the anterior (ANT), 45° left anterior oblique (LAO), and 30° right anterior oblique (RAO) positions. These outlines demonstrate the relationship of the right atrium and right ventricle in multiple positions. This is particularly relevant to analysis of first-pass and multiple-gated blood pool imaging studies. (Modified with permission from Dotter, C. T., and Steinberg, I.: Angiocardiography. Annals of Roentgenology, Volume 20. Paul D. Hoeber, Inc., New York, 1951, pages 51–52.)

nificant operator interaction and standardization. Quantification of the degree of the left-to-right shunt represents an important clinical application of radionuclide techniques in congenital heart disease.

The same first-pass study can be used to determine both right and left ventricular ejection fractions.[6] After definition of an appropriate region of interest, radioactivity is analyzed only at the time when it is in the chamber being evaluated (that is, right or left ventricles). In this way, activity from overlapping structures can be excluded (Figs. 3–10 and 3–11). A high frequency, high count rate time-activity curve is generated from the region of interest. Ventricular activity is corrected from noncardiac background activity using one of several standardized approaches. Following background correction, a representative cardiac cycle is created using either the R wave of the electrocardiogram or the peak of the ventricular volume curve to align the end-diastoles of several beats (usually three to six cycles). The ejection fraction can be determined from this summed cardiac

ANT

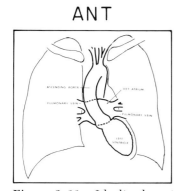

LAO

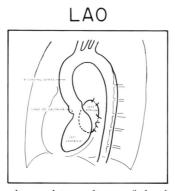

LLAT

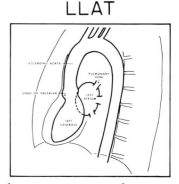

Figure 3–11. Idealized angiocardiographic outlines of the left heart structures in the anterior (ANT), 45° left anterior oblique (LAO), and left lateral (LLAT) positions. Note that in the left anterior oblique position, the left atrium is superior and posterior to the left ventricle. This is particularly relevant to multiple gated equilibrium blood pool studies, which are routinely performed in this position. There is relatively little overlap between these two left heart structures. (Modified with permission from Dotter, C. T., and Steinberg, I.: Angiocardiography. Annals of Roentgenology, Volume 20. Paul D. Hoeber, Inc., New York, 1951, pages 51–52.)

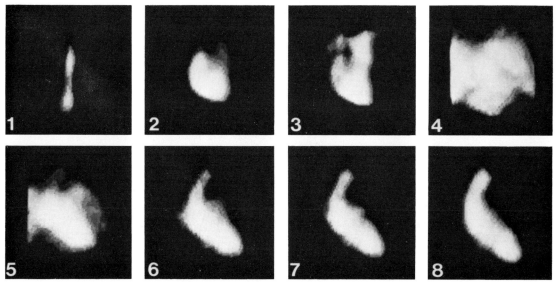

Figure 3–12. Normal first-pass radionuclide angiocardiogram obtained with the computerized multicrystal scintillation camera. Each frame represents a one-second accumulation. The right ventricle is best seen in frame 3, while the left ventricle is best seen in frames 7 and 8. Note the rapid disappearance of radioactivity from the lungs. This display can be used to identify specific regions of interest for computerized quantitative analysis. (Reproduced with permission from Berger, Matthay, Pytlik, et al.[6])

cycle. The peak of the curve represents end-diastolic counts (volume) and the valley of the curve represents end-systolic counts (volume) (Figs. 3–12 and 3–13). These values are used to determine ejection fraction in the conventional manner. Relatively high count density images are available from the summed representative cycle,

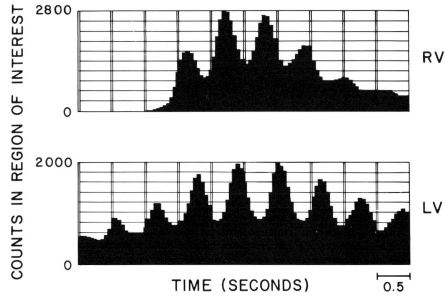

Figure 3–13. High frequency, high count rate regional time-activity curves generated from right ventricular (RV) and left ventricular (LV) regions of interest. The areas of interest were determined from the display shown in the previous figure. The peaks of each curve represent end-diastole, and the valleys end-systole. Ejection fraction can be determined from the summed end-diastolic and end-systolic count rates using the conventional equation of end-diastolic counts minus end-systolic counts divided by end-diastolic counts times 100. (Reproduced with permission from Berger, Matthay, Pytlik, et al.[6])

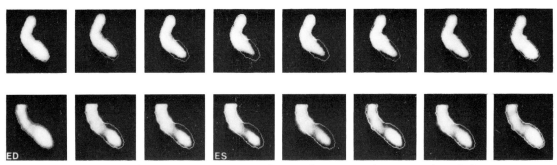

Figure 3–14. Levo phase representative cardiac cycles at rest (upper row) and during exercise (lower row) in a patient with coronary artery disease. The first frame represents end-diastole (ED) and the fourth frame end-systole (ES). The end-diastolic perimeter is shown superimposed on serial images from end-diastole through end-systole returning back to end-diastole. At rest, regional wall motion is normal. With exercise, the patient develops inferior wall hypokinesis. The two series are displayed at the same heart rate. (Reproduced with permission from Berger, Matthay, Pytlik, et al.[6])

especially obtained with the multicrystal camera. These images can also be used for evaluation of regional wall motion. The entire representative cycle can be viewed as a continuous endless loop cinematic display (Fig. 3–14). Alternatively, the end-diastolic perimeter can be superimposed upon the end-systolic image, and wall motion can be evaluated from the difference between these two images. Finally, an ejection fraction functional image can be obtained that displays the regional contributions to global ejection fraction. This latter approach may provide further insights into nontangential wall motion.

It is important to note that the first-pass method is also well suited for determination of right ventricular ejection fraction.[6, 17] This is due to the temporal and anatomic separation of radioactivity within the heart, as well as the lack of dependence of this approach upon geometric assumptions concerning the shape of the right ventricle[18] (Fig. 3–13). From a right ventricular region of interest, a right ventricular time-activity curve is generated, allowing direct determination of right ventricular ejection fraction from the peaks and valleys of this curve.

Quantitative first-pass radionuclide angiocardiography can be performed not only at rest, but also during various forms of physiologic stress, such as upright bicycle exercise.[6, 19] In many clinical situations, cardiac performance may be normal at rest, and only during exercise stress will an abnormal functional response of either ventricle be detected (Fig. 3–14).

MULTIPLE-GATED EQUILIBRIUM CARDIAC BLOOD POOL IMAGING

General Description

This technique provides a means of imaging the entire equilibrium cardiac blood pool at various times during cardiac contraction by synchronizing the collection of scintillation data with an independent marker of cardiac contraction.[7, 20] Since electrocardiographic events bear a relatively fixed relationship to the mechanical activity of the heart, continuous sampling of the specific phases of the cardiac cycle from each of several hundred beats can be performed until the composite image has an adequate count density. The gated blood pool study allows qualitative assessment of the relative size and configuration of individual cardiac structures and quantitative evaluation of global and regional ventricular performance.

Radionuclides

As noted earlier, either technetium-99m labeled human serum albumin or labeled autologous red blood cells (achieved either in vivo or in vitro) can be used (Table 3–1). The target-to-background ratio with technetium-99m red blood cells is better than with the human serum albumin, allowing improved definition of cardiac borders. Administration of perchlorate is not required.

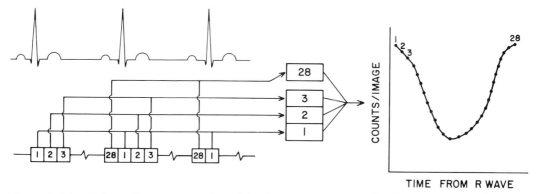

Figure 3–15. Schematic representation of the data processing involved in generation of a summed left ventricular time-activity curve from the multiple-gated equilibrium technique. In this example, the cardiac cycle has been divided into 28 equal segments. Data occurring during the specific time intervals shown below are stored in the computer memory for several hundred individual cardiac cycles. Following background correction, these individual data points are displayed as a relative ventricular volume curve as indicated on the right.

Instrumentation and Data Acquisition

In general, gated blood pool imaging is performed with a single crystal scintillation camera interfaced directly to a computer system. Either a high resolution or an all-purpose parallel hole collimator is employed. Many laboratories use a high sensitivity parallel hole collimator for imaging during exercise. The benefit gained by using a collimator with a higher intrinsic resolution may be partially offset by the more prolonged imaging time and the potential for resultant patient motion.

Scintillation data are collected temporally in synchrony with the electrocardiographic trigger (R wave). The RR interval is divided into 16 to 24 equal subdivisions, depending upon the patient's heart rate (Fig. 3–15). In

Figure 3–16. Serial cardiac images obtained with a 16 frame multiple-gated blood pool study. The first frame represents end-diastole (ED), and the seventh frame end-systole (ES). This study was obtained in the 45° left anterior oblique position. Note the normal contraction pattern for the right and left ventricles. Using computer techniques, the global left ventricular ejection fraction was 61 per cent. Activity is demonstrated in the entire blood pool, including the great vessels and the spleen. (Reproduced with permission from Berger, Gottschalk, and Zaret.[20])

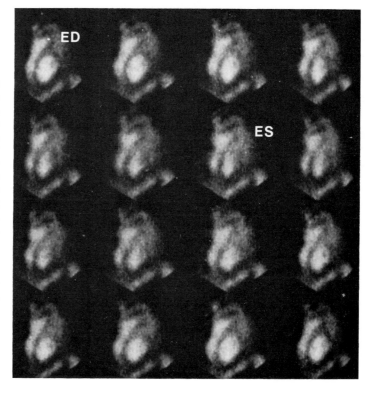

general, a framing interval of 40 to 50 msec is employed at rest and 20 to 40 msec during exercise. Scintillation data occurring during consecutive time intervals are segregated in sequence according to the elapsed time from the R wave. When the following R wave is reached, the sorting process is reset to the first interval. The result is a composite single-image sequence spanning the entire cardiac cycle, which is composed of data from several hundred individual cardiac cycles (Fig. 3–16). Gated blood pool data are interpretable after approximately 30 seconds of acquisition. However, acquisition of high spatial resolution data necessary for accurate analysis of wall motion generally requires at least two to three minutes, depending upon the choice of collimation. At rest, studies usually are acquired for 6 to 10 minutes. The imaging time may need to be modified based upon the cooperation of the patient, particularly in children who may be unable to lie quietly under the camera. In comparison to the first-pass method, this long acquisition time is a potential disadvantage in the pediatric age group.

Qualitative Analysis

Because the entire intravascular blood pool is labeled, imaging can be performed in multiple positions after a single radionuclide injection (Figs. 3–10 and 3–11). Although this allows visual assessment of the cardiac chambers and great vessels from various obliquities, accurate interpretation may be hampered by overlapping structures. Therefore, in a patient suspected of having congenital heart disease, it is preferable to start with a first-pass radionuclide angiocardiogram to define the intracardiac flow pattern and position of the various chambers. After this, the gated blood pool study can be performed to answer specific questions. It is important to point out that, as opposed to assessment in adults with acquired disease, unique obliquities tailored to the individual lesion may be required in a patient with congenital heart disease. In these instances, conventional anatomic relationships are frequently distorted. The gated blood pool study should begin with the obliquity in which the two ventricles are best separated. The study should then be performed in the anteropos-terior and either the left lateral or left posterior oblique position. Each cardiac chamber should be analyzed carefully in terms of relative position, size, and synchrony of contraction. This is best performed using the endless loop cinematic display. The field of view of the camera should be large enough to include major portions of the great vessels, a frequent site of additional congenital or acquired malformations (Fig. 3–17).

Quantitative Analysis

The left ventricular time-activity curve should be obtained from the individualized position (as opposed to the routine 45° left anterior oblique) that best separates the right and left ventricles (Fig. 3–18). It is critical that the time-activity curve be generated from a position without overlap of the two ventricles. Activity in the left ventricular region of interest also includes radioactivity from overlapping structures, such as the chest wall, lungs, and atria, as well as from scattered radiation from adjacent structures, such as the spleen and descending aorta. Therefore, to account for noncardiac activity, a background region of interest is chosen lateral to the left ventricle. Background counts, normalized for the left ventricular area, are subtracted from the left ventricular image frame. A variable region of interest, corresponding to the left ventricular edges throughout the cardiac cycle, is determined either manually or by using an automated program. Most available nuclear medicine computer programs calculate the left ventricular ejection fraction and ejection rate automatically from the background-corrected end-diastolic and end-systolic count rates.[19, 20]

Because externally detected counts are proportional to intravascular blood volume, determination of changes in counts in a region of interest can be used to assess relative changes in the respective chamber volumes. As long as the intravascular distribution of the radiotracer remains constant and the physical decay of technetium-99m is taken into account, the relative effect of acute interventions on these parameters can be determined. Using a similar approach, the degree of valvular regurgitation can be estimated from the ratio of left ventricular to

Figure 3–17. Multiple-gated cardiac blood pool imaging in a patient with an ascending aortic aneurysm. Images are shown at end-diastole (ED) and at end-systole (ES) in the anterior (ANT) and 45° left anterior oblique (LAO) positions. The large ascending aortic aneurysm is well visualized in both views. The left ventricle also is enlarged with a depressed global left ventricular ejection fraction. (Reproduced with permission from Berger, Gottschalk, and Zaret.[20])

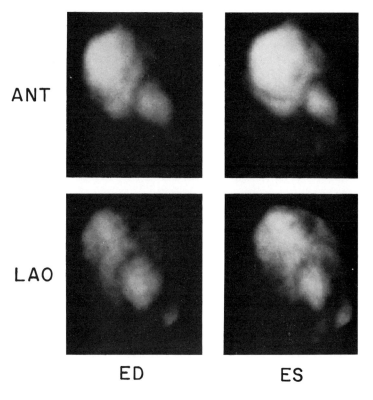

ANT

LAO

ED   ES

the right ventricular stroke counts.[21] Measurement of the change in counts between end-diastole and end-systole in the right and left ventricles reflects the respective stroke volume variations. In the absence of intracardiac shunting, the right ventricular stroke volume is normally equal to the left ventricular stroke volume, and the left-to-right ventricular stroke count ratio should be unity. In patients with aortic or mitral regurgitation, the left ventricular stroke volume increases, and the ratio exceeds unity. Measurement of the left-to-right ventricular stroke count ratio may also be useful to

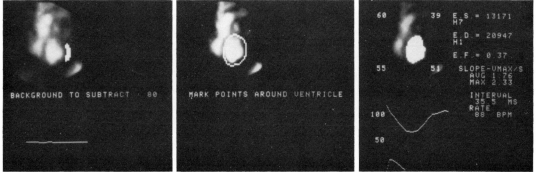

Figure 3–18. Computerized method employed for analysis of a 45° left anterior oblique gated equilibrium blood pool study. In the panel on the left, the background region of interest is defined adjacent to the left ventricle. The average count per pixel is 80. As shown below in this panel, this background remains constant throughout the cardiac cycle. In the central panel, the general region corresponding to the left ventricle has been identified. In the panel on the right, using frame-by-frame threshold analysis, the left ventricular region of interest has been identified. A background-corrected time-activity curve has been generated. The global left ventricular ejection fraction (EF) is 37 per cent. The number of counts in the summed end-diastolic (ED) and end-systolic (ES) frames also are shown. The average RR interval was 35.5 milliseconds, corresponding to a heart rate of 88 beats per minute. (Reproduced with permission from Berger, Gottschalk, and Zaret.[20])

evaluate right-sided valvular regurgitation, unidirectional shunts, anomalous pulmonary venous return, and the relative contribution of each circuit in complete transposition of the great vessels. Each of these volumetric parameters depends upon accurate definition of the true ventricular counts. This analysis must take into account not only background activity, but also activity from the atria contaminating the ventricular regions of interest (Figs. 3–10 and 3–11).

As noted earlier for first-pass radionuclide angiocardiography, multiple-gated cardiac blood pool imaging can be obtained during various forms of physiologic stress, such as supine bicycle exercise.[22] Evaluation of left ventricular ejection fraction and regional wall motion during various levels of exercise has already been applied to the study of patients with congenital, coronary, and rheumatic heart disease.[20]

PULMONARY PERFUSION IMAGING

General Description

Labeled particles have been used extensively to study regional pulmonary blood flow. The principle underlying their use depends upon the observation that blood flow to an organ can be determined when a tracer is completely removed from the bloodstream in a single passage through the organ. In these circumstances, if a tracer is evenly mixed with blood flowing to the lungs and then is virtually completely extracted by the lungs, its distribution within the lungs is proportional to pulmonary blood flow. Following intravenous injection, macroaggregates of albumin (10 to 50 μ) are too large to pass through the pulmonary capillaries and become impacted in the terminal arterioles and other precapillary vessels. In adults, there are approximately 300 million pulmonary arterioles with a diameter of 15 to 35 μ.[23, 24] These adult levels may be reached in children as early as five years of age. If an extracardiac or right-to-left shunt is present, a number of labeled particles will reach the systemic capillaries, and the shunt can be quantified (Fig. 3–19). Thus, pulmonary perfusion imaging can be used for the quantification of right-to-left shunting, as well as detection of intrapulmonary and segmental perfusion differences.[25–27]

Radionuclides

Technetium-99m macroaggregated human serum albumin is the radiotracer most commonly used (Table 3–1). In children, the administered dose is approximately 30 μCi/kg body weight, with a minimal dose of 200 μCi in infants, while in adults 4 mCi are used. The number of particles injected is also important. Injection of less than 30,000 particles in adults results in apparent perfusion defects in normal subjects, because of inhomogeneous or uneven distribution of the radionuclide. Injection of a minimum of 50,000 particles avoids random inhomogeneities in distribution. In adults, using commercial kits to produce technetium-99m macroaggregates, 200,000 to 300,000 particles are used. Care should be taken when administering this radiopharmaceutical to patients with right-to-left shunts, because the albumin particles will lodge in organs supplied by the systemic circulation. Although there appears to be a wide margin of safety involving the use of particles in patients with right-to-left shunts, there still is some concern regarding microembolization of systemic organs, especially the brain.

Instrumentation and Data Acquisition

Imaging routinely is performed with a high resolution parallel hole collimator on a conventional gamma scintillation camera. High-count density images are obtained in static mode. Images are obtained in the anterior and posterior positions, as well as in the left and right lateral positions and the left and right posterior oblique positions. When possible, the camera should be aligned to include not only the lungs, but also both kidneys.

Qualitative and Quantitative Analysis

The normal pulmonary perfusion scan demonstrates equal homogeneous perfusion to both lungs, with no subdiaphragmatic activity (Fig. 3–19). Both acquired and congenital abnormalities of the pulmonary circulation cause unequal perfusion of the two lungs.[24, 26] Congenital causes of inter-

LUNG　　　　　LUNG　　　　　BRAIN

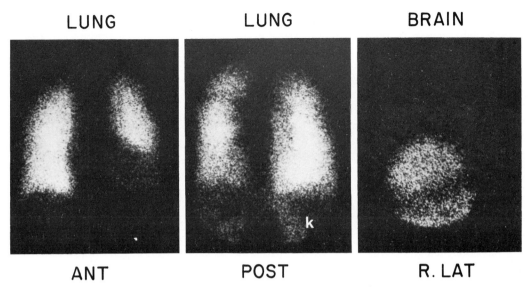

ANT　　　　　POST　　　　　R. LAT

Figure 3–19. Pulmonary perfusion imaging obtained using technetium-99m macroaggregated albumin in a patient with a right-to-left shunt. Note the relatively homogeneous uptake of radionuclide particles in the lungs. However, subdiaphragmatic radionuclide uptake is demonstrated in the kidneys (K). Because of this systemic distribution of radionuclide particles, imaging of the brain was performed in the right lateral (R. LAT) position. Uniform uptake in the brain is demonstrated. This is consistent with a right-to-left shunt located proximal to the takeoff of the brachiocephalic vessels. This patient has tetralogy of Fallot and had undergone palliative shunting. A definitive surgical correction had not been performed, thus the residual right-to-left shunt.

pulmonary perfusion differences (left vs right lung) are uncommon and rarely require the lung scan as a part of the diagnostic evaluation. Pulmonary artery stenosis or pulmonary valvar stenosis may result in differential radionuclide uptake in each lung. In addition, although uncommon, absence or complete interruption of a major pulmonary artery branch may occur in association with tetralogy of Fallot or as an isolated defect. In either case, pulmonary perfusion imaging demonstrates decreased uptake on the affected side.

The major use of the pulmonary perfusion scan in congenital heart disease is in the evaluation of acquired interpulmonary perfusion differences in patients who have had palliative shunts for cyanotic lesions associated with diminished pulmonary blood flow.[26] The relative distribution of the radionuclide particles is determined by the patency of the palliative shunt, the severity of right ventricular outflow stenosis, and the degree of development of the collateral circulation.

Quantification of the relative flow to both lungs and kidneys may be useful in the long-term follow-up of patients with palliative shunts. This can be accomplished by placing regions of interest over the right and left lungs, as well as over the right and left kidneys and determining the relative distribution of radionuclide particles. For example, in a superior vena cava to right pulmonary artery anastomosis (Glenn shunt), approximately 95 per cent of flow will be to the right lung after injection of the particles into the left arm (Fig. 3–20). Most of the blood flow through the surgically created venous shunt will pass to the lung on the side of the anastomosis. However, most of the right ventricular outflow obtained from the inferior vena cava passes to the lung opposite the shunt. In contrast, in a subclavian artery to pulmonary artery anastomosis (Blalock-Taussig shunt), most of the particles will distribute to the contralateral lung because of dilution of aggregates on the side of the shunt by the systemic arterial blood (in the absence of pulmonary atresia).

The magnitude of right-to-left shunting can also be determined by comparing pulmonary with systemic blood flows. Pulmonary blood flow is proportional to the radio-

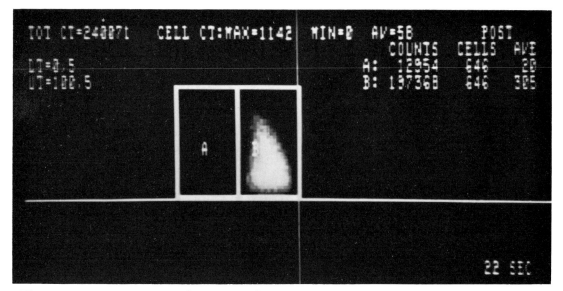

Figure 3–20. Quantitative pulmonary perfusion imaging in a patient with a patent superior vena cava to right pulmonary artery anastomosis (Glenn shunt). The image shown was obtained in the posterior position. Technetium-99m macroaggregated albumin was injected into the left arm and, after passage through the superior vena cava to the right pulmonary artery anastomosis, is distributed only to the right lung. The total counts (TOT CT) for the image is 240,071. Region of interest A corresponds to the left lung, while region of interest B corresponds to the right lung. The average counts per cell in each region of interest are determined by the computer. From these measurements, 94 per cent of the radioactivity within the lungs can be attributed to the right lung. This percentage can be used to serially follow patients with palliative venous shunts.

activity in the lungs, and systemic blood flow is proportional to the radioactivity in the whole body. This approach requires whole body imaging and is not routinely performed.[25-27] Furthermore, determination of oxygen saturations at the time of cardiac catheterization is still required for patient management and minimizes the need for this radionuclide approach.

MYOCARDIAL PERFUSION IMAGING

General Description

Thallium-201 myocardial perfusion imaging has been used widely in adults with coronary artery disease for defining areas of myocardial ischemia and is distributed according to regional myocardial blood flow, tissue viability, and myocardial mass. This radiopharmaceutical is an analog of the major intracellular cation, potassium.[29] The application of thallium-201 imaging to congenital heart disease has only recently been undertaken.

Radionuclides

Although original studies in patients with ischemic heart disease were performed with potassium-43, thallium-201 is the current myocardial perfusion tracer of choice (Table 3–1). Thallium-201 is administered intravenously in a dose of 30 μCi/kg of body weight, with a minimal dose of approximately 250 μCi in neonates. In adults, the usual dose is 1.5 to 2 mCi.

Instrumentation and Data Acquisition

Imaging should be begun within five minutes of intravenous injection and should be performed in multiple positions. The type of lesion suspected should determine the actual positions employed, but a minimum of three positions is suggested (anterior, 45° left anterior oblique, and left lateral). In a patient with complex congenital heart disease, in whom thallium-201 imaging is performed to evaluate cardiac morphology, it may be advantageous to ob-

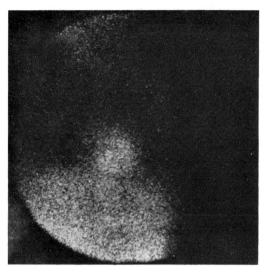 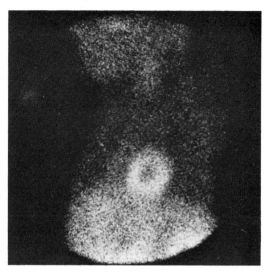

ANT   LAO

Figure 3–21. Resting thallium-201 images in a normal infant. Images are shown in the anterior (ANT) and 45° left anterior oblique (LAO) positions. Note the normal homogeneous perfusion in both positions. Subdiaphragmatic thallium-201 uptake in the liver and spleen is apparent. The overall left anterior oblique image extends from the midportion of the head to the lower abdomen.

tain images in additional positions, because the normal intracardiac relationships may be altered. Gated thallium-201 imaging, employing a technique similar to that used with gated equilibrium blood pool imaging, may also be of value in this setting. To evaluate cardiac anatomy using thallium-201 imaging, visualization of the image either in motion or at end-diastole may enhance the interpretability of the study. In addition, a preliminary study has suggested that single photon transaxial emission computed tomography may be applicable to myocardial perfusion imaging in children.[30] By using a three-dimensional reconstruction, this approach may allow better definition of perfusion defects. Greater experience with this technique is needed.

Qualitative and Quantitative Analysis

The normal thallium-201 image demonstrates uniform homogeneous perfusion throughout the left ventricular myocardium. In the left anterior oblique position, the interventricular septum and lateral free wall are visualized best (Figs. 3–21 and 3–22). At rest, the right ventricle is usually not seen

because its mass is markedly less than that of the left in the older child and young adult. When coronary blood flow to the right ventricle is augmented (for example, during exercise), the right ventricle is usually demonstrated. In an animal model with right ventricular hypertrophy, the degree of right ventricular myocardial thallium-201 uptake has been shown to directly reflect myocardial mass[31] (Fig. 3–23). Using computer techniques, the degree of right ventricular uptake relative to background or left ventricular uptake can be determined. In adults, several studies have demonstrated that right ventricular visualization on thallium-201 images is associated with elevated right ventricular systolic pressures and increased pulmonary vascular resistances, as well as right ventricular dysfunction determined by radionuclide angiocardiography.[32-35] However, because the right ventricle may be visualized in acute right ventricular volume overload prior to development of hypertrophy or with resting tachycardias, the significance of right ventricular thallium-201 uptake in an individual patient must be carefully qualified with respect to clinical and pathophysiologic implications.

Thallium-201 imaging can be performed not only at rest, but also immediately fol-

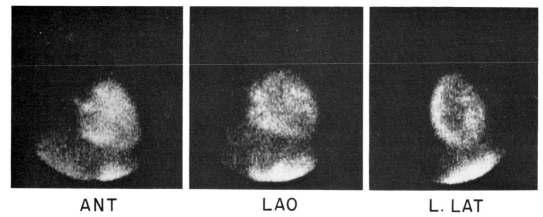

ANT   **LAO**   **L. LAT**

Figure 3–22. Resting thallium-201 images in a child with transposition of the great arteries. The child had undergone a Mustard procedure (placement of an intracardiac baffle) approximately 24 months prior to this study. Images are shown in the anterior (ANT), 45° left anterior oblique (LAO), and left lateral (L. LAT) positions. Note that the systemic and venous ventricles cannot be delineated from either the anterior or left anterior oblique images. However, in the left lateral position, the cavity of the systemic chamber can be appreciated. The free wall of the systemic ventricle is anterior. The cavity of the venous chamber cannot be seen because this chamber is relatively small. The interventricular septum and posterior wall cannot be differentiated from this scan. These findings are consistent with the known postoperative anatomy in this condition.

lowing exercise.[29] This application has been used predominantly in adults with atherosclerotic coronary artery disease. However, in the pre- and postoperative evaluation of older children with anomalous coronary arteries originating from the pulmonary artery, rest and exercise thallium-201 imaging may be useful. These studies provide both physiologic evidence of myocardial ische-

mia and a means of assessing the effects of surgical intervention[36] (Fig. 3–24). In addition, in infants with anomalous coronary arteries, myocardial infarction may occur owing to inadequate oxygenated blood flow through the anomalous coronary artery.[37-41] In these cases, perfusion defects may be identified and residual myocardial viability evaluated. Thallium-201 imaging in con-

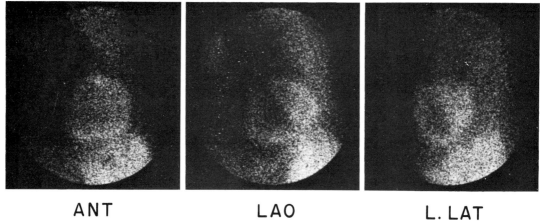

ANT   **LAO**   **L. LAT**

Figure 3–23. Resting thallium-201 images in a patient with mitral stenosis. Images are shown in the anterior (ANT), 45° left anterior oblique (LAO), and left lateral (L. LAT) positions. There is substantial right ventricular thallium-201 uptake, best seen on the left anterior oblique image. In addition, there is marked dilatation of the right ventricular chamber. The left ventricular cavity is not well delineated, as the interventricular septum and lateral left ventricular wall appear to be contiguous. This also is apparent on the left lateral image. These findings are consistent with marked right ventricular hypertrophy and enlargement.

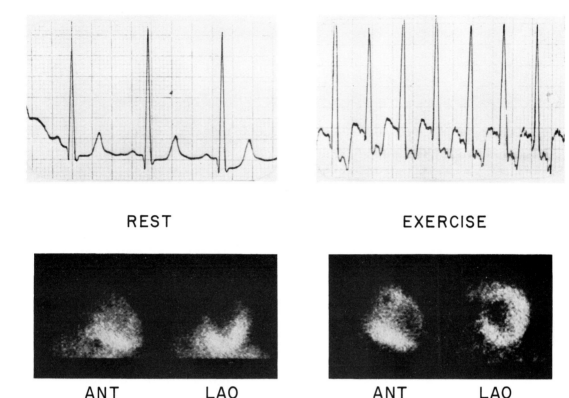

REST   EXERCISE

ANT   LAO   ANT   LAO

Figure 3–24. Rest and exercise thallium-201 imaging and electrocardiography in an adolescent with an anomalous coronary artery originating from the pulmonary artery. The patient had been relatively asymptomatic throughout childhood, but recently had developed limitation of exercise and dyspnea. The exercise study was performed first; thallium-201 was injected intravenously during the peak exercise load on the treadmill. Note the marked ST segment depression on the electrocardiogram. Decreased perfusion is demonstrated in the anterior and septal distributions. The resting images were obtained following a second intravenous injection of thallium-201. A subtle decrease in perfusion of the anterior wall still is present. However, there is marked improvement compared with the exercise study. These findings are consistent with substantial exercise-induced myocardial ischemia. ANT = anterior. LAO = 45° left anterior oblique. (This case was provided by Dr. David Johnstone.)

junction with the electrocardiogram may be helpful in directing cardiac catheterization and the need for coronary angiography in this clinical setting.

SURVEY OF CLINICAL APPLICABILITY

Diagnostic Assessment of Patients with Heart Murmurs

In certain patients, whether children or adults, it may be difficult to determine the etiology or the relevance of a cardiac murmur to clinical findings. Radionuclide angiocardiography provides a complement to the chest radiograph and to echocardiography[42] in this clinical setting. Cardiac scintigraphy has its major virtue in detecting the presence and defining the magnitude of left-to-right shunts.[2]

Evaluation of the asymptomatic patient with an apparently physiologic flow murmur or the differentiation between pulmonic stenosis and an atrial septal defect in an infant are two examples of the clinical applicability of first-pass radionuclide angiocardiography. Another situation is the choice of the appropriate time for cardiac catheterization in a patient with an atrial or ventricular septal defect, especially in the asymptomatic adult (Figs. 3–25 to 3–27). Serial evaluation of shunt flow (Qp:Qs) may demonstrate clinically inapparent changes in the magnitude of the shunt as well as spontaneous closure of small intracardiac or great vessel shunts. [2, 3]

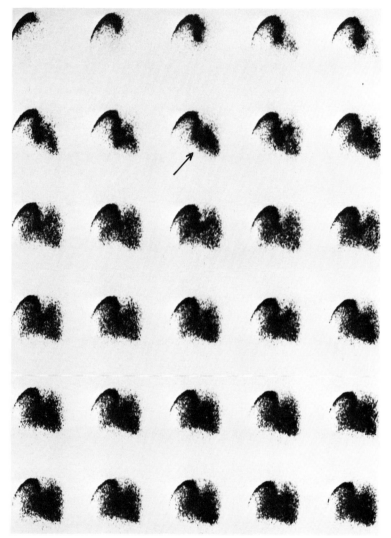

Figure 3–25. First-pass radionuclide angiocardiogram obtained in the anterior position in a 28-year-old patient with a large atrial septal defect. The bolus was injected through the right antecubital vein. Images are displayed at three per second. A markedly enlarged right ventricle is demonstrated (arrow). There is persistent radioactivity in the lungs, consistent with a left-to-right shunt. The left ventricle and the aorta are not visualized on this study.

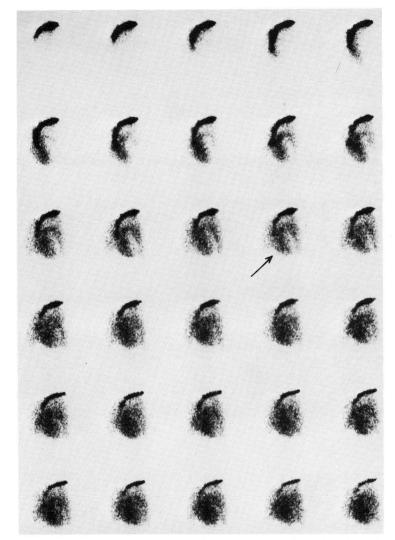

Figure 3–26. First-pass radionuclide angiocardiogram obtained in the 45° left anterior oblique position in the same patient as in the previous figure. The radioactive bolus was injected through the left antecubital vein, to evaluate the possibility of a duplicated superior vena cava. However, a normal right-sided superior vena cava is demonstrated. The presence of an enlarged right ventricle is confirmed by this study. The interventricular septum is well delineated. Radioactivity is seen in the main pulmonary artery and in the lungs at a time when activity is still in the right ventricle and superior vena cava (arrow). Note the persistent recirculation of radioactivity within the lungs, again consistent with a large left-to-right shunt.

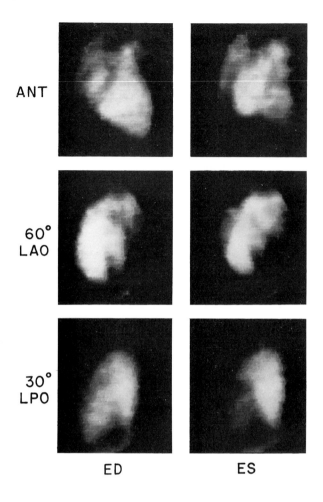

ANT

60°
LAO

30°
LPO

ED   ES

Figure 3–27. Multiple-gated cardiac blood pool imaging in the same patient as in the previous two figures. Studies were obtained in the anterior (ANT), 60° left anterior oblique (LAO), and 30° left posterior oblique (LPO) positions. Images are shown at end-diastole (ED) and at end-systole (ES). Note the markedly enlarged and diffusely hypokinetic right ventricle. On the left anterior oblique image, it is clear that the left ventricle is of normal size and contracts vigorously. The global left ventricular ejection fraction is 61 per cent. In the left posterior oblique study, the well-contracting left ventricle is closest to the detector and clearly functions well. The large hypokinetic right ventricle is furthest away from the detector, but at end-systole, when the left ventricle has contracted, there is still substantial radioactivity in the right ventricle.

Analysis of pulmonary time-activity curves from both lungs can be used to separate intracardiac and extracardiac shunts. For example, in a patient with a patent ductus arteriosus, the distribution of pulmonary artery blood flow is usually asymmetric, favoring the left lung. Thus, the degree of left-to-right shunting in the left lung region of interest will be larger than from the right lung region.[3] In patients with truncus arteriosus, first-pass radionuclide angiocardiography or pulmonary perfusion imaging can be used to determine relative shunt flow and pulmonary perfusion in each lung, respectively.[26]

In approaching a patient with suspected congenital heart disease, determining the visceroatrial situs and the presence and/or location of the spleen(s) may be helpful in the noninvasive diagnostic evaluation. As noted in Chapter 1, specific intracardiac lesions are frequently associated with situs ambiguus and the polysplenia or the asple-

nia syndromes. The chest radiograph and cross-sectional echocardiography provide the necessary data concerning situs in many patients, but at times the radionuclide liver-spleen scan may be required to provide definitive confirmation (Fig. 3–28).

Evaluation of the Newborn Infant

In the newborn infant, it may be difficult to differentiate between the cardiac and pulmonary etiologies of cyanosis and tachypnea, especially when they coexist (Figs. 3–29 and 3–30). Radionuclide angiocardiography can be used to help establish the presence or absence of a congenital cardiac lesion. When respiratory distress syndrome predominates, the radionuclide angiocardiogram should be normal. However, in patients with augmented pulmonary vascular resistance due to severe hypoxic pulmonary disease, the radionuclide angio-

ANT

POST

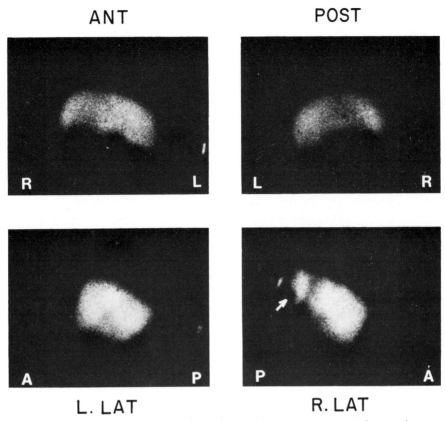

L. LAT

R. LAT

Figure 3–28. Technetium-99m sulfur colloid liver-spleen scan in an infant with an endocardial cushion defect and situs inversus. Images are shown in the anterior (ANT), posterior (POST), left lateral (L. LAT), and right lateral (R. LAT) positions. The radioactive tracer is technetium-99m sulfur colloid, which normally is taken up by the reticuloendothelial system. Although the chest radiograph usually provides the necessary information concerning the situs, at times liver-spleen scanning can be extremely helpful. It is important to determine the position of the spleen and to rule out polysplenia. In situs solitus, the spleen is best demonstrated on the left in the posterior position image or posteriorly in the left lateral image. However, in this case, the spleen is clearly demonstrated on the *right* on the posterior (POST) image and posteriorly on the right lateral image, consistent with situs inversus. In addition, there appears to be a small splenic defect, suggestive of a splenic infarct (arrow).

cardiogram may demonstrate right-to-left shunting through a patent foramen ovale, ductus arteriosus, or both.[2]

In neonates with documented patent ductus arteriosus, radionuclide angiocardiography allows quantification of the size of the shunt and therefore may aid in the selection of appropriate patients for surgical closure or medical therapy with prostaglandin synthetase inhibitors (Figs. 3–31 and 3–32). In both cases, the radionuclide study can be used to follow the results and potential complications of therapy as well as to document spontaneous closure of the ductus. This approach is preferable to M-mode echocardiographic evaluation of left

atrial dimension, because the radionuclide technique provides direct quantitative data on shunt size. Several studies have demonstrated that even in premature infants with large left-to-right shunts, the echocardiographic left atrial to aortic dimension ratio may be normal.[43, 44] Administration of oxygen can also be used to evaluate pulmonary vascular reactivity in an infant with a left-to-right shunt. Because oxygen is a potent pulmonary vasodilator, the magnitude of the shunt (Qp:Qs) would be expected to increase after oxygen.[5]

In newborn infants with a ventricular septal defect, pulmonary vascular resistance may be elevated. However, as the infant

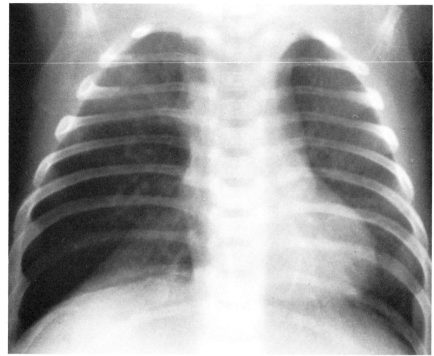

Figure 3–29. Anteroposterior chest radiograph in an infant with congenital lobar emphysema. Note the hyperlucent right lower lobe.

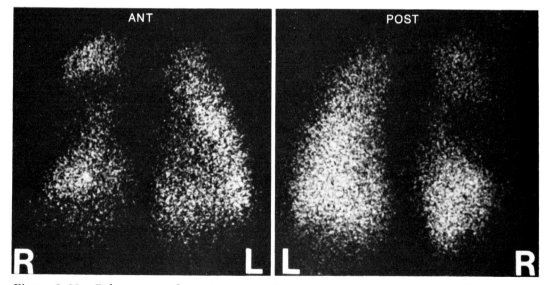

Figure 3–30. Pulmonary perfusion imaging in the same patient as in the previous figure. Imaging was performed using technetium-99m macroaggregated albumin. Note the substantial right lower lobe perfusion defect seen in the anterior (ANT) and posterior (POST) position images. Prior to performance of the technetium-99m perfusion scan, a xenon-133 ventilation scan was performed. This study demonstrated substantial air trapping with diminished washout corresponding to the area of decreased perfusion. This is the classic finding in congenital lobar emphysema and corresponds to what would be seen in an adult with chronic obstructive pulmonary disease (emphysema). In this patient, determination of the cause of the hyperlucent right lower lobe and the concomitant respiratory distress was of critical importance in management of the patient.

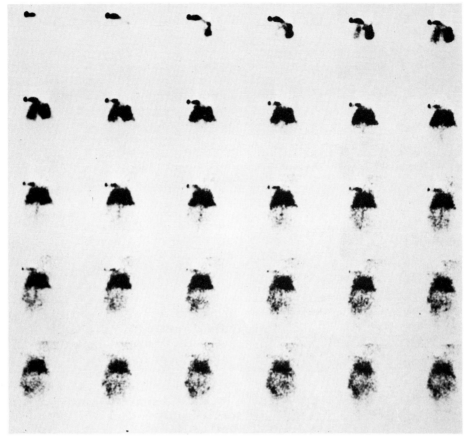

Figure 3–31. First-pass radionuclide angiocardiogram obtained in the anterior position in a premature infant with a patent ductus arteriosus. The study is displayed at three frames per second. Note the persistent pulmonary activity throughout the study, consistent with a left-to-right shunt. There is rapid clearance of the radionuclide from the right heart. In the third row, radioactivity is demonstrated in the descending aorta.

grows and pulmonary vascular resistance falls toward normal levels, the degree of left-to-right shunting may increase and become evident on the first-pass radionuclide study. In both instances, the two-dimensional echocardiographic examination may demonstrate the anatomic lesion directly; however, the radionuclide angiocardiogram will provide further assessment of its physiologic significance. Contrast echocardiographic techniques provide additional insights into the presence of intracardiac or extracardiac shunts.[45] This is a good example of how the two techniques can be employed in a complementary manner. In addition, cyanotic newborn infants can be evaluated with radionuclide angiocardiography. For example, in transposition of the great arteries or a right-to-left shunt with pulmonic stenosis,

the radionuclide appears early in the aorta after a peripheral injection.

An additional problem in the newborn, although uncommon, is transient myocardial dysfunction and respiratory distress in the absence of known congenital heart disease.[37] There may be fairly prompt improvement and complete resolution of pulmonary insufficiency, but electrocardiographic evidence of myocardial ischemia may persist for several months after clinical resolution. Myocardial perfusion imaging in these patients has been reported to show very poor cardiac uptake of thallium-201 relative to the lungs, suggestive of global myocardial ischemia. An alternative explanation of the imaging pattern is augmented lung uptake relative to the heart, suggestive of severe left ventricular dysfunction, as has been

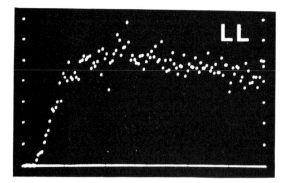

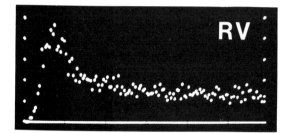

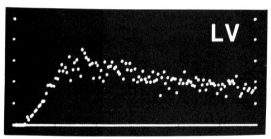

Figure 3-32. Regional time-activity curves obtained in the same patient as in the previous figure. Data are shown for the left lung (LL), right ventricle (RV), and for the left ventricle (LV). Note the marked recirculation of radioactivity demonstrated in the left lung time activity curve. This should be compared to the normal curve illustrated in Figure 3-5. The right ventricular time activity curve in the present example is consistent with a patent ductus arteriosus. There is decreased wash-out of radioactivity from the left ventricle, probably due to overlap between the left ventricular and left lung regions of interest.

demonstrated recently in adults during exercise.[46] This pattern differs from that seen in patients with myocarditis or congenital heart disease, in whom uptake is generally normal. In patients with idiopathic congestive cardiomyopathy or endocardial fibroelastosis, the left ventricular cavity may be dilated and uptake inhomogeneous (Figs. 3-33 to 3-35). Left ventricular hypoplasia as seen in the hypoplastic left heart syndrome

(aortic atresia) results in compensatory right ventricular hypertrophy, which can be documented on thallium-201 imaging (Figs. 3-36 to 3-39). In children with anomalous left coronary arteries originating from the pulmonary artery, extensive segmental perfusion defects are seen (Fig. 3-39). In these instances, there are regions of myocardial scar similar to those encountered in adults with myocardial infarction.[38-41] Assessment of right and left ventricular performance with first-pass or equilibrium techniques may be of clinical utility in these patients, especially to evaluate the effects of therapy directed at the congestive heart failure that accompanies this lesion.[47]

Evaluation of the Postoperative Patient

In patients who have had cardiac surgery for congenital heart disease, radionuclide angiocardiography allows accurate detection of residual shunts or unexpected changes in intracardiac flow patterns in the immediate postoperative period or at long-term follow-up. Congestive heart failure,

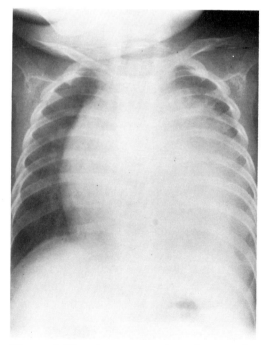

Figure 3-33. Anteroposterior chest radiograph in a three-month-old infant with congestive heart failure. There is marked cardiomegaly and indistinct pulmonary vasculature.

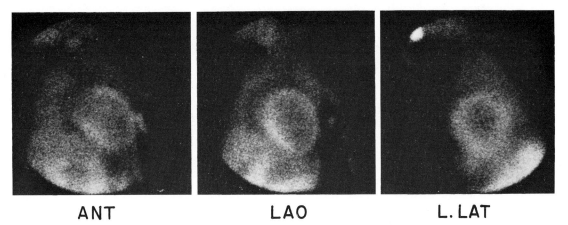

ANT LAO L. LAT

Figure 3–34. Resting thallium-201 myocardial imaging in the same infant as illustrated in the previous figure. Images are shown in the anterior (ANT), 45° left anterior oblique (LAO), and left lateral (L. LAT) positions. The field of view includes the entire thorax and upper abdomen. The ventricular myocardium is thin, and there is a large anterolateral perfusion defect. This is best appreciated on the left anterior oblique image. The left ventricle occupies approximately two-thirds of the thorax. These images should be compared with the normal study depicted in Figure 3–21. The magnification and displays are comparable. The electrocardiogram in this child demonstrated anterolateral transmural myocardial infarction. At autopsy, an anomalous coronary artery originating from the pulmonary artery was demonstrated. In addition, there was substantial evidence of endocardial fibroelastosis. This would help explain the marked left ventricular dilatation and thinning of the left ventricular myocardium in addition to the large perfusion defect.

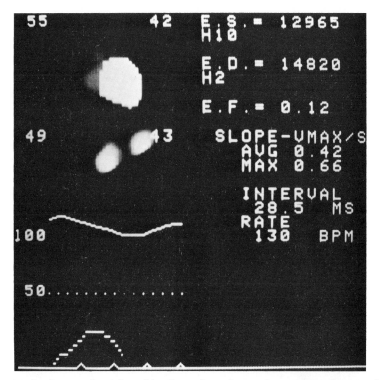

Figure 3–35. Multiple-gated cardiac blood pool study in the same infant as the previous two figures. The summed time activity curve is shown. The approximate region of interest used to generate this curve also is shown in the upper left hand corner. This study was obtained in the 45° left anterior oblique position and required approximately five minutes for data acquisition. Note that the left ventricular ejection fraction (EF) was 12 per cent. The resting heart rate was 130 beats per minute (BPM). Analysis of regional wall motion in multiple positions demonstrated diffuse left ventricular hypokinesis. These findings are consistent with marked left ventricular dysfunction.

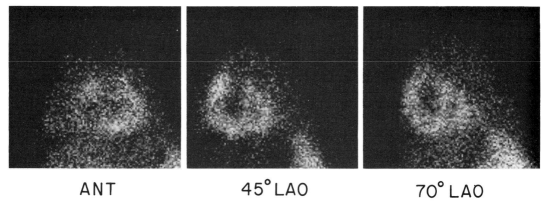

ANT   45° LAO   70° LAO

Figure 3–36. Resting thallium-201 imaging in a newborn infant with congestive heart failure. Images are shown in the anterior (ANT), 45° left anterior oblique (LAO), and 70° left anterior oblique positions. The infant had electrocardiographic evidence of myocardial ischemia. There was no evidence of congenital heart lesions. Note in the anterior position image the heart is difficult to distinguish from the pulmonary background. In the 45° and 70° left anterior oblique position images, there is marked right ventricular thallium-201 uptake. In addition, the right ventricular cavity is dilated, and the left ventricular cavity is difficult to identify. These findings are consistent with marked right ventricular dilatation and hypertrophy. There are no discrete left ventricular perfusion defects seen. These images differ substantially from those in the previous figures. In this setting, the right ventricle must bear much of the hemodynamic burden usually undertaken by the left ventricle.

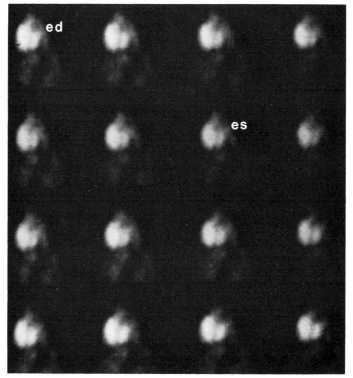

Figure 3–37. Serial images obtained from a multiple-gated blood pool study in the same infant as in the previous figure. The RR interval has been subdivided into 16 equal image positions. The end-diastolic (ed) and end-systolic (es) frames are indicated. Note the marked right ventricular dilatation. Diffuse hypokinesis of both ventricles is demonstrated. Neither ventricle appears to contract well.

ANT

LAO

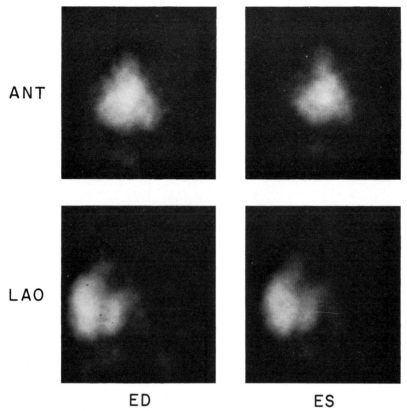

ED   ES

Figure 3–38. Multiple-gated cardiac blood pool study in the same infant as in the previous two figures. Images are shown in the anterior (ANT) and 45° left anterior oblique (LAO) positions at end diastole (ED) and end-systole (ES). Note once again that there is markedly diminished biventricular performance. In the anterior position, it is difficult to separate the enlarged overlapping right ventricle from the left ventricle.

persistent cyanosis, persistent murmurs, or the appearance of a new murmur postoperatively may imply residual lesions, detachment of a patch, or intrinsic valvular abnormalities. Repeat cardiac catheterization may be undesirable in the immediate postoperative period, and radionuclide angiocardiography may be helpful in deciding whether or not to reoperate or to recatheterize these patients.[48]

The use of radionuclide angiocardiography in postoperative evaluation of a patient with transposition of the great arteries is illustrated in Figure 3–40. Corrective surgery is performed early in life with the use of an intracardiac baffle (Mustard procedure). Residual shunting through the atrial baffle or obstruction to systemic or pulmonary venous flow by the baffle are known postoperative complications that can be documented from assessment of the flow patterns obtained with radionuclide angiocardiography.

As noted earlier, patency or occlusion of palliative shunts can be demonstrated by careful assessment of pulmonary dilution curves or by pulmonary perfusion imaging. For example, in a patent Blalock-Taussig shunt (subclavian artery to pulmonary artery), the radionuclide dilution curve obtained over the lung on the side of the anastomosis should reflect a larger early pulmonary recirculation than that of the contralateral lung.[2] This can clearly be quantified using radionuclide angiocardiography and may be useful in the early postoperative period when shunt murmurs may be inaudible.

The status of a Glenn shunt (superior vena cava to right pulmonary artery) can be evaluated using pulmonary perfusion imaging.[26] After left arm injection, patients with

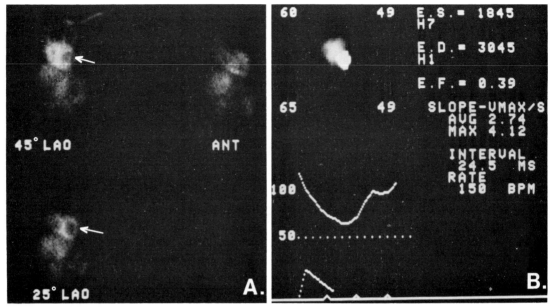

Figure 3–39. Resting thallium-201 myocardial perfusion imaging (in panel A) and multiple gated cardiac blood pool imaging (in panel B) in an infant with mitral insufficiency and anterior myocardial infarction. In the thallium-201 study, images are shown in the 45° and 25° left anterior oblique (LAO) and anterior (ANT) positions. The arrows point to the area of marked anterior wall hypoperfusion. There also appears to be some right ventricular thallium-201 uptake. These perfusion defects are consistent with anterior wall myocardial infarction. The gated blood pool study demonstrates a left ventricular ejection fraction (EF) of 39 per cent at a resting heart rate of 150 beats per minute (BPM). Considering the presence of mitral insufficiency, probably due to infarction of the papillary muscles, the 39 per cent ejection fraction may be an overestimation of the true left ventricular function. At autopsy, there was pathologic confirmation of these findings.

patent systemic to pulmonary artery shunts will demonstrate unilateral pulmonary visualization. An increase in the degree of right-to-left shunting due to progressive pulmonary artery stenosis, occlusion of a shunt, or arteriovenous fistula formation in the right lower lobe will result in more uniform bilateral distribution of macroaggregates. In addition, macroaggregates injected in the left upper extremity will pass through the collateral channels to the kidneys and gut (Figs. 3–20 and 3–41). Computer quantification of relative flow to each organ allows standardization and long-term follow-up. Although Glenn shunts are not commonly performed today, they may be included in the Fontan procedure for tricuspid atresia in addition to the valved conduit from the right atrium to the left pulmonary artery. Postoperative evaluation of patients with this new surgical procedure represents another potential application of quantitative pulmonary perfusion imaging.

In patients who have undergone corrective surgery for various congenital cardiac lesions, evaluation of right and left ventricular performance in the long-term follow-up period may be helpful in determining prognosis and relating postoperative symptoms to residual functional impairment.[49, 50] In these cases, either first-pass radionuclide angiocardiography or multiple-gated cardiac blood pool imaging can be performed at rest and during exercise. Numerous studies have demonstrated that the normal ventricular response to exercise is an augmentation in right and left ventricular ejection fraction (Fig. 3–42). This approach already has been applied to the study of patients with surgical correction for tetralogy of Fallot.[49] Even when an effective surgical procedure has been performed and the patient has improved symptomatically, the chronically pressure overloaded and hypertrophied right ventricle may not function normally under conditions of exercise stress. In this prototype study, right ventricular performance generally was normal at rest, but 13 of 16 asymptomatic patients manifested abnormal right ventricular ejection fraction

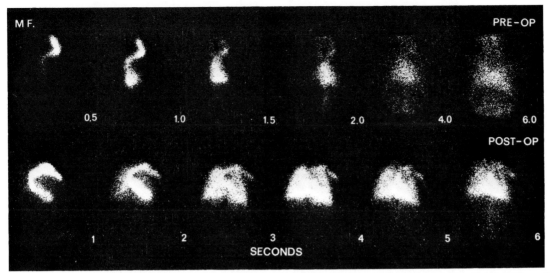

Figure 3-40. First-pass radionuclide angiocardiograms obtained preoperatively (PRE-OP) and postoperatively (POST-OP) in a six-month-old child with a right-to-left shunt. The child had transposition of the great arteries with an intact interventricular septum. The postoperative studies were obtained following the placement of an intracardiac baffle (Mustard procedure). In the preoperative study, radioactivity appears early in the ascending aorta and arch at 1.5 seconds and in the descending aorta at two seconds. The radionuclide appears in the pulmonary circulation after its occurrence in the aorta. These findings demonstrate the presence of a right-to-left shunt. In the postoperative study, the left ventricle fills from the right atrium, which is evident at one and two seconds. After radioactivity appears in the pulmonary circulation, the left atrium, right ventricle, and ascending aorta are seen at five and six seconds. Right ventricular activity is not seen in the first three seconds. Radioactivity in the aorta appears early in the preoperative study, but substantially later in the postoperative study. (Reproduced with permission from Treves, Maltz, and Adelstein.[4])

responses to exercise at long-term follow-up (Fig. 3–43). In contrast, the left ventricular exercise responses were normal. Thallium-201 myocardial imaging demonstrated evidence of substantial residual right ventricular hypertrophy in these patients (Fig. 3–44).

Evaluation of Cardiac Performance in Acquired Heart Disease in Children

Assessment of ventricular performance has been employed widely in adults with primary myocardial disease, coronary artery disease, and valvular heart disease. In many instances, lessons learned in adults with acquired heart disease can be applied to the pediatric population. For example, radionuclide techniques have been shown to be useful in the evaluation of patients with aortic insufficiency.[51, 52] On clinical and radiographic grounds, choice of the appropriate time for valve replacement often is difficult and may result in irreparable myocardial damage that cannot be modified by subsequent surgical intervention. It is important to note that an abnormal ejection fraction response to exercise does not necessarily indicate intrinsic myocardial disease. The stress of an abnormally augmented ventricular volume as seen in aortic regurgitation or increased outflow impedance associated with aortic stenosis may, by itself, modify the ejection fraction response. Nevertheless, assessment of the ventricular response to exercise provides clinically important physiologic data. Evaluation of exercise reserve prior to valvular replacement and in the postoperative period provides a means of assessing surgical results.

In children with myocarditis or acute rheumatic carditis, assessment of biventricular performance at rest should allow appropriate categorization of patients in terms of therapy and prognosis. In some cases, it may be helpful to combine this with thallium-201 perfusion imaging. In both cases, left ventricular dysfunction would be expected. Symptoms of congestive heart

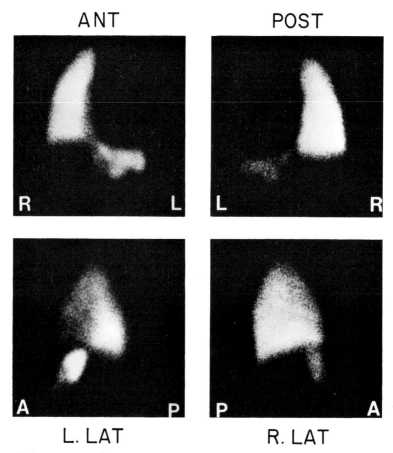

ANT POST

L. LAT R. LAT

Figure 3–41. Pulmonary perfusion imaging in a patient with a partially occluded superior vena cava to right pulmonary artery (Glenn) shunt. Technetium-99m macroaggregated albumin was injected into the left antecubital vein. Radioactivity is demonstrated in the right lung, as well as in subdiaphragmatic structures. Images are shown in the anterior (ANT), posterior (POST), left lateral (L. LAT) and right lateral (R. LAT) positions. Radionuclide particles pass through collateral veins and distribute to the stomach and gut. In a patient with a patent Glenn shunt, there should be no subdiaphragmatic activity. The relative distribution of radionuclide particles to the right lung and to the subdiaphragmatic region can be quantified using computer techniques.

NORMAL CONTROL SUBJECTS

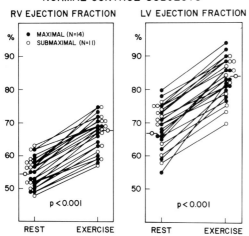

Figure 3–42. Rest and exercise right ventricular (RV) and left ventricular (LV) ejection fractions in 25 normal control subjects. Patients who exercised maximally are shown by closed circles, while patients who exercised at 50 per cent of their maximum are shown by open circles. Patients exercised on an upright bicycle ergometer. Ejection fraction was determined using first-pass radionuclide angiocardiography. Note that both right and left ventricular ejection fractions increased by at least 5 per cent (absolute ejection fraction units), irrespective of exercise protocol. Therefore, normal exercise ventricular reserve is defined as an increase of at least 5 per cent above resting values. (Reproduced with permission from Berger, Matthay, Pytlik, et al.[6])

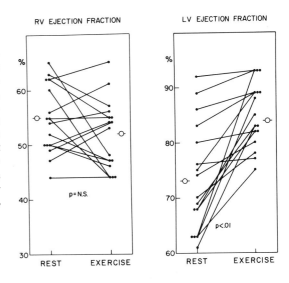

RV EJECTION FRACTION   LV EJECTION FRACTION

Figure 3–43. Rest and exercise right ventricular (RV) and left ventricular (LV) ejection fractions in 16 asymptomatic adolescents who had undergone surgical correction of tetralogy of Fallot. These studies were obtained at long-term follow-up. Note that abnormal right ventricular exercise reserve was present in 13 of 16 patients. For the group, right ventricular ejection fraction was not significantly different at rest and exercise. In contrast, left ventricular exercise reserve was normal, with the mean values rising significantly. (Reproduced with permission from Reduto, Berger, Johnstone, et al.[49])

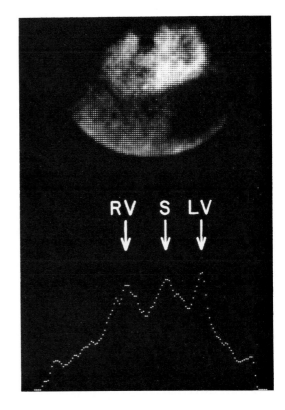

Figure 3–44. Resting thallium-201 image in the 45° left anterior oblique position in a patient who had undergone total surgical correction for tetralogy of Fallot. Note the right ventricular thallium-201 uptake, comparable to the uptake in the left ventricle. A profile through the midportion of the heart is shown below. The number of counts within the profile is on the vertical axis. The peak activity in the right ventricular (RV) and left ventricular (LV) free walls is comparable. The septum (S) also is demonstrated. These findings are consistent with marked right ventricular hypertrophy. (Reproduced with permission from Reduto, Berger, Johnstone, et al.[49])

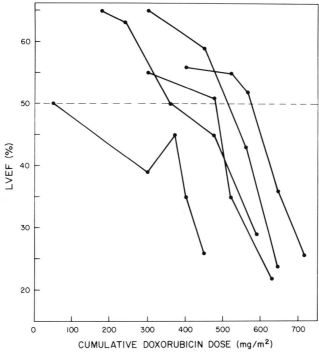

Figure 3–45. Sequential measurements of left ventricular ejection fraction (LVEF) in five adult patients who developed severe doxorubicin cardiotoxicity with congestive heart failure. Note that each of these patients initially passed through a phase of moderate cardiotoxicity that was detected with serial ejection fraction measurements. At the time when patients developed congestive heart failure, left ventricular ejection fraction was always less than 30 per cent. In a parallel group of six patients in whom doxorubicin was discontinued after demonstration of moderate cardiotoxicity, there was no further fall in ejection fraction. In fact, ejection fraction increased modestly after discontinuation of doxorubicin. (Reproduced with permission from Alexander, Dainiak, Berger, et al.[53])

failure may also complicate sickle cell crisis. Differentiation of right ventricular and left ventricular dysfunction can be obtained using radionuclide techniques. Since therapy for sickle cell crisis includes administration of large volumes of fluid, determination of left ventricular performance may have major clinical implications. Two additional cardiomyopathies relevant to the pediatric population should be mentioned. First, children receiving doxorubicin chemotherapy for treatment of certain malignancies have a tendency to develop an often irreversible cardiomyopathy. Although highly effective in the treatment of numerous cancers, the efficacy of doxorubicin depends upon high cumulative doses that often lead to congestive heart failure. Serial assessment of left ventricular performance allows identification of adult patients at risk for subsequent development of congestive heart failure and of those who can receive

therapy safely at higher than conventionally recommended cumulative doses.[53] A series of guidelines has been developed in adults on the basis of sequential ejection fraction measurements that allow for improved therapy with this drug (Fig. 3–45). Second, in patients receiving long-term blood tranfusions, such as those with thalassemia, myocardial iron deposition may result in a cardiomyopathy. This may result in decreased left ventricular performance both at rest and during exercise[54, 55] (Fig. 3–46). Some patients with this condition also may demonstrate small segmental perfusion defects on thallium-201 imaging.

In patients with cystic fibrosis, the major hemodynamic burden is on the right ventricle[56] (Fig. 3–47). Although cystic fibrosis is noted primarily for marked clinical abnormalities in pulmonary function, a substantial number of patients die secondary to cardiac complications. Right heart failure and right

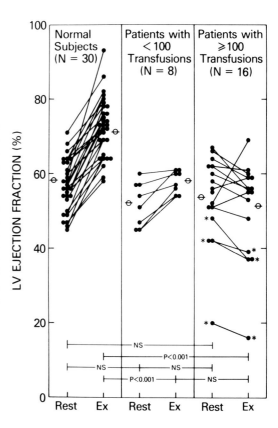

Figure 3–46. Rest and exercise (Ex) left ventricular (LV) ejection fractions in 30 normal subjects and in 24 patients with transfusion-dependent congenital anemias. Note that ejection fraction rose significantly in all normal subjects. These data were obtained using multiple-gated blood pool imaging. Approximately 75 per cent of the patients studied with congenital anemias had abnormal ejection fraction responses to exercise. The patients with asterisks also had regional functional abnormalities. Functional left ventricular impairment during exercise appears to be related to the cumulative blood transfusion load and subsequent iron deposition in the heart. (Reproduced with permission from Leon, Borer, Bacharach, et al.[54])

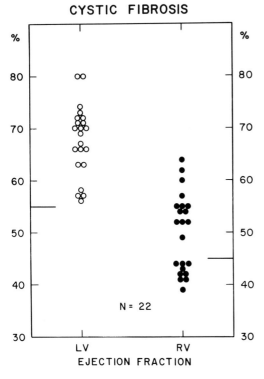

Figure 3–47. Right ventricular (RV) and left ventricular (LV) ejection fraction at rest in 22 young adults with cystic fibrosis. Note that left ventricular ejection fraction was normal in all 22 ambulatory patients. However, in nine of 22 patients, right ventricular ejection fraction was abnormal (less than 45 per cent). Five of these nine patients developed decompensated cor pulmonale during a subsequent two year follow-up. In contrast, none of the patients with normal right ventricular ejection fraction developed cardiopulmonary decompensation. (Reproduced with permission from Matthay, Berger, Loke, et al.[56])

ventricular hypertrophy frequently are difficult to identify prior to overt cardiopulmonary decompensation, and these usually occur very late in the course of the disease and have been found to be a harbinger of imminent death. Abnormalities in right ventricular performance are predictive of subsequent cardiopulmonary decompensation.[56] Radionuclide angiocardiography may provide a means for selecting appropriate patients with cystic fibrosis for therapy and for following their hemodynamic responses.[57]

Future Directions

The use of technetium-99m as a radioisotope is not ideal, especially in children. Although it emits gamma photons with energy suitable for external imaging, its physical half-life is substantially longer than necessary (Table 3–1). The isotope exposes the patient to radiation after completion of the study. It would be preferable to have ultrashort-lived radionuclides. Two such radiotracers undergoing clinical trials include tantalum-178,[58, 59] which has a half-life of 9.3 minutes, and iridium-191m,[60, 61] which has a half-life of 4.9 seconds. Utilization of these radiotracers would permit serial imaging with extremely high doses but markedly diminished overall radiation burden. An alternative approach involves the use of short-lived positron-emitting radioactive gases.[62, 63] By inhalation of oxygen-15 labeled carbon dioxide, a compact bolus of radionuclide indicator can be delivered directly to the left heart. The inhaled carbon dioxide passes freely across the alveolar membrane and is transferred into water in the pulmonary venous blood. In this way, the radioindicator is input directly into the left heart at a rate limited only by pulmonary blood flow. However, at present, clinical application of this technique is limited to medical centers with the capability for online cyclotron production of the short-lived gases.

REFERENCES

1. Prinzmetal, M., Corday, E. Spritzer, R.: Radiocardiography and its clinical applications. JAMA 139:617, 1949.

2. Parker, J., Treves, S.: Radionuclide detection, localization, and quantification of intracardiac shunts and shunts between the great vessels. Prog Cardiovasc Dis 20:121, 1977.
3. Treves, S., Collins-Nakai, R. L.: Radioactive tracers in congenital heart disease. Am J Cardiol 38:711, 1976.
4. Treves, S., Maltz, D., Adelstein, S.: Intracardiac shunts. In Pediatric Nuclear Medicine. James, A. E., Wagner, H. N., Cooke, R. E. (eds.). W. B. Saunders Co., Philadelphia, 1974, pp. 231–246.
5. Treves, S.: Detection and quantification of cardiovascular shunts with commonly available radionuclides. Sem Nucl Med 10:16, 1980.
6. Berger, H. J., Matthay, R. A., Pytlik, L., et al.: First-pass radionuclide assessment of right and left ventricular performance in patients with cardiac and pulmonary disease. Sem Nucl Med 9:275, 1979.
7. Strauss, H. W., McKusick, K. A., Boucher, C. A., et al.: Of linens and laces — The eighth anniversary of the gated blood pool scan. Sem Nucl Med 9:296, 1979.
8. Hayden, W. G., Kriss, J. P.: Scintiphotographic studies of acquired cardiovascular disease. Sem Nucl Med 3:177, 1973.
9. Graham, J. P., Goodrich, J. K., Robinson, M., et al.: Scintiangiocardiography in children: Rapid sequence visualization of the heart and great vessels after intravenous injection of radionuclide. Am J Cardiol 25:387, 1970.
10. Mason, D. T., Ashburn, W. L., Harbert, J. C., et al.: Rapid sequential visualization of the heart and great vessels in man using the wide-field. Anger scintillation camera: Radioisotope-angiography following the injection of technetium-99m. Circulation 39:19, 1969.
11. Greenfield, L. D., Bennett, L. R.: Comparison of heart chamber and pulmonary dilution curves for the diagnosis of cardiac shunts. Radiology 111:359, 1974.
12. Alazraki, N. P., Ashburn, W. L., Hagan, A.: Detection of left-to-right cardiac shunts with the scintillation camera pulmonary dilution curve. J Nucl Med 13:142, 1972.
13. Maltz, D. L., Treves, S.: Quantitative radionuclide angiocardiography: determination of Qp:Qs in children. Circulation 47:1049, 1973.
14. Askenazi, J., Ahnberg, D. J., Korngold, E., et al.: Quantitative radionuclide angiocardiography: Detection and quantification of left to right shunts. Am J Cardiol 37:382, 1976.
15. Jones, R. H., Sabiston, D. C., Bates, B. B., et al.: Quantitative radionuclide angiocardiography for determination of chamber to chamber cardiac transit times. Am J Cardiol 30:855, 1972.
16. Anderson, P. A. W., Jones, R. H., Sabiston, D. C.: Quantitation of left-to-right cardiac shunts with radionuclide angiography. Circulation 49:512, 1974.
17. Berger, H. J., Matthay, R. A., Loke, J., et al.: Assessment of cardiac performance with quantitative radionuclide angiocardiography: Right ventricular ejection fraction with reference to findings in chronic obstructive pulmonary disease. Am J Cardiol 41:897, 1978.

18. Fisher, E. A., Dubrow, I. W., Hastreiter, A. R.: Right ventricular volume in congenital heart disease. Am J Cardiol 36:67, 1975.

19. Berger, H. J., Reduto, L. A., Johnstone, D. E., et al.: Global and regional left ventricular response to bicycle exercise in coronary artery disease. Assessment by quantitative radionuclide angiocardiography. Am J Med 66:13, 1979.

20. Berger, H. J., Gottschalk, A., Zaret, B. L.: Radionuclide assessment of left and right ventricular performance. Radiol Clin North Am 18:441, 1980.

21. Rigo, P., Alderson, P. O., Robertson, R. M., et al.: Measurement of aortic and mitral regurgitation by gated cardiac blood pool scans. Circulation 60:306, 1979.

22. Borer, J., Bacharach, S., Green, M., et al.: Realtime radionuclide cineangiography in the noninvasive evaluation of global and regional left ventricular function at rest and during exercise in patients with coronary artery disease. N Engl J Med 296:839, 1977.

23. Neumann, R. D., Sostman, H. D., Gottschalk, A.: Current status of ventilation-perfusion imaging. Sem Nucl Med 10:198, 1980.

24. Papanicolaou, N., Treves, S.: Pulmonary scintigraphy in pediatrics. Sem Nucl Med 10:259, 1980.

25. Gates, G. F., Orme, H. W., Dove, E. K.: Cardiac shunt assessment in children with technetium-99m macroaggregate albumin. Radiology 112:649, 1974.

26. Haroutunian, L. M., Neill, C. A. Wagner, H. N., et al.: Preoperative and postoperative assessment of congenital heart disease. In Pediatric Nuclear Medicine. James, A. E., Wagner, H. N., Cooke, R. E. (eds.). W. B. Saunders Co., Philadelphia, 1974, pp. 265–276.

27. Strauss, H. W., Hurley, P. J., Rhodes, B. A., et al.: Quantification of right to left transpulmonary shunts in man. J Lab Clin Med 74:597, 1969.

28. Gates, G. F., Orme, H. W., Dove, E. K.: Surgery of congenital heart disease assessed by radionuclide scintigraphy. J Thor Cardiovasc Surg 69:767, 1975.

29. Zaret, B. L.: Myocardial imaging with radioactive potassium and its analogs. Prog Cardiovasc Dis 20:81, 1977.

30. Treves, S., Hill, T. C., Van Praagh R., et al.: Computed tomography of the heart using thallium-201 in children. Radiology 133:707, 1979.

31. Rabinovitch, M., Fisher, K., Gamble, W., et al.: Thallium-201: Quantitation of right ventricular hypertrophy in chronically hypoxic rats. Radiology 130:223, 1979.

32. Cohen, H. A., Baird, M. G., Rouleau, J. R., et al.: Thallium-201 myocardial imaging in patients with pulmonary hypertension. Circulation 54:790, 1976.

33. Khaja, F., Alam, M., Goldstein, S., et al.: Diagnostic value of visualization of the right ventricle using thallium-201 myocardial imaging. Circulation 59:182, 1979.

34. Wackers, F., Klay, J., Laks, H., et al.: Thallium-201 myocardial imaging in experimental right ventricular hypertrophy: Comparison to acute pulmonary banding. Circulation 62:III–230, 1980 (Abstract).

35. Berger, H. J., Wackers, F., Mahler, D., et al.: Right ventricular visualization on thallium-201 myocardial images in chronic obstructive pulmonary disease: Relationship to right ventricular function and hypertrophy. Circulation 62:III–103, 1980 (Abstract).

36. Verani, M. S., Marcus, M. L., Ehrhardt, J. C., et al.: Demonstration of improved myocardial perfusion following aortic implantation of anomalous left coronary artery. J Nucl Med 19:1032, 1978.

37. Finley, J. P., Howman-Giles, R. B., Gilday, D. L., et al.: Transient myocardial ischemia of the newborn infant demonstrated by thallium myocardial imaging. J Pediatr 94:263, 1979.

38. Finley, J. P., Howman-Giles, R. B., Gilday, D. L., et al.: Thallium-201 myocardial imaging in anomalous left coronary artery arising from the pulmonary artery: Application before and after medical and surgical treatment. Am J Cardiol 42:675, 1978.

39. Rabinovitch, M., Rowland, T. W., Castenada, A. R., et al.: Thallium-201 scintigraphy in patients with anomalous origin of the left coronary artery from the main pulmonary artery. J Pediatr 94:244, 1979.

40. Gutgesell, H. P., Pinsky, W. W., DePuey, E. G.: Thallium-201 myocardial perfusion imaging in infants and children. Value in distinguishing anomalous left coronary artery from congestive cardiomyopathy. Circulation 61:596, 1980.

41. Moodie, D. J., Cook, S. A., Gill, C. C., et al.: Thallium-201 myocardial imaging in young adults with anomalous left coronary artery arising from the pulmonary artery. J Nucl Med 21:1076, 1980.

42. Botvinick, E. H., Schiller, N. B.: The complementary roles of M-mode echocardiography and scintigraphy in the evaluation of adults with suspected left-to-right shunts: Additional observations on the role of two-dimensional echocardiography. Circulation 62:1070, 1980.

43. Higgins, C. B., Rausch, J., Friedman, W. F., et al.: Patent ductus arteriosus in preterm infants with idiopathic respiratory distress syndrome. Radiology 124:189, 1977.

44. Lester, L. A., Vitullo, D., Sodt, P., et al.: An evaluation of the left atrial/aortic root ratio in children with ventricular septal defect. Circulation 60:364, 1979.

45. Sahn, D. J., Allen, H. D., George, W., et al.: The utility of contrast echocardiographic techniques in the care of critically ill infants with cardiac and pulmonary disease. Circulation 56:959, 1977.

46. Boucher, C. A., Zir, L. M., Beller, G. A., et al.: Increased lung uptake of thallium-201 during exercise myocardial imaging: Clinical, hemodynamic and angiographic implications in patients with coronary artery disease. Am J Cardiol 46:189, 1980.

47. Gilday, D. L., Howman-Giles, R., Rowe, R., et al.: Combined thallium-201 myocardial imaging and multiple gated blood pool studies in children. Am J Cardiol 41:442, 1978 (Abstract).

48. Keane, J. F., Williams, R., Treves, S., et al.: Assessment of the postoperative patient by noninvasive techniques. Prog Cardiovasc Dis 18:57, 1975.

49. Reduto, L. A., Berger, H. J., Johnstone, D. E., et al.: Radionuclide assessment of right and left ventricular exercise reserve after total correction of tetralogy of Fallot. Am J Cardiol 45:1013, 1980.

50. Rosing, D. R., Borer, J. S., Kent, K. M., et al.: Long-term hemodynamic and electrocardiographic assessment following operative repair of tetralogy of Fallot. Circulation 58 (Suppl. 1):209, 1978.

51. Borer, J. S., Bacharach, S. L., Green, M., et al.: Exercise-induced left ventricular dysfunction in symptomatic and asymptomatic patients with aortic regurgitation: Assessment with radionuclide cineangiography. Am J Cardiol 42:351, 1978.

52. Lewis, S., Riba, A., Berger, H., et al.: Relationship of ventricular geometry at rest to exercise left ventricular performance in aortic regurgitation. Am Heart J (in press).

53. Alexander, J., Dainiak, N., Berger, H. J., et al.: Serial assessment of doxorubicin cardiotoxicity with quantitative radionuclide angiocardiography. N Engl J Med 300:278, 1979.

54. Leon, M. B., Borer, J. S., Bacharach, S. L., et al.: Detection of early cardiac dysfunction in patients with severe beta-thalassemia and chronic iron overload. N Engl J Med 301:1143, 1979.

55. Hellenbrand, W. E., Berger, H. J., O'Brien, R. T., et al.: Left ventricular performance in thalassemia: Combined noninvasive radionuclide and echocardiographic assessment. Circulation 56:III–49, 1977.

56. Matthay, R. A., Berger, H. J., Loke, J., et al.: Right and left ventricular performance in ambulatory young adults with cystic fibrosis. Br Heart J 43:474, 1980.

57. Chipps, B. E., Alderson, P. O., Roland, J. A., et al.: Noninvasive evaluation of ventricular function in cystic fibrosis. J Pediatr 95:379, 1979.

58. Holman, B. L., Harris, G. I., Neirinckx, R. D., et al.: Tantalum-178: A short-lived nuclide for nuclear medicine — Production of the parent W-178. J Nucl Med 19:510, 1978.

59. Holman, B. L., Neirinckx, R. D., Treves, S., et al.: Cardiac imaging with tantalum-178. Radiology 131:525, 1979.

60. Treves, S., Kulprathipanja, S., Hnatowich, D. J.: Angiography with iridium-191m. An ultra-short-lived radionuclide (T ½ 4.9 sec.). Circulation 54:275, 1976.

61. Treves, S., Cheng, C., Samuel, A., et al.: Iridium-191m angiocardiography for the detection and quantification of left-to-right shunting. J Nucl Med 21:1151, 1980.

62. Watson, D. D.: Shunt detection with the short-lived radioactive gases. Sem Nucl Med 10:27, 1980.

63. Boucher, C. A., Ahluwalia, B., Block, P. C., et al.: Inhalation imaging with oxygen-15 labeled carbon dioxide for detection and quantification of left-to-right shunts. Circulation 56:632, 1977.

Chapter 4

THE ANGIOCARDIOGRAM

TECHNICAL ASPECTS

In the past few years angiographic techniques for the delineation of intracardiac and great vessel anatomy have changed in three important ways. First, the concept of compound angulated projections (axial cineangiography), originally conceived by Bargeron and his colleagues,[1,2] has evolved and become an accepted and, in fact, necessary prerequisite to the precise depiction of cardiac anatomy. The precision needed to depict congenital cardiac lesions, with the ultimate goal being optimal surgical therapy, has also resulted in the use of larger volumes of contrast material delivered over a shorter period of time. A third, though indirect, effect on the way that the angiocardiogram is performed relates to the fact that M-mode and two-dimensional echocardiography frequently provide information regarding the presence of major cardiac anomalies prior to cardiac catheterization and angiography. This allows physicians to tailor the catheterization and angiographic procedures to (1) more accurately depict the suspected lesions and (2) search for unexpected variations or associated malformations.

Contrast Material

Generally, most laboratories use Renografin 76 in children and Renografin 60 in neonates. The latter has the theoretic advantage of causing less increase in serum osmolality. Nonionic materials such as metrizamide have been used in pediatric angiography in Europe.[3] Investigations in an infant experimental model have shown that metrizamide causes less alteration in hemodynamic parameters and less increase in osmolality than Renografin 76. With newer angiographic exams employing larger volumes of contrast material, the use of nonionic contrast materials may become an important consideration, especially in the sick neonate.

Contrast Volumes and Injection Rates

In the absence of a left-to-right shunt or a valvular regurgitant lesion, our laboratory currently uses approximately 1.5 cc of contrast per kilogram of body weight for ventriculography. When large shunts or regurgitant lesions are present, we increase this to 2 cc per kilogram. In the presence of semilunar valve stenosis, we reduce the volume for ventriculography to approximately 1 cc per kilogram. This same volume is used for aortography. The volume for ventriculography may be further reduced in the presence of severe myocardial dysfunction or a hypoplastic ventricle.

An attempt should be made to deliver the contrast material within one heartbeat (that is, if the heart rate is 120 beats/min, the injection rate for 10 cc would be 20 cc/sec). In order to accomplish this safely and to reduce the possibility of intramyocardial injection, two methods may be employed. One may either use a balloon angiographic catheter of suitable French size to deliver the volume required or use large caliber, short length, standard (NIH) catheters. The French size and length vary, depending on the age of the child: infants—5 to 6 F, 50 cm; children less than two years of age—6 to 7 F, 60 cm; older children—8 F, 60 cm. Although Bargeron advocates rapid hand injection through larger catheters,[1] we have safely employed an automatic pressure injector with PSI settings in the 600 to 700 range.

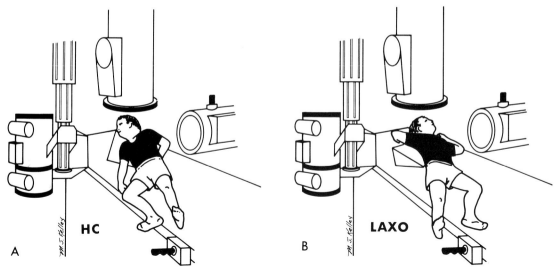

Figure 4–1. Patient positioning for the two most commonly used axial views. The diagrams illustrate a fixed biplane radiographic unit. *A,* Patient positioned for hepatoclavicular (HC) view. The patient is slanted 15 to 20° to the right side of the table, is rotated into a 45° left anterior oblique position, and the head and shoulders are elevated 30 to 40° off the table. The vertical image intensifier records the most important information in this projection. *B,* Patient positioned for long-axial oblique (LAXO) view. The patient is again slanted to the right on the table, is rotated into a 15 to 20° right anterior oblique projection, and the head and shoulders are elevated 20 to 30° off the table. The lateral image intensifier records the most important information in this projection. (Reproduced with permission from Kelley et al.[6])

Axial Angiocardiography

Until recently, the angiocardiographic diagnosis in children with suspected heart disease (whether acquired or congenital) depended upon frontal (vertical tube) and lateral (horizontal tube) projections. Except for the pioneering work of Bargeron,[1] the use of oblique and caudal or cranial "axial" views was limited by fixed biplane angiographic units and by a reluctance of some angiographers to turn or reposition infants and children who were sedated and had catheters in place. Recent reports have documented the usefulness of angled views in patients with acquired[5] and congenital[2, 6] heart disease. Some laboratories have employed U-arm or C-arm cineangiocardiographic units to achieve caudal or cranial and compound caudal-cranial-oblique views without moving the patient from the supine position. However, our experience (like Bargeron's) has involved a fixed system with horizontal and vertical x-ray tubes and image intensifiers. Using this system, we have found three angled views to be a crucial part of the angiocardiographic diagnosis. There are (1) a 30 to 40° caudal-cranial

view ("the sitting up" view); (2) a 40° cranial/45° left anterior oblique view (hepatoclavicular [HC] view); and (3) a long-axial 20° right anterior oblique view (long-axial oblique [LAXO] view).

Patient positioning for these views is well described elsewhere[1] and is illustrated in Figures 4–1 and 4–2D. Prior to positioning in the 40° cranial/45° left anterior oblique and the long-axial 20° right anterior oblique view, it is important to remember to slant the patient to the right approximately 15 to 20° in the horizontal plane (feet to the right side of the table). This will align the long axis of the heart perpendicular to the vertical tube for the left anterior oblique and the horizontal tube for the right anterior oblique view.

The *30 to 40° caudal-cranial (PA) view* ("sitting up" view) is obtained by placing a 30° wedge under the patient's shoulders and filming with the vertical imaging intensifier (Fig. 4–2D). It places the pulmonary trunk almost perpendicular to the x-ray beam, as opposed to the standard PA view, which foreshortens it (Fig. 4–2A). Angiograms using this view may be obtained with the vertical tube alone or biplane. The

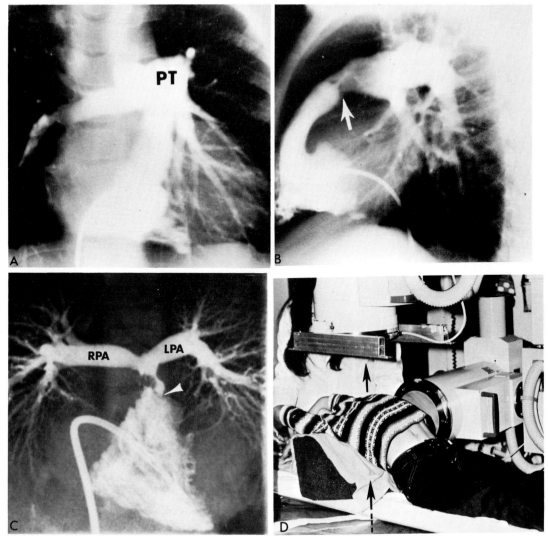

Figure 4–2. Standard posteroanterior (A) and lateral (B) projections of a patient with valvar pulmonary stenosis. The PA view (A) foreshortens the right ventricular outflow tract and pulmonary trunk (PT). Only the lateral view (B) demonstrates the thickened pulmonary valve (arrow). 30° caudal-cranial view ("sitting up" view) (C) shows right ventricular outflow tract, thickened pulmonary valve (arrow), and the origin of both pulmonary arteries (RPA, LPA) from the pulmonary trunk. Patient positioning for the "sitting up" view is shown in D. A 30° wedge is placed under the child's shoulders and the vertical tube and image intensifier are used. Direction of x-ray beam is indicated by arrows.

"sitting up" projection is most useful for evaluating: (1) the pulmonary trunk and its bifurcation into right and left pulmonary arteries; (2) the pulmonary valve and annulus; and (3) the right ventricular outflow tract (Fig. 4–2C). It is the view of choice in patients with peripheral pulmonic stenosis, as it shows the origins of the main pulmonary arteries as well as more distal stenoses. It is helpful in patients with tetralogy of Fallot for evaluating possible pulmonary

artery bifurcation stenosis (usually the left), and pulmonary artery size. In patients with pulmonary atresia with ventricular septal defect (pseudotruncus), who derive their lung flow from systemic collaterals, it is helpful in defining continuity between peripheral pulmonary arteries and the pulmonary trunk. Table 4–1 lists those lesions in which this view is useful.

The *40° cranial/45° left anterior oblique view* (hepatoclavicular [HC] view) is an-

TABLE 4–1. Common Anomalies and Preferred Angled Views

ANOMALY	AXIAL VIEW	INJECTION SITE
Aortic stenosis	HC or LAXO	LV
Atrial septal defect	HC	RULPV
Endocardial cushion defect	LAXO	LV
	HC	LV
Pulmonic stenosis	Caudal-cranial PA/Lat	RV
Subvalvar aortic stenosis	HC or LAXO	LV[6]
Tetralogy of Fallot	LAXO	LV
	Caudal-cranial PA/Lat	RV
	HC or LAO	Asc Ao
Transposition (DORV)	HC	LV, RV
Transposition with PS	LAXO	LV

Asc Ao = ascending aorta
DORV = double-outlet right ventricle
HC = hepatoclavicular
Lat = lateral
LAXO = long axial oblique
LV = left ventricle
PA = posteroanterior
PS = pulmonic stenosis
RULPV = right upper lobe pulmonary vein
RV = right ventricle

other useful angled angiographic projection. Angiograms using it may be obtained with the vertical tube alone or biplane (Fig. 4–3A and B). In the latter situation, the lateral image intensifier provides information usually obtained with the vertical image intensifier in the standard RAO projection (Fig. 4–3B). The HC view places the vertical tube perpendicular to the long axis of the heart and additionally aligns the atrial septum and the posterior interventricular septum parallel to the beam. A left ventriculogram performed in this projection allows visualization of the posterior portion of the ventricular septum—a region that is not seen using conventional views (Fig. 4–3A). Characteristic of this view is a bulge occurring in systole that represents the junction of the anterior and posterior mitral leaflets and the junction of the left ventricular free wall and posterior septum. The muscular septum, the left ventricular outflow tract, and the anterior leaflet of the mitral valve are also well seen in this view (Fig. 4–3A). The aortopulmonary window and the coronary arteries may also be evaluated (Fig. 4–3A). In addition, the atrial septum is seen in its entirety in this projection (Fig. 4–4). Defects in it are best found with injections made in the right upper pulmonary vein (Fig. 4–4). Tables 4–1 and 4–2 list those entities that may be clarified using this useful view.

The *long-axial 20° right anterior oblique view* (long axial oblique [LAXO] view) may be filmed using the horizontal tube alone or biplane. This projection places the anterior interventricular septum in profile when viewed with the lateral image intensifier (Fig. 4–5A). In addition to profiling the anterior interventricular septum, the long-axial oblique emphasizes the left ventricular outflow tract and the subaortic valve area (Fig. 4–5A). Below this region, the muscular septum is seen in profile. Between these two regions, the anterior leaflet of the mitral valve and its relationship to the left ventricular outflow tract are visualized (Fig. 4–5A). In this view, the vertical image intensifier gives information that is very similar to that obtained in the conventional right anterior oblique view (Fig. 4–5B). It profiles the atrioventricular septum (which is absent in most endocardial cushion abnormalities) and can be used to quantitate the degree of mitral regurgitation (Fig. 4–5B).

A right ventriculogram may be performed in either the hepatoclavicular or long-axial oblique projection. The horizontal image intensifier in the HC projection and the vertical image intensifier in the LAXO projection (Fig. 4–6A) provide information that is similar to that seen with the standard RAO view. The tricuspid valve, the inflow and sinus regions of the right ventricle, as well as the infundibulum, pulmonary valve, and

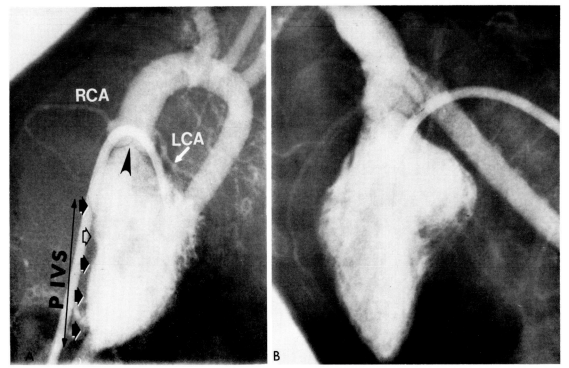

Figure 4–3. Left ventriculogram — hepatoclavicular (HC) view. *A,* The vertical image intensifier gives an elongated LAO projection that profiles the *posterior* interventricular septum (PIVS — arrows). This diastolic frame (note closed aortic valve — arrowhead) of a normal left ventricle shows a hint of the normally prominent systolic septal bulge (open arrowhead). This bulge represents the junction of the anterior and posterior mitral leaflets as well as the junction of the left ventricular free wall and posterior septum. Note that the left ventricular outflow tract (beneath arrowhead) and the coronary arteries (RCA and LCA) are well seen in this view. *B,* The lateral (horizontal) image intensifier gives a view that is very similar to the standard right anterior oblique projection. Therefore, left ventricular function (ejection fraction) and mitral regurgitation can be assessed in this view.

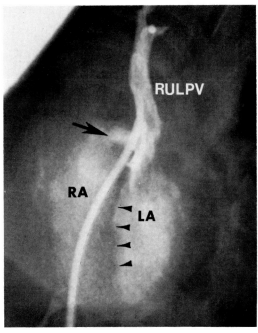

Figure 4-4. Hepatoclavicular view—right upper lobe pulmonary venogram (RULPV). The atrial septum is profiled in its entirety (arrowheads) and contrast is seen streaming across a high atrial septal defect (arrow) between the left atrium (LA) and right atrium (RA).

TABLE 4–2. Anatomy Depicted by Axial Views

ANATOMY	ANOMALIES IDENTIFIED
40° Cranial/45° LAO View (Hepatoclavicular View) *(Vertical Tube)*	
LEFT VENTRICULOGRAM	
Posterior ventricular septum	VSDs of the AV canal type
Left ventricular outflow tract	IHSS; subvalvar aortic stenosis; tunnel aortic stenosis; membranous and supracristal VSDs; LV outflow obstruction in d-TGV
Left ventricular/right atrial region	Left ventricular to right atrial communications
Anterior leaflet of mitral valve	Cleft in partial endocardial cushion defects
Mitral valve–left ventricular outflow	Subvalvar obstruction in d-TGV
Mitral valve–aortic valve relationship	Double outlet right ventricle
Aortic valve region and coronary arteries	Sinus of Valsalva aneurysm, anomalous coronary origin (esp. LAD from RCA)
Transverse aorta/ductus region	PDA
Pulmonary valve, pulmonary trunk, and bifurcation	d-TGV, tetralogy of Fallot (T/F)
LEFT ATRIOGRAM	
Left atrium	Sinus venous ASD, cor triatriatum
RIGHT UPPER PULMONARY VENOGRAM/RIGHT ATRIOGRAM	
Atrial septum	ASD size, location, and type (secundum and primum); atrial septum in tricuspid atresia
Right upper pulmonary vein/SVC	Partial anomalous pulmonary venous return to right atrium, pulmonary varix
Tricuspid valve/ventricular septum	Straddling tricuspid valve
RIGHT VENTRICULOGRAM	
Ventricular septum	VSD, location, and size in right-to-left shunt, origin of left pulmonary artery
Right ventricular sinus portion and infundibulum	Anomalous muscle bundle in right ventricle
Pulmonary trunk	Bifurcation
40° Cranial/45° LAO View (Hepatoclavicular View) *(Horizontal Tube)*	
Left ventriculogram	Similar information as conventional RAO view (mitral valve, papillary muscles, aortic valve, high ventricular septum, LV function)
Right ventriculogram	Right ventricular infundibulum (T/F), tricuspid valve (tricuspid prolapse); inflow and sinus regions of right ventricle (Ebstein's malformation of TV; RV muscle bundle); pulmonary valve (T/F); right pulmonary artery origin
Long Axial 20° RAO View (Long Axial Oblique View) *(Horizontal Tube)*	
LEFT VENTRICULOGRAM	
Anterior ventricular septum	Membranous, supracristal, and muscular VSDs; relationship of aorta to anterior interventricular septum
Left ventricular outflow tract	IHSS, subvalvar aortic stenosis, tunnel aortic stenosis
Mitral-left ventricular outflow	IHSS, prolapse of anterior leaflet of mitral valve
RIGHT VENTRICULOGRAM	
Anterior ventricular septum	VSD in tetralogy
Left pulmonary artery	Origin in tetralogy
Long Axial 20° RAO View (Long Axial Oblique View) *(Vertical Tube)*	
Left ventriculogram	Atrioventricular membrane in endocardial cushion defects; similar information as shallow RAO
Right ventriculogram	Similar information as shallow RAO and horizontal tube HC view

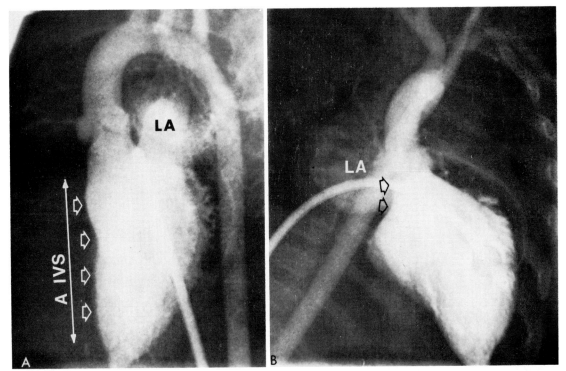

Figure 4–5. Left ventriculogram — long-axial oblique (LAXO) view. *A*, The lateral image intensifier gives an elongated LAO projection that profiles the *anterior* interventricular septum (AIVS — arrows) and provides information about the relationship of the anterior mitral leaflet to the left ventricular outflow tract. Some regurgitation occurs into the left atrium (LA). *B*, The vertical image intensifier shows the left ventricle in an RAO projection and additionally profiles the atrioventricular septum (arrows) — a region that is absent or deficient in endocardial cushion defects. Note again that there is faint visualization of the left atrium (LA).

right pulmonary artery are all well visualized (Fig. 4–6A). The vertical image intensifier in the HC view and the horizontal image intensifier in the LAXO projection (Fig. 4–6B) profile the interventricular septum, the infundibulum and pulmonary valve, and the origin of the left pulmonary artery (Fig. 4–6B). This view is especially useful in locating and sizing VSDs when there is a right-to-left shunt. Tables 4–1 and 4–2 list the entities that may be delineated by the LAXO view.

NORMAL ANGIOCARDIOGRAPHIC AND MORPHOLOGIC FEATURES OF THE CARDIAC CHAMBERS AND THE GREAT VESSELS

The key anatomic landmarks of the four cardiac chambers are outlined in Table 4–3.

The Atria

In patients with normal atrial morphology and position (situs solitus), each atrium has unique anatomic characteristics. It so happens that the atria in this situation are the bellwether organs for the remainder of the noncardiac viscera, especially the spleen. This fact has been elaborated in the discussion on abnormalities of situs (see Chapter 1). Anatomically, the right atrium consists of a posterior, smooth-walled portion that receives the superior and inferior venae cavae and a thin-walled trabeculated portion that gives rise to the triangular-shaped right atrial appendage (Fig. 4–7A–D). A ridge of muscle, the crista terminalis, separates these two regions. The body of the normal right atrium is an ovoid structure that extends from approximately two thoracic segments below the carina to the medial aspect of the right hemidiaphragm. The right atrial

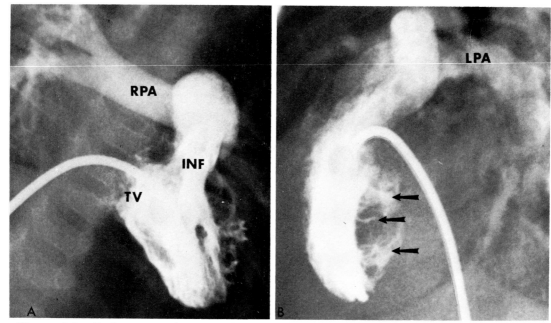

Figure 4–6. Right ventriculogram — long-axial oblique (LAXO) view. *A,* The vertical image intensifier shows the right ventricle in an RAO projection. The tricuspid valve (TV), inflow and sinus portions, and infundibulum (INF) are well seen. Note that the origin of the right pulmonary artery (RPA) is also well delineated. *B,* The horizontal image intensifier profiles the anterior interventricular septum and in this patient demonstrates multiple small muscular ventricular septal defects (arrows). Note that the origin of the left pulmonary artery (LPA) is well seen.

appendage is filled with coarse parallel pectinate muscles and extends in an anterior and lateral direction from the body of the right atrium (Fig. 4–7*D*) and forms the upper portion of the right heart border. The tip of the appendage may reach to the level of the carina. The coronary sinus enters the base of the right atrium anterior and medial to the inferior vena cava (Fig. 4–7*C*). The orifice of the coronary sinus and the orifice of the inferior vena cava are guarded by folds of tissue, the eustachian and the thebesian valves, respectively.

The body of the left atrium is more round-

TABLE 4–3. Anatomic Landmarks of Cardiac Chambers*

	MORPHOLOGIC RIGHT	MORPHOLOGIC LEFT
ATRIA	Situated on same side as trilobed lung	Situated on same side as bilobed lung
	Receives inferior vena cava	
	Contains crista terminalis	
	Triangular atrial appendage with parallel pectinate muscles	Irregular atrial appendage with small pectinate muscles
	Fossa ovalis on right side of atrial septum	Ostium secundum on left side of atrial septum
VENTRICLES	Contains tricuspid valve	Contains mitral valve
	Septum has coarse, parallel trabeculations	Septum is smooth with fine, oblique trabeculations
	Crista supraventricularis separates tricuspid from semilunar valve	Fibrous continuity exists between mitral and semilunar valve
	Contains septal papillary muscle (papillary muscle of the conus)	Contains no septal papillary muscle
	Contains right branch of bundle of His	Contains left branch of bundle of His

*Modified from Stanger.[7]

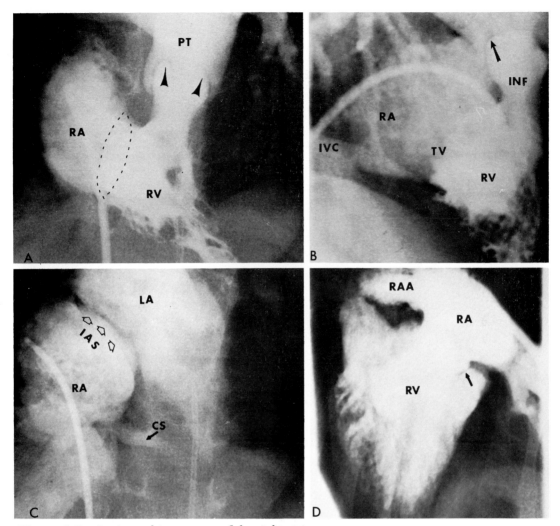

Figure 4–7. Angiographic anatomy of the right atrium.

A, "Sitting up" view, right atriogram shows catheter entering the right atrium (RA) and contrast filling the right ventricle (RV) and pulmonary trunk (PT). A thickened pulmonary valve (arrows) is present. The region of the tricuspid valve annulus is indicated (dotted lines).

B, Lateral view demonstrates relationship of inferior vena cava (IVC) to posterior smooth-walled body of the right atrium (RA). The tricuspid valve (TV), right ventricle (RV) and infundibulum (INF) are indicated. Note the thickened pulmonary valve (arrow).

C, HC view (vertical image intensifier), right atriogram in a patient with tricuspid atresia. Note the position of the interatrial septum (IAS — arrows) separating the inferiorly located right atrium (RA) from the left atrium (LA). The coronary sinus (CS — arrow) is faintly opacified.

D, HC view (lateral image intensifier), right atriogram, showing smooth-walled body of the right atrium (RA) and the triangular-shaped right atrial appendage (RAA). The posterior leaflet of the tricuspid valve (arrow) is seen opening into the right ventricle (RV).

ed than that of the right atrium, although its transverse axis is somewhat larger than its vertical and anteroposterior axes (Fig. 4–8A and B). It is located in a relatively midline position, with its roof one thoracic segment below the carina and its base well above the hemidiaphragms (Fig. 4–8A). On the lateral

projection, the wall of the left atrium makes up the upper two-thirds of the posterior cardiac silhouette (Fig. 4–8B). In contrast to the right atrial appendage, the left atrial appendage has a waist-like origin, is much more irregular and elongated in shape, and has small pectinate muscles (Fig. 4–9A and B).

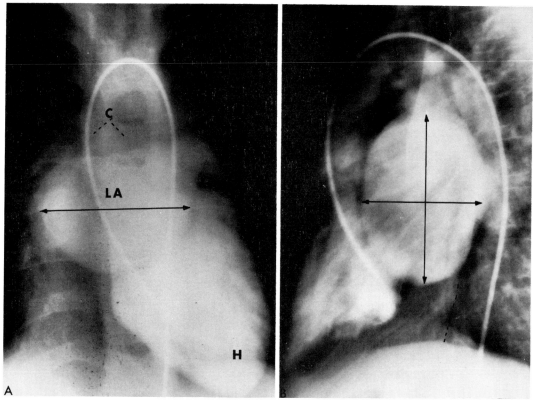

Figure 4–8. Left ventriculogram in anteroposterior (A) and lateral (B) projections in a patient with severe mitral regurgitation, demonstrating the anatomy of the left atrium. The body of this enlarged left atrium (LA) is approximately as large in the transverse axis (horizontal arrow — A) as it is in the vertical axis (vertical arrow — B). The anteroposterior dimension is the smallest (horizontal arrow — B). The left atrium is located in a midline position with its roof just below the carina (C). The base is situated well above the hemidiaphragms (H). When enlarged, the left atrium forms the upper two-thirds of the posterior cardiac silhouette (B).

The number of pulmonary veins that enter the left atrium varies. There are usually two (occasionally three) on the right and two (occasionally one) on the left (Fig. 4–10). The entrance of pulmonary veins into an atrium should not be used to distinguish it morphologically, since variation in pulmonary venous return is not uncommon.

From the aforementioned, one can see that the right atrium is not only to the right but also inferior and anterior to the left atrium. The interatrial septum formed between these two structures is oriented in a slightly oblique manner as it passes from right posterior to left anterior (Fig. 4–7C). In the center of this muscular septum there is a shallow thin fibrous depression, the fossa ovalis, which is visible from the right atrium.

Ventricles and Atrioventricular Valves

The right ventricular cavity as seen angiographically consists of a relatively smooth posteroinferior inflow portion that contains the tricuspid valve. This leads to the larger and heavily trabeculated sinus portion. The trabeculae are coarse and are oriented in a parallel fashion. The sinus region gives rise to a smooth anterosuperior outflow region or infundibulum (Fig. 4–11A and B). It is not unusual for contrast material to pass from the inflow portion to the infundibulum and exclude opacification of the heavily trabeculated apical region (Fig. 4–11A). The roof of the inflow portion of the right ventricle is made up of a muscular fold (the ventriculo-infundibular fold), which exists between

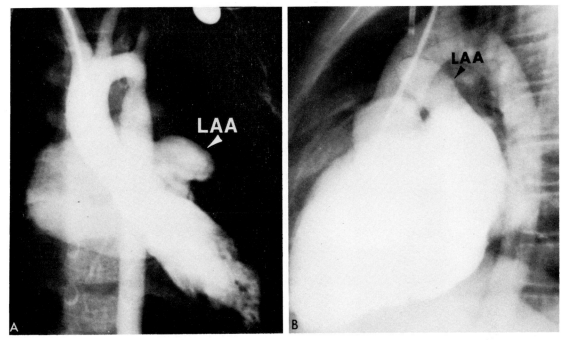

Figure 4-9. Left ventriculogram in two patients with severe mitral regurgitation demonstrating the left atrial appendage (LAA) in the anteroposterior (A) and lateral (B) projections.

Figure 4-10. Levophase venous angiogram showing right and left pulmonary veins entering the left atrium (LA). On the right, two main venous channels are present (arrows), while on the left a single confluence is seen (arrow).

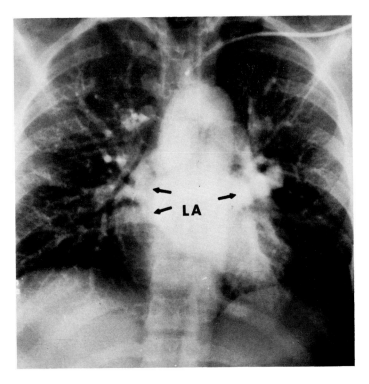

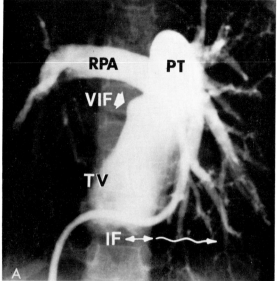

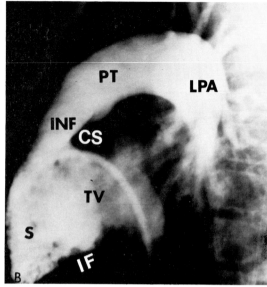

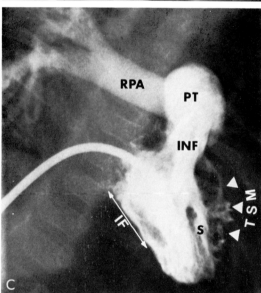

Figure 4–11. Right ventricular angiograms in (A) postero-anterior, (B) lateral, and (C) right anterior oblique projections. The smooth inflow portion (IF); the heavily trabeculated sinus region (S); and the outflow region, or infundibulum (INF), are indicated. Note that contrast fails to opacify the apical region (wavy arrow) in (A). The ventriculo-infundibular fold (VIF) is indicated in A, while the position of crista supraventricularis (CS) is best seen in the lateral view (B). The prominent trabeculae in the septal region are termed the trabecula septomarginalis (TSM). The right pulmonary artery (RPA) is best visualized in the RAO view (C), while the pulmonary trunk (PT) and left pulmonary artery (LPA) are viewed optimally in the lateral projection (B).

the aortic valve and the tricuspid valve (Fig. 4–11A). There is often one prominent trabecula in the septal region, which is termed the trabecula septomarginalis (Fig. 4–11C). The medial and anterior papillary muscles, which are reasonably constant in position, arise from this prominent trabecula and attach via delicate chordae tendinae to the anterior and septal cusps of the tricuspid valve. The posterior wall of the outflow tract of the right ventricle is formed by a muscular body, the crista supraventricularis. This muscle separates the two semilunar valves and is best viewed in the lateral projection

as an ovoid structure posterior to the infundibulum (Fig. 4–11B). The tricuspid valve is situated just to the right of the thoracic spine and is obliquely oriented in both the anteroposterior and lateral planes (Figs. 4–11A and B). It is actually misnamed in that the leaflets vary both in number and size. Usually there is a long septal leaf that lies adjacent to the ventricular septum. The tricuspid valve is separated from the infundibulum and pulmonary valve by the ventriculo-infundibular fold (Fig. 4–11A).

The interventricular septum is obliquely oriented from right posterior to left anterior (see Fig. 4–16). This creates a most important relationship between the two chambers — namely, that the right ventricle is anterior to the left ventricle. In addition, the apex of the right ventricle is just inferior to the apex of the left ventricle and a small portion of the left ventricle extends to the left of the right ventricle in the anteroposterior projection.

The left ventricle, like the right ventricle, has three portions, although the first and third are less well developed. The short, smooth inflow portion lies beneath the posterior leaflet of the mitral valve (Fig. 4–12A and B). The fornix is a small portion of left ventricular myocardium located at the junction of the posterior mitral leaflet insertion into the mitral annulus (Fig. 4–12B). The sinus portion differs considerably from that of the more heavily trabeculated right ven-

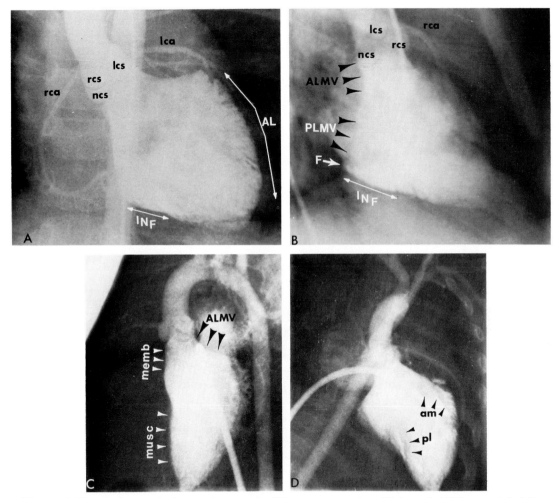

Figure 4–12. Left ventricular angiograms in (A) posteroanterior, (B) lateral, (C) long-axial oblique (cranial LAO), and (D) long-axial (RAO) projections. The short, smooth inflow portion (INF) lies beneath the posterior leaflet of the mitral valve (PLMV — arrowheads). The fornix (F) of the left ventricle is located at the junction of the inflow portion and the posterior leaflet insertion. The fine trabecular pattern is appreciated in all projections. The muscular (musc — arrowheads) and membranous (memb — arrowheads) portions of the interventricular septum are best visualized in the LAO view (C). In the posteroanterior projection (A) one can see that the anterolateral (AL) wall makes up the lateral margin of the cardiac silhouette. In the lateral (B) and LAO (C) views, the anterior leaflet of the mitral valve (ALMV — arrowheads) forms a curvilinear region of continuity with the noncoronary sinus (ncs) of the aortic valve. The posterolateral (PL) and anteromedial (AM) papillary muscles are visualized in the right anterior oblique projection (D). The relationships between the right and left coronary arteries (rca, lca) and the right, left, and noncoronary sinuses (rcs, lcs, ncs) are depicted in the posteroanterior (A) and lateral (B) projections.

tricle (Fig. 4–12A and B). The trabeculae are relatively fine and "flattened" (Fig. 4–12A–D) into the wall of the left ventricle and tend to run in an oblique orientation. The short, smooth outflow portion of the left ventricle takes a somewhat horizontal and sigmoid course before terminating at the aortic valve. Beneath the aortic valve is a small area on the medial wall of the left ventricular outflow tract made up of fibrous tissue, the membranous septum (Fig. 4–12C). The apex of the left ventricle does not extend as far inferiorly as the right ventricle. A small portion of the anterolateral wall of the left ventricle forms the lateral border of the cardiac silhouette in the posteroanterior projection (Fig. 4–12A). In the lateral projection, the left ventricle forms the inferior third of the posterior border of the cardiac silhouette (Fig. 4–12B).

The mitral valve consists of two leaflets: a large anteromedial leaflet and a smaller posterolateral leaflet connected to two well-developed papillary muscles—the anteromedial and posterolateral papillary muscles. These papillary muscles are best visualized in the RAO projection (Fig. 4–12D). In the normal heart, there is usually fibrous conti-

nuity between the anterior leaflet of the mitral valve and the semilunar valve, forming a portion of the left ventricular outflow tract (Fig. 4–12B and C). The mitral valve is situated not only to the left of the tricuspid valve but also superior and posterior to it.

Semilunar Valves and Great Vessels

The pulmonary valve has three distinct cusps and it is located above the infundibulum of the right ventricle, superior to the major cardiac mass. It gives origin to the pulmonary trunk, which courses in a slightly leftward and posterior direction before giving rise to the right and left pulmonary arteries (Fig. 4–11A–C). The right pulmonary artery originates from the pulmonary trunk at approximately a 90° angle (Fig. 4–11A and C), while the left pulmonary artery continues as a direct posterior extension of the trunk as it passes over the left mainstem bronchus (Fig. 4–11B).

The aortic valve, situated above the short outflow tract of the left ventricle, gives rise to right and left coronary arteries above its

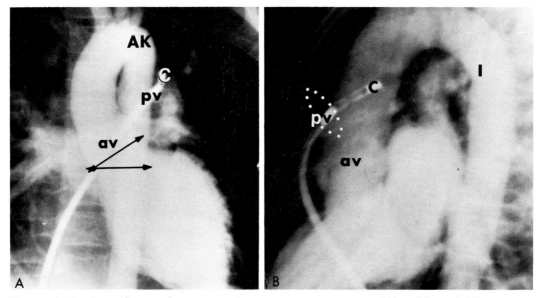

Figure 4–13. Levophase pulmonary angiogram in posteroanterior (A) and lateral (B) projections demonstrating the relationship between the aortic valve and aorta to the pulmonary valve and pulmonary trunk. The catheter (C) is situated with its tip in the pulmonary trunk just distal to the pulmonary valve (pv). The aortic annulus is elevated 30° in the horizontal plane (arrows). The aortic valve (av) is located to the right and posterior to the pulmonary valve (pv). The aortic knob (AK) is that portion of the transverse aorta in continuity with the descending aorta, while the isthmus (I) is the slight narrowing of the descending aorta just distal to the left subclavian artery.

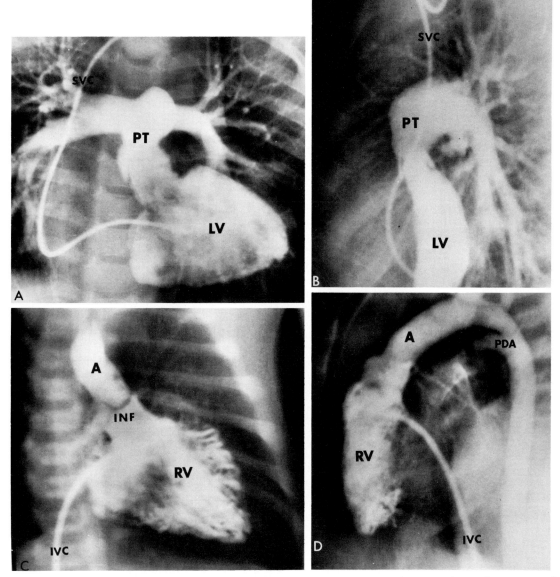

Figure 4–14. Morphologic characteristics of the left ventricle and right ventricle are demonstrated in these angiograms of a child with complete transposition of the great vessels. Note that the morphologic left ventricle (LV) is smooth in these posteroanterior (A) and lateral (B) ventriculograms. This ventricle, however, gives rise to the pulmonary trunk (PT) and supplies blood to the lungs. The morphologic right ventricle (RV) in the posteroanterior (C) and lateral (D) ventriculograms is more heavily trabeculated and has a smooth-walled outflow tract, the infundibulum (INF). This ventricle gives rise to the anteriorly positioned aorta (A). There is a patent ductus arteriosus (PDA). Note that the venous catheter entering from the inferior vena cava (IVC) enters the RV from the right atrium, while the venous catheter from the superior vena cava (SVC) enters the LV by crossing from the right atrium, through a patent foramen ovale, to the left atrium and then across the mitral valve.

sinuses of Valsalva (Fig. 4–12A). In the posteroanterior projection, the right coronary sinus is located anteriorly and medially (Fig. 4–12A). The left coronary sinus is located to the left and posteriorly and is superior to the right and noncoronary sinus-

es. The inferior-most sinus (and often the most rightward) is the noncoronary sinus. These relationships are constant in all views. In the lateral view, the left sinus is above the noncoronary and the right is anterior to both (Fig. 4–12B). The axis of the aortic annulus is elevated 30° above the horizontal plane (Fig. 4–13A). The aortic valve is located in a more intracardiac location than the pulmonary valve and is situated to the right and posterior to it (Fig. 4–13A and B). The ascending aorta courses to the right and posterior to the pulmonary trunk before giving rise to the great vessels, the transverse arch, and the left descending aorta (Fig. 4–13A and B). The "aortic knob" is that portion of the transverse aorta seen on end in the posteroanterior projection that is distal to the subclavian artery and in continuity with the descending aorta (Fig. 4–13A). The isthmus of the aorta is a narrowing in its caliber located just distal to the subclavian artery (Fig. 4–13B). The side of the aortic arch (left or right) is determined by the side of the trachea to which the arch relates.

The criteria one uses for distinguishing the morphologic right from the morphologic left ventricle take on particular importance when ventricular positions and/or great vessel relationships are altered (Fig. 4–14A–D). In general, the morphologic left ventricle has a smooth contour (less well developed trabeculae) than the right ventricle (Fig. 4–14A and B). The right ventricle is more heavily trabeculated and has a smooth-walled outflow tract — the infundibulum (Fig. 4–14C and D).

INTERPRETATION OF THE ANGIOCARDIOGRAM

Practically speaking, interpretation of the angiocardiogram begins in the catheterization laboratory as the study is proceeding. Appreciation of the various catheter positions assumed during the performance of the cardiac catheterization (Fig. 4–14A–D) and the pressure and oxygen saturation values obtained from typical positions within the cardiac silhouette provide important clues to the expected cardiac pathology at the time of angiocardiography. Once the angiogram has been obtained and recorded on 35mm cine film or serial "cut" films, final interpretation of the angiocardiogram begins. During the short interval before contrast is injected, the position of the catheter is noted (Fig. 4–15) and calcification in the contrast-free cardiovascular silhouette is sought. After contrast is injected,

and using the anatomic clues previously described, one identifies the chamber or great vessel being studied. A series of mental exercises ensues. In summary, one is attemping to gain as much information as possible from the contrast bolus.[8] Information is gained in the ways described in the following paragraphs.

The Presence of Contrast Material

The presence of contrast material can delineate an intracardiac lesion, such as a ventricular septal defect, merely by its presence in a region where contrast is normally not seen (Fig. 4–16). It should be remembered when attempting to opacify left-to-right shunts that the injection of contrast should be made as close to the suspected lesion as possible. This is due to the fact that nonopacified blood may dilute the contrast material and, if the injection is made at a distance from the suspected lesion, a potential defect can be missed.

The Absence of Contrast Material

When contrast material leaves a chamber or great vessel it usually does so as a broad column. Therefore, linear areas of absent or diluted contrast material may suggest pathology. For instance, the contrast column in the ascending aorta in a patient with aortic valve stenosis often demonstrates a linear lucency as nonopacified blood projects through the narrow orifice of the stenotic valve (Fig. 4–17). In addition, the interface between the contrast material and the area that does not contain contrast often delineates an abnormal structure, such as the domed and thickened valves associated with aortic and pulmonary valve stenosis (Fig. 4–18).

Flow of Contrast Material

The *direction* of flow of contrast can be of great help in evaluating an angiocardiogram. Retrograde visualization of a chamber from either a great vessel or ventricular injection may suggest insufficiency of the semilunar valve or atrioventricular valve located between the site of injection and the chamber — for example, the opacification of

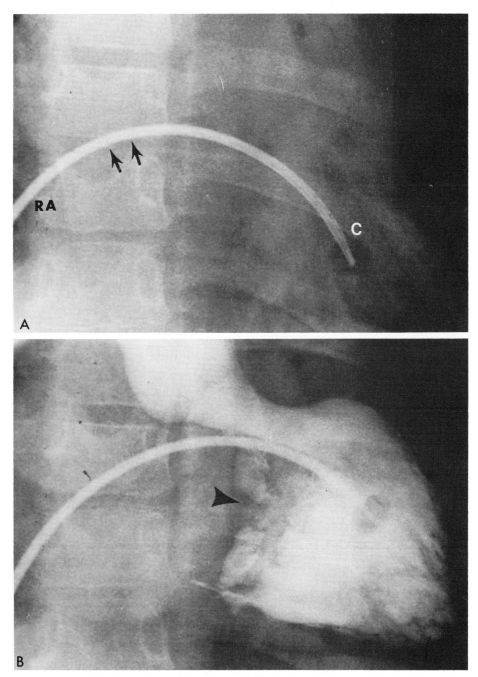

Figure 4–15. A, Balloon catheter (C) positioned in a posteroanterior projection prior to left ventricular angiogram. The catheter has entered the right atrium (RA) from the inferior vena cava, has crossed a low atrial septal defect (in the approximate position of the arrows), and enters the left ventricle after traversing the mitral valve. This "low pass" is typical of endocardial cushion defects. *B,* Left ventriculogram performed through catheter shown in Figure 4–15A demonstrates the "goose-neck" deformity of the left ventricle typical of endocardial cushion defects. Note the cleft (arrowhead) in the mitral valve and the elongated, horizontal left ventricular outflow tract.

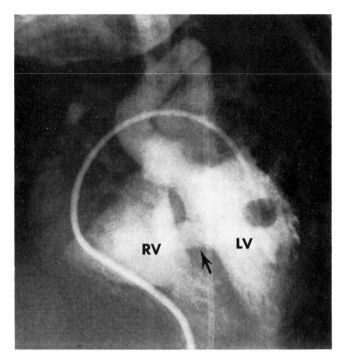

Figure 4–16. Hepatoclavicular (LAO) left ventriculogram showing a posterior defect (arrow) in the mid muscular ventricular septum allowing communication of contrast between the left ventricle (LV) and right ventricle (RV). This angiogram also demonstrates the normal orientation of the interventricular septum.

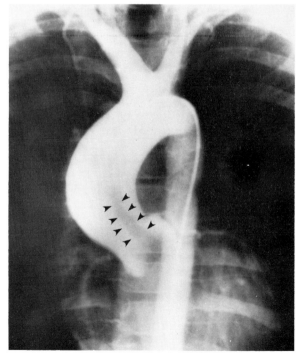

Figure 4–17. Posteroanterior ascending aortogram demonstrates a linear lucency (arrowheads) in the contrast column in this child with aortic stenosis.

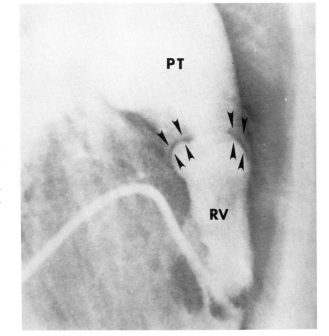

Figure 4–18. Lateral view, right ventriculogram in a patient with pulmonary valve stenosis. Note how the interface between the contrast in the right ventricle (RV) and the pulmonary trunk (PT) delineates the thickened valve leaflets (arrowheads).

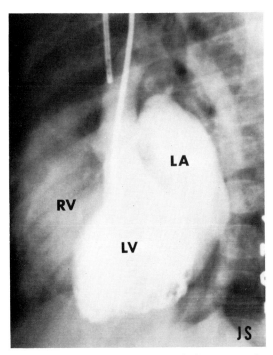

Figure 4–19. Lateral view left ventriculogram (LV) demonstrates retrograde opacification of the left atrium in this child with an endocardial cushion deformity and severe mitral regurgitation. Note that there is some contrast in the right ventricle (RV). This indicates that there is either a ventricular septal defect or that there is left-to-right flow of contrast from the left atrium to the right atrium and into the right ventricle.

the left atrium from a left ventricular injection in a patient with mitral regurgitation (Fig. 4–19). Catheterization of the left ventricle in infants and young children is often accomplished by catheters passed across the foramen ovale and mitral valve. This may interfere with valve closure, so that assessment of mitral regurgitation must be tempered by this fact. Angiographic evaluation of suspected tricuspid regurgitation is also made with a catheter positioned across the tricuspid valve; thus the same problem of interference with valve closure arises. Regurgitation of the tricuspid and pulmonary valves is usually "organic" when it is severe. For example, when a right ventricular injection results in opacification of the right atrium as well as the superior and/or inferior vena cava, the regurgitation is usually hemodynamically significant.

Another clue offered by the flow of the contrast is *early* visualization of a chamber or great vessel. For instance, the visualization of the aorta from a right ventricular injection (Fig. 4–20A and B) suggests the presence of a ventricular septal defect and significantly elevated right ventricular pressures (classically seen in tetralogy of Fallot). Visualization of the left atrium from a right atrial injection is used to diagnose tricuspid atresia (Fig. 4–21).

The *sequence* of opacification of chambers

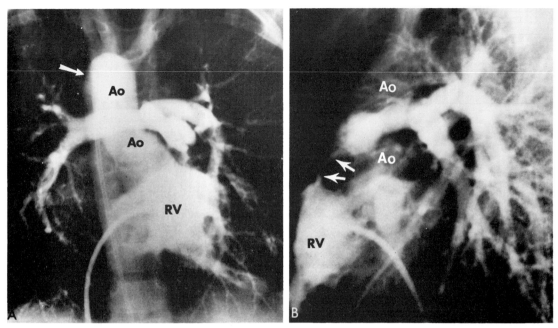

Figure 4–20. Posteroanterior (A) and lateral (B) views of a right ventriculogram performed in a child with tetralogy of Fallot. Note that the aorta (Ao) opacifies shortly after the right ventricle (RV), indicating the presence of a ventricular septal defect and significant elevation of right ventricular pressure. The lateral view (B) shows some contrast in the left ventricle beneath the aorta (Ao). Note the stenotic infundibulum (arrows) and the right aortic arch (single arrow).

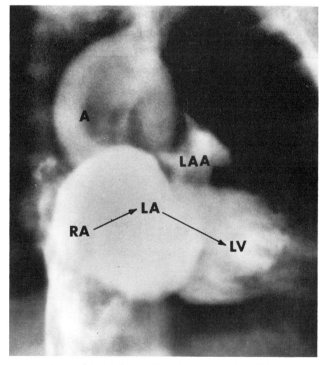

Figure 4–21. Posteroanterior right atrial injection in a patient with tricuspid atresia. Contrast flows from the right atrium (RA), to the left atrium (LA) (Note the left atrial appendage [LAA]), to the left ventricle (LV), and from there into the aorta (A).

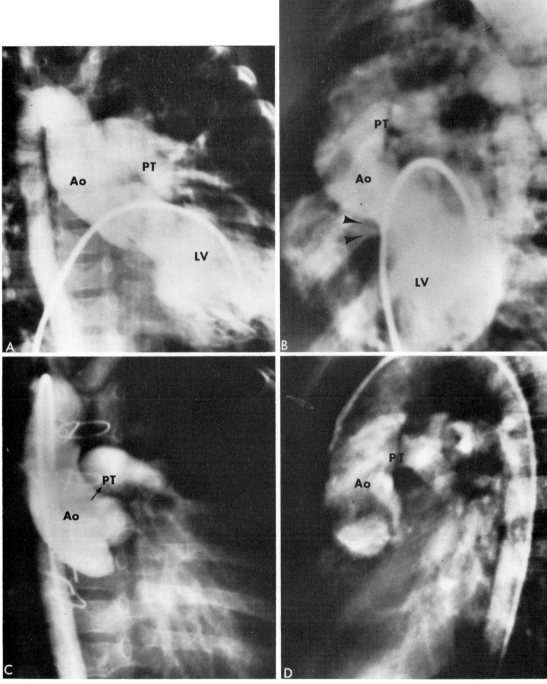

Figure 4-22. Posteroanterior (*A*) and lateral (*B*) left ventriculograms (LV) show opacification of both the aorta (Ao) and the pulmonary trunk (PT) in this acyanotic child. While this may suggest a ventricular septal defect (present here — arrowheads), one cannot exclude a more distal (great vessel) left-to-right shunt. Following repair of the VSD in this child, a continuous murmur was heard. An ascending aortogram in posteroanterior (*C*) and lateral (*D*) projections demonstrates a communication (arrow) between the ascending aorta (Ao) and the pulmonary trunk (PT) — an aorto-pulmonary window. Note the right aortic arch.

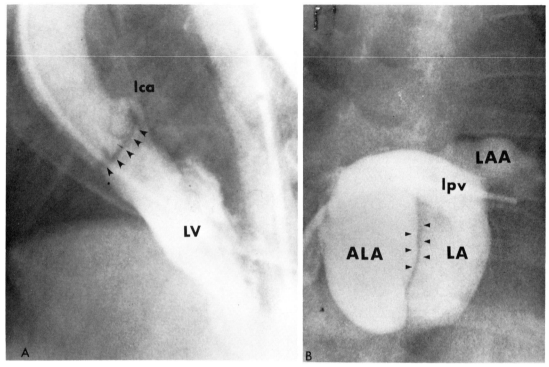

Figure 4-23. *A,* Long-axial oblique (LAO) view, left ventriculogram showing a lucent filling defect (arrowheads) in the subaortic region of the left ventricle (LV). This represents a subaortic membrane. The left coronary artery (lca) arises above the left sinus of Valsalva. *B,* Left pulmonary venogram (lpv) demonstrates a lucent partition (arrowheads) between the true left atrium (LA) and an accessory left atrial chamber (ALA). This is an example of cor triatriatum. Note that the left atrial appendage (LAA) relates to the true left atrium (LA).

and great vessels by the contrast material will offer additional diagnostic clues. An injection in the left ventricle that opacifies both the ascending aorta and pulmonary trunk suggests a left-to-right communication at the ventricular or great vessel level (Fig. 4–22A and B). While this may be a ventricular septal defect, one cannot rule out a more distal left-to-right shunt (aortopulmonary window or patent ductus arteriosus) without an aortic injection (Fig. 4–22C and D).

Defects in Contrast Material or Chamber Contour

One should look for unusual protrusions or filling defects within the chambers as might be seen in membranous subaortic stenosis (Fig. 4–23A) or cor triatriatum (Fig. 4–23B). Filling defects on valves or in chambers may be seen with vegetations,

clots, or tumors. An abnormal left ventricular contour may indicate intrinsic disease of the ventricle such as hypertrophy (Fig. 4–24A and B) or deranged left ventricular morphology as seen with endocardial cushion defects (Fig. 4–25A). Left ventricular contour abnormalities may reflect the secondary effects of dilated right heart structures (Fig. 4–26A) or suggest right heart volume or pressure overload (Fig. 4–26C).

Function

The function of ventricular chambers can also be evaluated by means of contrast material. The left ventricle is typically studied in the posteroanterior or right anterior oblique projection (Fig. 4–27A). The left anterior oblique provides additional information (Fig. 4–27B). Cineangiography is most valuable in this regard and allows assessment of both global and regional abnormalities of contractility. Left ventricular

Text continued on page 181

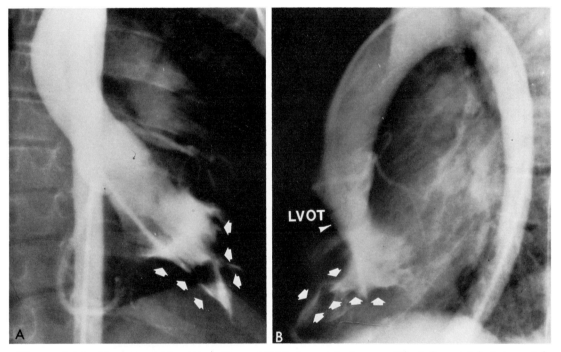

Figure 4-24. Posteroanterior (*A*) and lateral (*B*) left ventriculogram. The left ventricle is in systole in both views. Note that the ventricular cavity is almost obliterated by the markedly hypertrophied ventricular wall and papillary muscles (arrows). There is no obstruction (either membranous or muscular) in the left ventricular outflow tract (LVOT) in this child with a hypertrophic cardiomyopathy.

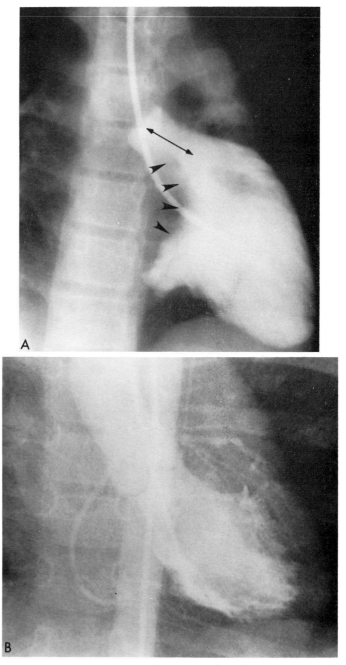

Figure 4–25. *A,* Posteroanterior left ventriculogram in diastole showing the abnormal and classic left ventricular contour of a patient with endocardial cushion defect. Compare this with Figure 4–25*B* and note the "scooped out" appearance of the medial left ventricular outflow tract (arrowheads) and the narrowed and horizontal outflow tract (arrow). *B,* Normal posteroanterior left ventriculogram in diastole for comparison with Figure 4–25*A.*

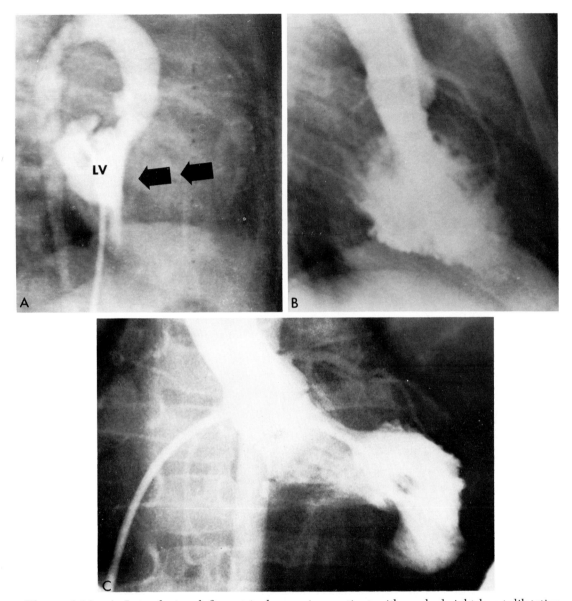

Figure 4-26. A, Lateral view left ventriculogram in a patient with marked right heart dilatation (secondary to total anomalous pulmonary venous return). Not only is the left ventricle (LV) small, but it is pushed posteriorly from its usual location (arrows) by the dilated right ventricle. Compare the position of this ventricle with that in Figure 4–26B. *B*, Normal lateral view left ventriculogram. *C*, Posteroanterior left ventriculogram in a patient with Ebstein's anomaly of the tricuspid valve. The unusual shape of the left ventricle is secondary to distortion of its free walls and septum by a deformed right ventricle.

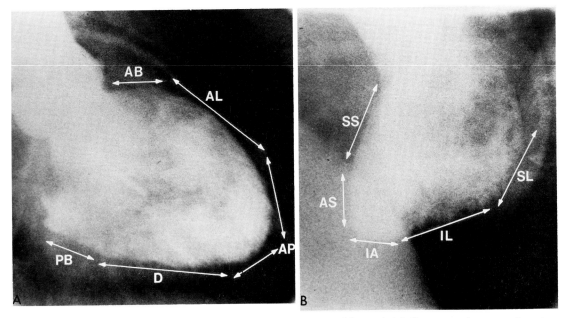

Figure 4-27. Right anterior oblique (A) and left anterior oblique (B) left ventriculograms showing five wall segments in each view: anterobasal (AB), anterolateral (AL), apical (AP), diaphragmatic (D), posterobasal (PB), superior septal (SS), apical septal (AS), inferior apical (IA), inferior lateral (IL), and superior lateral (SL). These regions correspond to specific myocardial segments perfused by the right and left coronary arteries and may show abnormal motion in association with pressure overload lesions of the left ventricle.

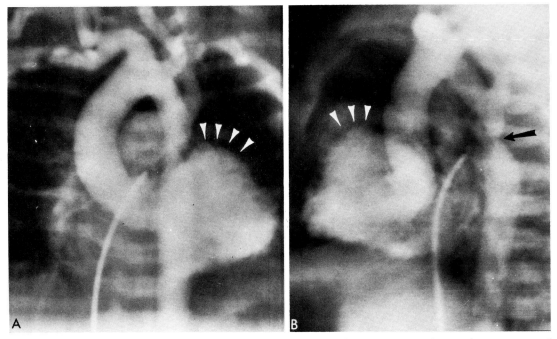

Figure 4-28. Posteroanterior (A) and lateral (B) left ventriculograms in an infant with coarctation of the aorta (arrow). Note the prominent anterolateral wall of the left ventricle (arrowheads). This region moved poorly during systole (hypokinesis), indicating probable myocardial ischemia due to pressure overload.

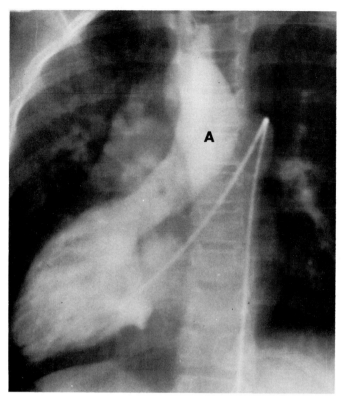

Figure 4–29. Posteroanterior ventriculogram. Note that although the apex is on the right, the ventricle has all the characteristics of a left ventricle and gives origin to the aorta (A). In fact, this angiogram (except for the position of the ventricle) is essentially identical to the ventriculogram in Figure 4–25A. Both patients have endocardial cushion deformities — one with a "gooseneck" looking to the right and one looking to the left.

volumes and ejection fraction can be calculated using standard methods. The contour of the left ventricle in the right anterior oblique and left anterior oblique projections involves clear delineation of five segments in each view (Fig. 4–27A and B). These ventricular segments are commonly evaluated in adult patients with ischemic heart disease. It is helpful to recognize, however, that certain ventricular segments correspond to specific regions perfused by the right and left coronary arteries and that they may be abnormal in various pressure or overload lesions involving the left ventricle (Fig. 4–28A and B). Global assessment of right ventricular contractility can be made, but methods of circulating volumes and ejection fraction suffer from the nonmathematical geometry of this ventricle.

Ventricular, Valvular, and Great Vessel Relationships

Finally, it should be mentioned that the relationships between the great vessels and the ventricles should be ascertained in evaluating an angiocardiogram. Although specific derangements of great vessels and ventricular relationships will be discussed in the following chapters, it should be remembered that when there are two ventricles, the atrioventricular valves remain with the ventricles (that is, the morphologic right ventricle contains a tricuspid valve and the morphologic left ventricle contains a mitral valve). Furthermore, the great vessels may have variable positions, both in an anteroposterior and mediolateral direction (see Fig. 4–14). The ventricles themselves may be inverted in position so that the left ventricle is rightward and anterior and the right ventricle is leftward and posterior (Fig. 4–29).

In summary, the presence of contrast material allows one to (1) detect intracardiac and great lesions by its presence; (2) demonstrate dilutional or interface abnormalities; (3) show abnormalities in direction, timing, or sequence of flow; (4) uncover unusual filling defects or contour abnormalities; and (5) allow an accurate assessment of ventricular function and the relationships of ventricles, valves, and great vessels.

REFERENCES

1. Bargeron, L. M., Elliott, L. P., Soto, B., et al.: Axial cineangiography in congenital heart disease. Circulation 56:1075, 1977.
2. Elliott, L. P., Bargeron, L. M., Bream, P. R., et al.: Axial cineangiography in congenital heart disease. Circulation 56:1084, 1977.
3. Kannen, M., Devloo-Blancquaert, A.: Comparative study in angiocardiography in children, evaluating the side effects of non-ionic and ionic contrast media. Diagn Imaging 48:228, 1979.
4. Kelley, M. J., Higgins, C. B., Schmidt, W. S., Newell, J. D.: Effects of ionic and nonionic contrast agents on left ventricular and extracellular fluid dynamics during angiography in an infant experimental model. Invest Radiol 15(4):335, 1980.
5. Sos, T. A., Baltaxe, H. A.: Cranial and caudal angulation for coronary angiography revised. Circulation 56:119, 1977.
6. Kelley, M. J., Higgins, C. B., Kirkpatrick, S. E.: Axial left ventriculography in discrete subaortic stenosis. Radiology 135:77, 1980.
7. Stanger, P., Rudolph, A. M., Edwards, J. E.: Cardiac malpositions: An overview based on the study of sixty-five necropsy specimens. Circulation 56:159, 1977.
8. Baron, M. G.: Angiography. Clin Symposia 17:91, 1965.

Section II

CLINICAL-RADIOGRAPHIC CLASSIFICATION OF HEART DISEASE IN INFANTS AND CHILDREN

Chapter 5

ACYANOTIC PATIENT WITH NORMAL VASCULARITY OR PULMONARY VENOUS HYPERTENSION

Cardiac lesions in this category generally present in two peak age groups. If the lesion leads to severe ("critical") obstruction to left ventricular inflow (for example, total anomalous pulmonary venous return below the diaphragm) or to left ventricular outflow (for example, critical aortic coarctation), the presentation is in the neonatal period (Table 5–1). The chest film in this group of patients shows signs of significant pulmonary venous hypertension (often frank pulmonary edema) and the heart is usually enlarged.[1] Less severe obstruction to the left ventricle is characterized by presentation later in life (with some lesions presenting in adulthood), often without evidence of congestive heart failure on clinical or radiographic grounds. Lesions causing severe obstruction to right ventricular outflow invariably lead to diminished pulmonary vasculature and to an early clinical presentation of cyanosis. These lesions will be discussed in the chapters dealing with cyanotic heart disease. Mild obstruction to pulmonary flow (for example, pulmonary valve stenosis) usually does not result in cyanosis and will be treated in this chapter. Two other anomalies require mention in this acyanotic–normal vascularity group — namely, mitral valve prolapse and congenitally corrected transposition of the great vessels.

It should be noted that any lesion that results in mild hemodynamic alterations, whether it be an intracardiac or great vessel left-to-right shunt, left or right ventricular obstruction, or mild mitral regurgitation, may present with minimal radiographic findings or with a normal chest radiograph.

TABLE 5–1. Cardiovascular Lesions Producing Pulmonary Venous Hypertension in the Neonate

---

First Week of Life
Hypoplastic Left Heart (Aortic Atresia)*
Critical Aortic Stenosis
Total Anomalous Pulmonary Venous Return
 (Obstructed)
Cor Triatriatum
Atresia of Pulmonary Veins
Noncardiac Arteriovenous Fistula
Intrauterine Myocarditis
Tachy- or Bradyarrhythmias

Second and Third Week of Life
Coarctation of the Aorta*
Interruption of Aortic Arch
Critical Aortic Stenosis
Cardiomyopathies
Cor Triatriatum
Congenital Mitral Stenosis, etc.
Noncardiac Arteriovenous Fistula

Fourth to Sixth Week of Life
Coarctation of the Aorta*
Critical Aortic Stenosis*
Cardiomyopathies
Anomalous Origin of Left Coronary Artery
 from the Pulmonary Trunk
Cor Triatriatum
Congenital Mitral Stenosis, etc.

Modified from Higgins, C. B.[2]
*Most common lesion in this age group.

THE ACYANOTIC NEO-NATE WITH PULMONARY VENOUS HYPERTENSION

The most common reason for congestive heart failure and radiographic findings of pulmonary venous hypertension (congestion) in the neonate is left ventricular failure due to outflow obstruction. Less frequently, pulmonary venous hypertension is secondary to obstruction of pulmonary venous return. The mechanism of failure in the former instance is the inability of the relatively underdeveloped left ventricle to withstand a severe pressure overload.

It should be recognized that certain noncardiac problems related to the birth process enter into the differential diagnosis of congestive failure in the acyanotic neonate.[2] These are associated with a volume overload of, or a hypoxic insult to, the underdeveloped left ventricle, with the subsequent development of pulmonary venous hypertension. These noncardiac problems are listed in Table 5-2. Their radiographic features are similar[1] and are illustrated in Figures 5-1 through 5-3. In general, the history attending the birth process will aid in differentiating these noncardiac problems from cardiac lesions that result in congestive heart failure in the first week of life.

There is a tendency for certain cardiac defects to produce congestive heart failure in infants at given times in the postnatal period. A rough guide to this age related-lesion presentation is given in Table 5-1,[2] with the most common lesions indicated by an asterisk. The radiographic, angiocardiographic, and echocardiographic features of these defects will be presented in the following paragraphs.

Radiographic and Angiocardiographic Features

The chest radiographic findings of all lesions listed in Table 5-1 tend to be quite similar and are therefore nonspecific. The radiographic manifestations of pulmonary venous hypertension (PVH) in the neonate include indistinctness of pulmonary vessels, perihilar haziness, and prominent interstitial markings (Figs. 5-1 to 5-3). Kerley B-lines are infrequently found in infants and when present suggest severe pulmonary venous hypertension. Cardiomegaly is the rule in all lesions listed in Table 5-1, except for the obstructed variety of total anomalous pulmonary venous return (Figs. 5-5A and 5-6A). A disproportionately large heart when compared with minor abnormalities of the vascularity (Figs. 5-7A and 5-9A) should also alert one to this group of lesions. The age of presentation, the clinical picture, and the chest radiograph should suggest the differential diagnostic possibilities listed in Table 5-1. Since the radiographic features are quite similar in this group of lesions (Figs. 5-4 through 5-12) we have included the typical angiographic findings next to the radiographs.

Pulmonary venous hypertension and cardiomegaly occurring in the first day or two of life are most frequently due to the *hypoplastic left heart syndrome (aortic atresia)*. Cardiogenic shock, metabolic acidosis, and poor peripheral pulses generally accompany this lesion. Aortic atresia is characterized by complete closure of the aortic valve by a fibrous membrane. The mitral valve is hypoplastic or atretic, and endocardial fibroelastotic changes are frequently found in the tiny left ventricular cavity.[3] The ascending aorta is hypoplastic and acts as a common coronary artery. Cyanosis, if present, is due to poor peripheral perfusion and lung congestion. Cardiomegaly in this lesion is due

TABLE 5-2. Noncardiac Causes of Pulmonary Venous Hypertension in the Neonate

Overhydration
Excess Stripping of Umbilical Cord
Delayed Clamping of Umbilical Cord
Twin to Twin Transfusion
Maternal to Fetal Transfusion
Neonatal Asphyxia
Infant of Diabetic Mother — Hypoglycemia

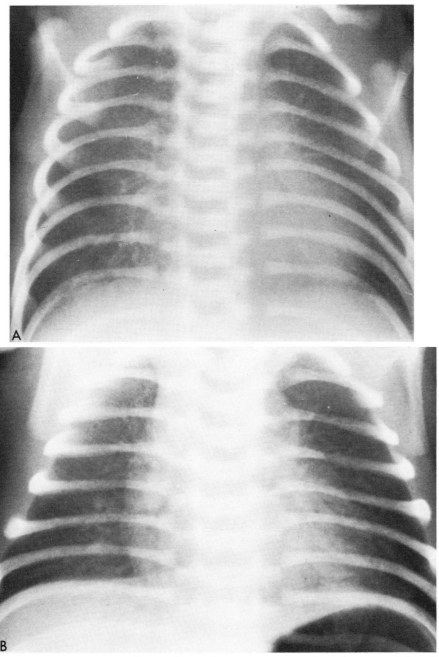

Figure 5–1.   A, Anteroposterior chest radiograph in a neonate in whom there was delayed clamping of the umbilical cord, resulting in transient volume overload of the underdeveloped left ventricle. Note the perivascular haziness, indistinct hilar regions, and ill-defined cardiac silhouette. *B*, Follow-up chest radiograph two days later shows clearing of interstitial edema in this infant.

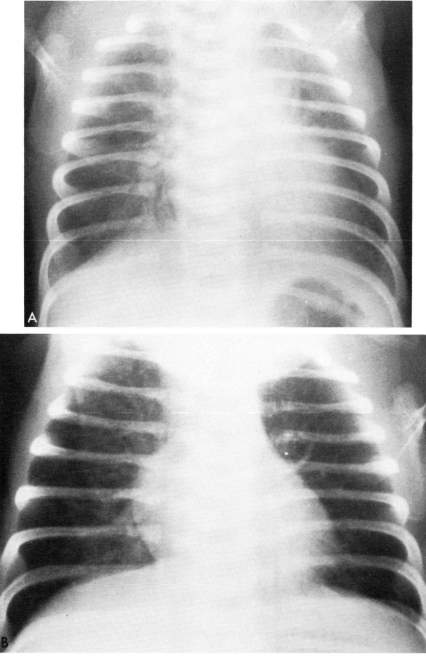

Figure 5–2. *A*, Anteroposterior chest radiograph in a neonate with polycythemia secondary to maternal-to-fetal transfusion. The appearance of the chest is very similar to that illustrated in Figure 5–1A. *B*, Follow-up chest film four days later shows that lung fields have cleared and that heart size has returned to normal.

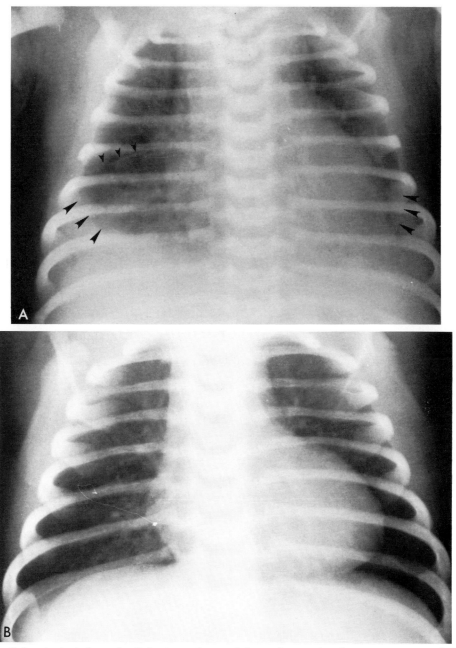

Figure 5–3. A, An infant of a diabetic mother with hypoglycemia and transient myocardial failure. Bilateral pleural effusions and fluid in the minor fissure (arrowheads) are consistent with significant pulmonary venous hypertension. B, Follow-up chest radiograph several days after therapeutic intervention shows normal lung fields but persistent cardiomegaly.

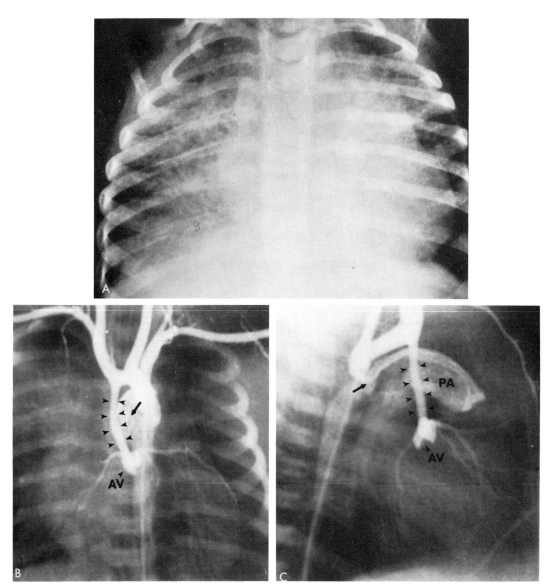

Figure 5–4. *A,* Anteroposterior chest radiograph in a one-day-old infant presenting with cardiogenic shock, acidosis, and poor peripheral pulses. Pulmonary edema, cardiomegaly, and a large pulmonary trunk in this clinical setting should suggest the diagnosis of aortic atresia ("hypoplastic left heart syndrome"). Descending aortogram in anteroposterior *(B)* and lateral *(C)* projections in this infant shows left-to-right flow of contrast through the ductus (arrow) into the pulmonary artery (PA) and retrograde flow into the diminutive ascending aorta (arrowheads), aortic valve (AV), and coronary arteries. These findings are typical of aortic atresia.

to the dilated right heart and pulmonary trunk (Fig. 5–4*A*). In the past, angiographic study of these infants has included a thoracic aortogram to show the typical features of the atretic aortic valve and hypoplastic ascending aorta (Figs. 5–4*B* and *C*). Currently, this may not be required if the echocardiographic features of this invariably fatal entity are present.

In the infant who presents in a similar clinical fashion as hypoplastic left heart syndrome but who has a normal cardiac size (Fig. 5–5*A*), one should consider the diagnosis of the *obstructed variety of total anomalous pulmonary venous connection.* In the most common variety of this anomaly, all of the pulmonary veins return to a common vertical channel that courses through the

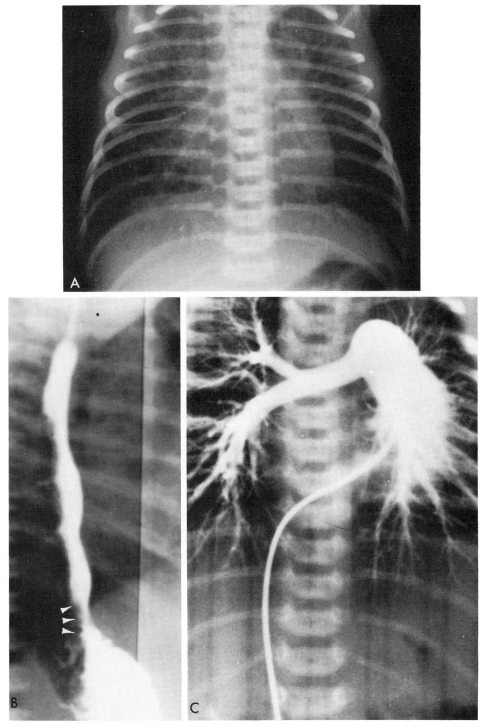

Figure 5–5. Anteroposterior chest radiograph *(A)* in a four-day-old infant with heart failure. Even though there are severe pulmonary venous hypertensive changes in the form of interstitial pulmonary edema, the heart is normal in size. The lateral barium swallow *(B)* shows a posterior indentation at the esophageal-gastric junction (arrowheads). A posteroanterior pulmonary angiogram *(C)* with delayed filming during venous phase in posteroanterior *(D)* and lateral projections *(E)* shows that all pulmonary veins (PVS — black arrowheads) enter a common channel (C — white arrowheads) that descends through the esophageal hiatus to join the portal vein (PV).

Illustration continued on following page

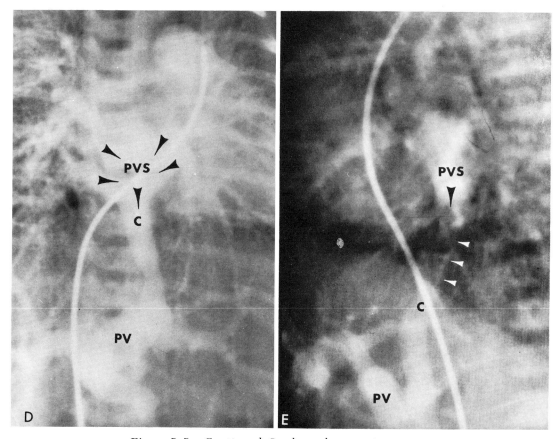

Figure 5–5. *Continued. See legend on previous page.*

esophageal hiatus to reach the portal vein. This anatomic arrangement results in severe diminution in flow to the left heart and marked pulmonary venous obstruction (Fig. 5–5A). The left heart structures are small, and a barium swallow may reveal a posterior indentation produced by the anomalous draining common venous channel (Fig. 5–5B). Less frequently, obstructed anomalous pulmonary venous return involves supracardiac venous structures (Fig. 5–6A–C). Pulmonary angiography will demonstrate the anomalous venous anatomy in these cases (Fig. 5–5C–E and Fig. 5–6B and C). Although this lesion causes severe distress in the neonate, it is potentially surgically correctable if surgery can be accomplished soon after birth.

In the infant with *critical aortic stenosis*, cardiomegaly and signs of pulmonary hypertension predominate (Fig. 5–7A).[4] By the end of the first week of life, or in infants who present in the first two months, cardiomegaly will invariably be present. In infants with critical aortic stenosis, the left ventriculogram demonstrates the most dramatic angiographic findings.[5] Left ventricular wall thickness is increased as are the end-systolic and end-diastolic volumes (Fig. 5–7B and C). The ejection fraction is invariably reduced (Fig. 5–7B and C). Trabecular effacement (indicative of subendocardial sclerosis) and myocardial segmental dysfunction (Fig. 5–7B and C) has been noted in these infants.[5] The aortic valve is thickened, showing the characteristics of the bicuspid aortic valve, and the ascending aorta may be dilated, even in infants studied in the first days of life (Fig. 5–7B and C).

Lesions resulting in obstruction to left ventricular inflow (pulmonary vein atresia and cor triatriatum) and the various forms of congenital mitral stenosis (supravalvar mitral stenosing ring, congenital mitral stenosis, and "parachute" mitral valve) are rare and tend to present in the second to sixth week of life (Table 5–1). They have similar plain film radiographic findings (Fig. 5–8A

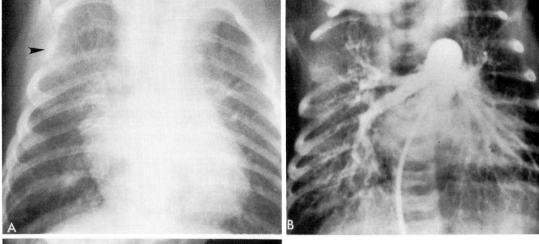

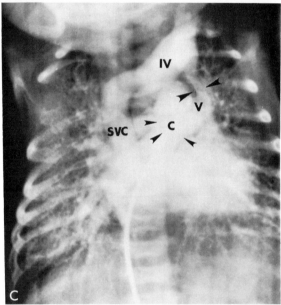

Figure 5–6. Anteroposterior chest radiograph *(A)* in a one-week-old infant, status/ postesophageal atresia repair (note resected right third rib — arrowhead). Persistent respiratory distress was thought to be related to cardiac failure. The radiograph shows signs of pulmonary venous hypertension (ill-defined vascular markings; perihilar haziness), a wide mediastinum, and normal heart size. Posteroanterior pulmonary arteriogram *(B)* with late film in venous phase *(C)* demonstrates that all pulmonary veins (three small arrowheads) enter a common horizontal channel (C) that ascends through vertical vein (V — large arrowheads) to join innominate vein (IV) and superior vena cava (SVC). A "vise effect" was created between the left bronchus and the vertical vein (V) leading to pulmonary venous obstruction.

and *B*). *Cor triatriatum* is defined as a membranous obstruction between the pulmonary veins and the true left atrium. This membrane significantly impedes pulmonary venous return, causing severe pulmonary venous hypertension (Fig. 5–8A). Frequently the membrane is incomplete or fenestrated (Fig. 5–8C). *Supravalvar mitral stenosing ring* is characterized by the presence of a fibrous membrane located proximal to the mitral valve and has hemodynamic consequences similar to cor triatriatum. In *congenital mitral stenosis*, the mitral apparatus (annulus, valve, chordae tendineae, and papillary muscles) is hypoplastic, fused and malformed, and creates an inflow obstruction to left ventricular filling (Fig, 5–9B and

C). The so-called *"parachute" mitral valve* is identified by the abnormal insertion of the anterior and posterior chordae tendineae into a single large papillary muscle (Fig. 5–9D). Although all of these inflow obstructive lesions may occur singly, they may also occur in combination. In summary, they result in the same hemodynamic derangement — namely, severe pulmonary venous obstruction and impaired left ventricular inflow.

Critical aortic coarctation is the most frequent cause of pulmonary venous hypertension in the second and third week of life (Fig. 10A–C) (Table 5–1).[6] More commonly, aortic coarctation presents in the older child (see next section for detailed discussion).

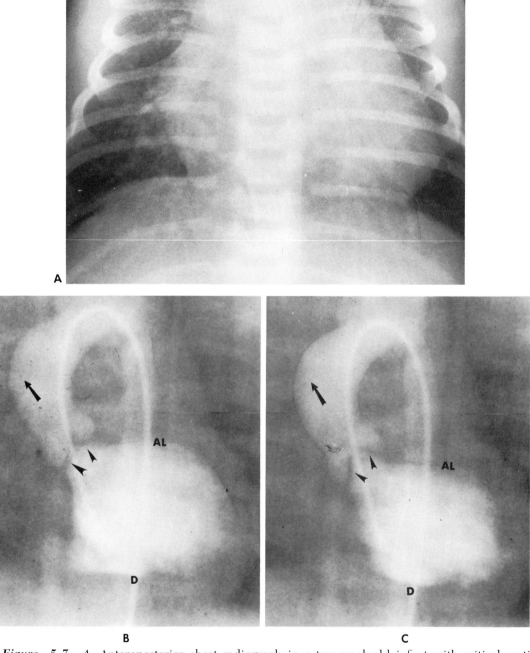

Figure **5–7.** *A,* Anteroposterior chest radiograph in a two-week-old infant with critical aortic stenosis. Mild pulmonary venous hypertension is out of proportion to the significant cardiomegaly. Posteroanterior left ventriculograms in diastole (*B*) and systole (*C*) in a two-week-old infant with critical aortic stenosis. The ejection fraction is reduced and there is severe hypokinesis of the anterolateral (AL) and diaphragmatic (D) wall segments. Note the thick aortic valve (arrowheads) and poststenotic dilatation of the ascending aorta (arrow) (Parts *B* and *C* reproduced with permission from Broderick, Higgins, Guthaner, et al.[5])

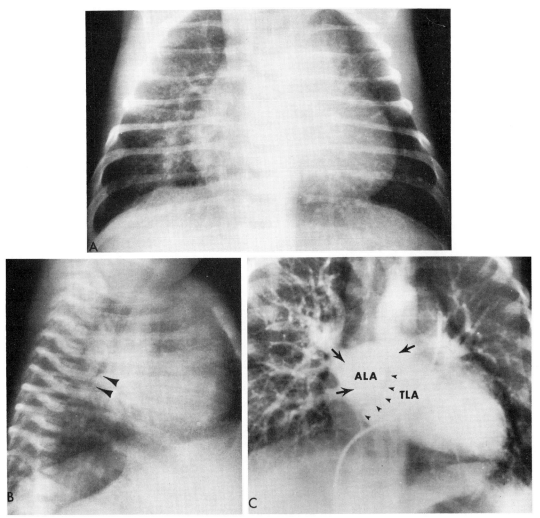

Figure 5–8. Anteroposterior *(A)* and lateral *(B)* chest radiographs in a one-month-old boy with congestive heart failure. Interstitial edema is present on the frontal film; left atrial enlargement on the lateral film is evident as posterior deviation of the left mainstem bronchus (arrowheads). The venous phase of a pulmonary angiogram *(C)* performed in this patient shows a lucent membrane (arrowheads) that partially obstructs pulmonary venous return. The membrane separates the accessory left atrium (ALA) and pulmonary veins (arrows) from the true left atrium (TLA).

Not infrequently, the chest radiograph will give a clue to the diagnosis of coarctation (Fig. 5–11A). In the infant this aortic lesion is often associated with a patent ductus arteriosus or ventricular septal defect (Fig. 5–11B and C).[7]

Interruption of the aortic arch is a rare anomaly that as an isolated lesion has a time course and manner of presentation similar to severe coarctation.[8] This anomaly is frequently associated with other cardiac anomalies, including a variety of intracardiac and great vessel shunts.[8] The clinical pre-

sentation in these cases is one of congestive heart failure. Cyanosis, if present, is usually mild, and pulse deficiencies in the extremities are frequent. Because of the common association of this lesion with a VSD, the chest radiograph shows shunt vascularity, with or without signs of pulmonary venous hypertension, and a large pulmonary trunk and descending aorta (Fig. 5–12A). Three varieties of this anomaly have been described and relate to the site of aortic interruption.[9] The site of interruption may be distal to the left subclavian artery (type A)

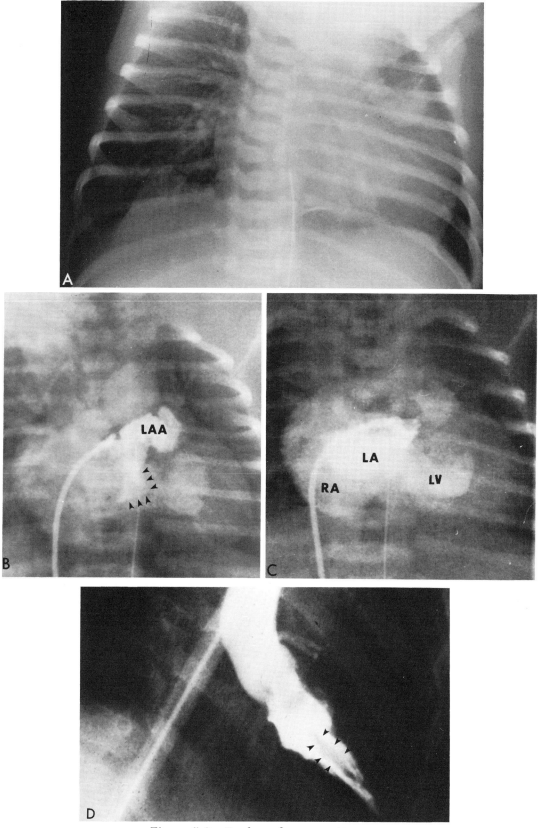

Figure 5–9. See legend on opposite page

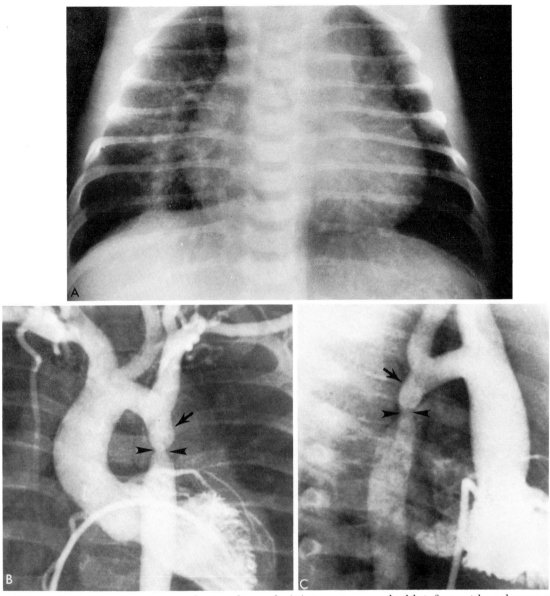

Figure 5–10. Anteroposterior chest radiograph *(A)* in a two-week-old infant with pulmonary venous hypertension and cardiomegaly. Anteroposterior *(B)* and lateral *(C)* projections of a left ventriculogram demonstrate critical aortic coarctation (arrowheads). The ascending aorta is dilated and the aortic isthmus (arrow) is hypoplastic.

Figure 5–9. Anteroposterior *(A)* chest radiograph in a three-week-old infant with congestive heart failure. There is cardiomegaly and mild pulmonary venous hypertension. Left atriogram performed in anteroposterior projections *(B and C)* demonstrates a funnel-shaped mitral valve (arrowheads) and left-to-right flow of contrast into the right atrium (RA). The left ventricle (LV) is small and poorly filled. The left atrium (LA) and left atrial appendage (LAA) are well visualized. The findings are consistent with congenital mitral stenosis. *D,* Right anterior oblique left ventriculogram in an infant who clinically and radiographically presented a picture similar to that of the infant in Figure 5–9A. Note the single centrally placed papillary muscle (arrowheads) in this infant with a "parachute" mitral valve.

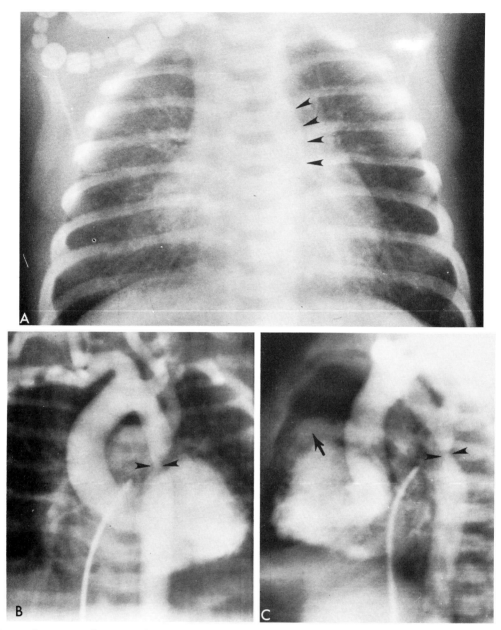

Figure 5–11. *A*, The area of poststenotic dilatation of the aorta is well visualized (arrowheads) in this infant with critical coarctation. The left atrial angiogram in anteroposterior *(B)* and lateral *(C)* projections shows the coarctation (arrowheads) and a frequently associated lesion— a VSD (arrow).

(Fig. 5–12*B* and *C*), between the left subclavian and left common carotid artery (type B), or between the left common carotid and innominate arteries (type C).

The term *cardiomyopathy* as used in Table 5–1 refers to a group of three entities: (1) endocardial fibroelastosis, (2) hypertrophic cardiomyopathy, and (3) glycogen storage disease. These abnormalities of heart muscle may present in the second through sixth week of life or in the older child. They mirror the three types of cardiomyopathy found in adults — namely, the congestive (dilated) cardiomyopathy, the hypertrophic obstructive cardiomyopathy, and the restrictive (infiltrative) cardiomyopathy. *Endocardial fibroelastosis* (EFE) as seen in infancy is usually not associated

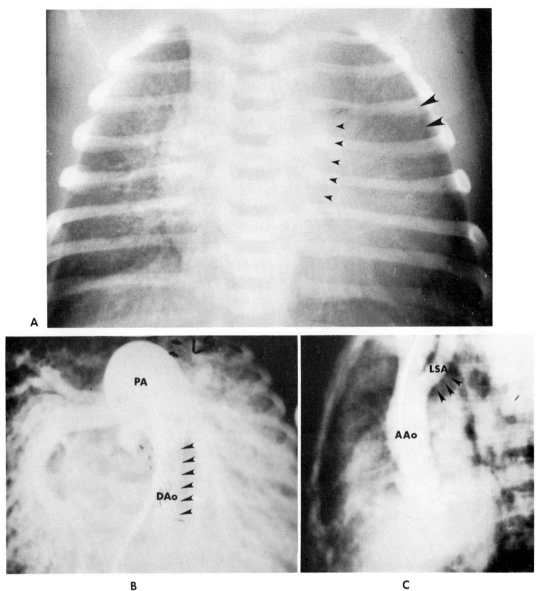

Figure 5–12. *A,* Anteroposterior chest radiograph in a three-week-old infant with congestive heart failure and pulse deficiencies in the lower extremities. Interstitial pulmonary edema, as well as shunt vascularity (note large lower lobe vessels), is present. The pulmonary trunk reaches to the left upper rib cage (arrowheads) and the descending aorta is prominent (small arrowheads). A critical aortic coarctation was suspected, but an interrupted aortic arch was present at cardiac catheterization. *B,* Posteroanterior pulmonary arteriogram (PA) in an infant with congestive heart failure and a large VSD. Note that the descending aorta (DAo — arrowheads) fills from this injection. *C,* A lateral ascending aortogram (AAo) demonstrates complete interruption of the aortic arch beyond the left subclavian artery (LSA).

with other cardiac defects. Pathologically, it is characterized by a diffuse, shiny, thickened endocardium due to a proliferation of elastic tissue. This same endocardial abnormality may also occur in association with other forms of critical left ventricular ob-

struction (aortic stenosis, coarctation of the aorta, and hypoplastic left heart syndrome) in which subendocardial fibrosis likely relates to subendocardial ischemia. In the most common variety of this lesion (the dilated type), the left ventricle is enlarged

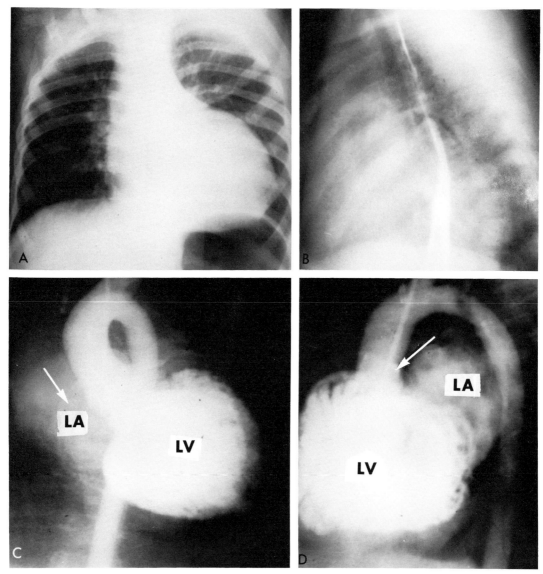

Figure 5–13. Anteroposterior *(A)* and lateral *(B)* chest radiographs in a six-week-old infant with congestive heart failure. There is mild pulmonary venous hypertension (redistribution) and massive left ventricular enlargement. Posteroanterior *(C)* and lateral *(D)* left ventriculograms in this infant show a massively dilated left ventricle (LV). There is significant mitral regurgitation with contrast seen in the left atrium (LA). Both right and left coronary arteries are faintly visualized (arrows). These findings are typical of endocardial fibroelastosis.

and hypertrophied and mitral regurgitation is frequently encountered. The etiology of this entity is not certain, but a variety of viral infections, including mumps, have been implicated.[10] The radiographic findings in EFE include a large left ventricle and left atrium that are dilated out of proportion to the degree of pulmonary venous hypertension (Fig. 5–13A and B). The left ventricular angiogram demonstrates a dilated, poorly contracting ventricle and mitral regurgitation (Fig. 5–13C and D).

Noncardiac arteriovenous fistulae of sufficient magnitude to produce symptoms in the first through third week of life generally involve the liver or brain. In the latter situation, an arteriovenous shunt of variable size exists between the cerebral arteries

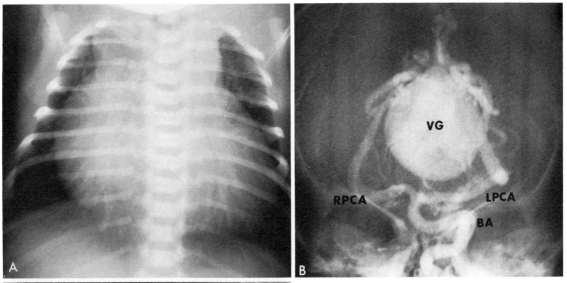

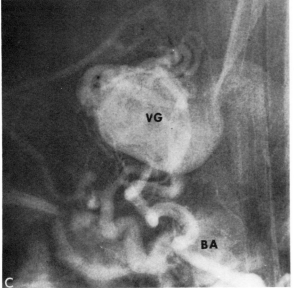

Figure 5–14. Anteroposterior *(A)* chest radiograph in an infant with congestive heart failure and decreased pulses. There is increased pulmonary vascularity and massive cardiomegaly with a huge right atrium. Posteroanterior *(B* and *D)* and lateral *(C* and *E)* views of the skull were recorded on cine film after thoracic aortogram in this infant. The basilar artery (BA) and the right and left posterior cerebral arteries (RPCA and LPCA) empty via multiple tortuous channels into a massively dilated vein of Galen (VG).

Illustration continued on following page.

(invariably the posterior circulation) and the vein of Galen, or venous channels approximal to it. This communication causes aneurysmal dilatation of the vein of Galen because the vein is the most proximal, distensible venous structure draining the shunts.[11] These defects may be responsible for intrauterine fetal distress and may cause congestive heart failure, cyanosis, and decreased pulses soon after birth. High output failure in the fetus results from the large shunt through the malformation producing a volume overload on the heart.[12] Although bruits over the head or liver may be expected in these arteriovenous malformations,

their absence due to congestive heart failure is not unusual.[13] The chest radiograph shows cardiomegaly with increased pulmonary flow or flow-failure pattern (Fig. 5–14A). Angiographic demonstration of the malformation (Fig. 5–14B–E) is imperative prior to therapeutic decision making.

Anomalous origin of the left coronary artery from the pulmonary trunk is a rare anomaly.[14] In this entity the left coronary artery rises from the pulmonary trunk and supplies a thin, scarred, frequently aneurysmal region of the left ventricle. The right coronary artery rises in a normal fashion from the aorta, is often dilated, and supplies

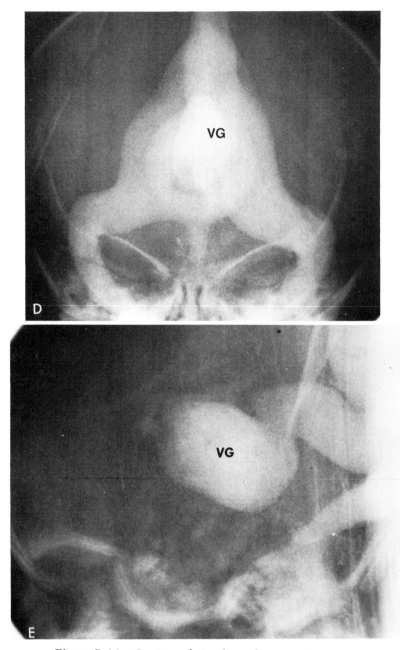

Figure 5–14. Continued. See legend on previous page.

a hypertrophied portion of the left ventricle.[15] Myocardial ischemia is an invariable accompaniment to this lesion. Interestingly, the ischemia is not due to the abnormal origin of the left coronary artery nor to the presence of venous blood in the left coronary system (remember that cyanotic heart disease is not usually associated with left ventricular ischemia). Rather, the insult to the myocardium is thought to be due to the

abnormal circulatory pattern created by the lesion. Elevated neonatal pulmonary artery pressure results in adequate perfusion of the left coronary artery shortly after birth. As the pressure in the pulmonary circuit (and thus, in the left coronary artery) declines, left coronary flow is reduced. Gradually, flow occurs from the high pressure right coronary artery, through intercoronary anastomoses, to the left coronary artery.

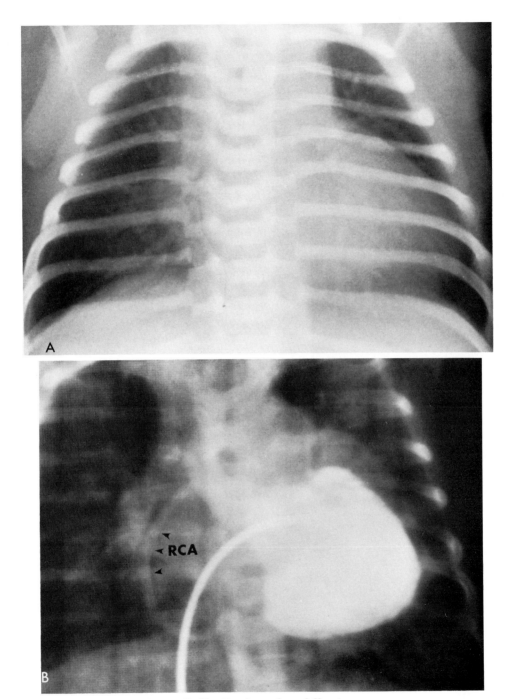

Figure 5–15. See legend on following page.

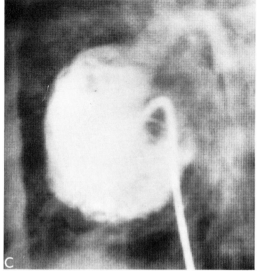

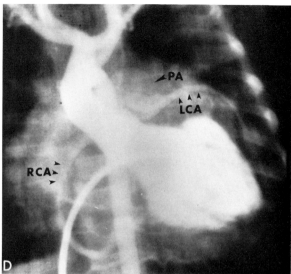

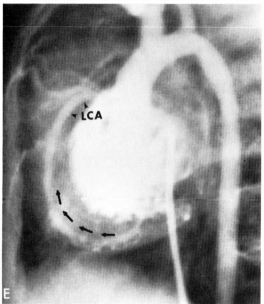

Figure 5–15. Anteroposterior *(A)* chest radiograph in a six-week-old infant with congestive failure and evidence of left ventricular ischemia on the electrocardiogram. There is massive cardiomegaly with left ventricular enlargement and mild pulmonary venous hypertension. Posteroanterior *(B* and *D)* and lateral *(C* and *E)* projections of left ventriculogram show a dilated, poorly contracting left ventricle. The right coronary artery (RCA) fills from the aorta but the left coronary artery (LCA) fills late in a retrograde manner through right coronary collaterals (arrows — *E*). The pulmonary artery (PA) is faintly opacified from the left coronary artery.

This has the positive effect of reestablishing left coronary flow but the negative effect of creating a low resistance channel that bypasses the myocardial capillary bed — a coronary "steal."[16] This abnormal flow pattern is thought to be the main cause of the myocardial ischemia in this entity. Infants with this lesion are usually normal at birth but present with symptoms of congestive failure from the sixth to eighth week of life.[17] The lesion may not be discovered until childhood[18] or even adulthood,[19] often in association with mitral regurgitation or a continuous murmur. In infants, the chest radiograph shows pulmonary venous hyper-

tension and massive cardiomegaly with left ventricular enlargement (Fig. 5–15A). Left atrial enlargement can also be expected because of the frequent presence of mitral regurgitation. Angiography to detect the lesion can usually be accomplished with an ascending aortogram or left ventriculogram (Fig. 5–15B–E).

Echocardiographic Features — Left Ventricular Outflow Tract Obstruction in the Neonate

Anatomic abnormalities of the left ventricular outflow tract may be visualized in infants presenting with critical ventricular outflow tract obstruction. These infants may present in low cardiac output states, making accurate anatomic diagnosis difficult on clinical grounds. Occasionally, such infants will present in a manner simulating neonatal sepsis. The presence of an ejection murmur should raise the possibility of critical left ventricular outflow tract obstruction (critical aortic stenosis or coarctation). Such obstruction may be found in association with other intracardiac abnormalities, such as left-to-right shunting at the atrial or ventricular level and left ventricular inflow tract obstruction. The association of aortic outflow tract obstruction at the valve or subvalvar level and malalignment interventricular septal defect has been frequently associated with other abnormalities of the aorta, including hypoplastic aortic isthmus, discrete

juxtaductal coarctation, and aortic arch interruption[7] (Fig. 5–16). The presence of left ventricular outflow obstruction and septal malalignment suggested from findings on the long-axis subxiphoidal view should raise the possibility of associated extracardiac abnormalities of the aortic arch. The association of these abnormalities with hypoparathyroidism and thymic aplasia should also be considered.[20]

Hypoplastic Left Heart (Aortic Atresia)

Patients with various forms of hypoplastic left heart syndrome may be readily identified on the basis of clinical and radiographic information and echocardiographic imaging. On two-dimensional echocardiog-

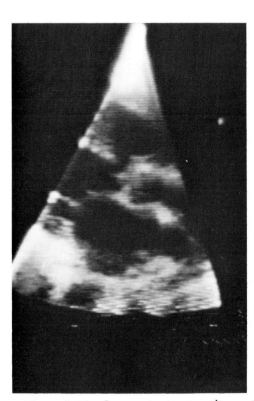
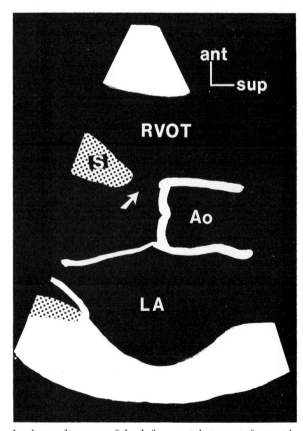

Figure 5–16. Long-axis view two dimensional echocardiogram of the left ventricle in an infant with an interventricular septal defect, a bicuspid aortic valve, and an associated type A interruption of the aortic arch (interruption distal to the left subclavian artery). Note the malalignment interventricular septal defect (arrow) and the large left atrial (LA) dimension. Because of increased pulmonary flow, the LA/Ao ratio is greater than 2.0. The aortic valve (Ao) is thickened and domed and the right ventricular outflow tract (RVOT) is enlarged. The presence of a malalignment interventricular septal defect in association with aortic valve thickening and eccentricity in a newborn infant is frequently found in association with abnormalities of the aortic arch, including hypoplasia of the aortic isthmus, discrete juxtaductal coarctation, and aortic arch interruption.

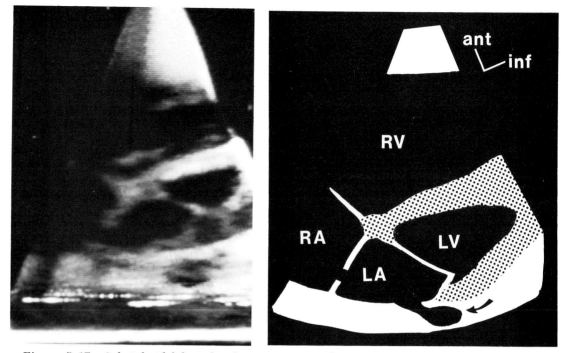

Figure 5–17. Subxiphoidal four-chamber view in an infant with a hypoplastic left ventricle. The right ventricle (RV) and atrium (RA) are markedly dilated with evidence of dilatation of the left lower pulmonary vein (curved arrow). The left ventricular cavity (LV) is "muscle bound," and dense echoes arising from the endocardium suggest the presence of endocardial fibrosis. The mitral valve apparatus is poorly developed. (LA = left atrium.)

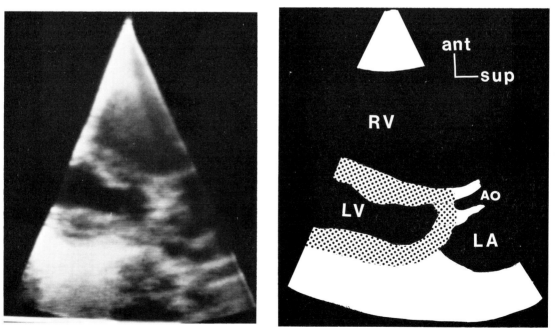

Figure 5–18. Long-axis view of a hypoplastic left ventricle (LV). There is no communication visualized between the left atrium (LA) and the muscle bound left ventricular cavity. In addition there is a hypoplastic aortic root (Ao) measuring less than 6 mm in diameter. No discernible aortic valve tissue was visualized. The right ventricular cavity (RV) is grossly dilated.

raphy, the left ventricular outflow tract, in the long-axis view, is miniscule. The aortic root is often seen as a solid structure with a "string-like" ascending aorta, measuring less than 6 mm in diameter. The left ventricular inflow tract is diminished in size. Dilated pulmonary veins can usually be seen posterior to the left atrium in the long-axis, apical, and subxiphoidal views (Figs. 5–17 and 5–18). In addition to the small, poorly contractile left heart structures, the right-sided structures are dilated. There is usually massive enlargement of the right ventricular cavity and pulmonary outflow tract (Fig. 5–18) and a ubiquitous pulmonic valve.

Echocardiographic Features — Left Ventricular Inflow Obstruction in the Neonate

The flow of blood into the left ventricle may be obstructed proximal to, at, or distal to the mitral valve. On two-dimensional echocardiography, left atrial enlargement and dilatation of the pulmonary veins may be seen on the long-axis, subxiphoidal, and apical examinations[21] of the left ventricular inflow tract. Restriction to blood flow at the supravalvar level results in left atrial enlargement best visualized from the subxiphoidal view as a bowing of the interatrial septum toward the right atrial cavity (Fig. 5–19).

In patients with *cor triatriatum*, optimal viewing of the obstructing membrane within the left atrial cavity proximal to the mitral valve may be obtained from the apical[21] or subxiphoidal views (Fig. 5–20). The membrane may also be seen prolapsing toward the left ventricular inflow tract in the long-axis view of the left atrium (Fig. 5–21). The motion and configuration of the mitral valve distal to the membrane can be evaluated on the same images.

In contrast to cor triatriatum, *supravalvar*

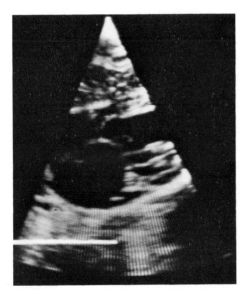
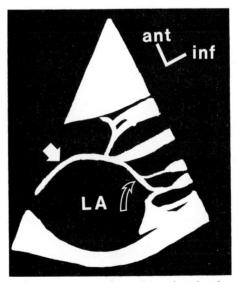

Figure 5–19. Left ventricular inflow obstruction. Short-axis view from the subxiphoid position demonstrates the ventricular inflow tract. The left atrium (LA) is enlarged with bowing of the interatrial septum (solid arrow) toward the right atrial cavity. There is no evidence of an interatrial communication. The mitral valve (open arrow) is thickened and restricts left ventricular inflow.

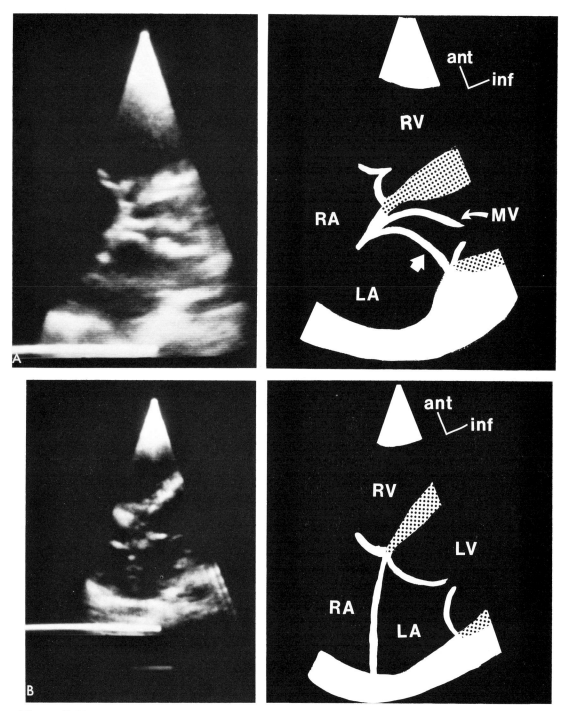

Figure 5–20. A, Cor triatriatum. Subxiphoidal four-chamber view. The mitral valve leaflets (MV) are seen and are on a plane that is distal to the obstructing abnormal intraatrial membrane (bold arrow). The interatrial septum appears to bulge into the right atrial cavity (RA), suggesting left atrial (LA) hypertension. *B,* Cor triatriatum (Postoperative). Postoperatively, the abnormal atrial membrane can no longer be seen in the subxiphoidal four-chamber view. The mitral leaflets appear normal. (LV = left ventricle; RV = right ventricle; RA = right atrium; LA = left atrium.)

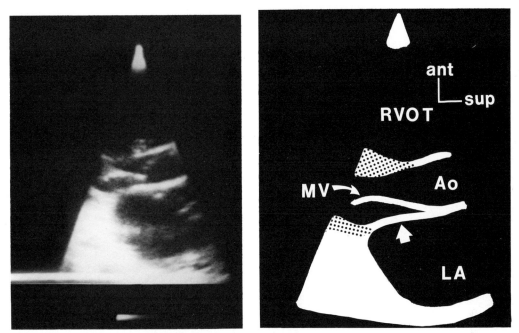

Figure 5–21. Cor triatriatum. Long-axis view of the left ventricle. The left atrium (LA) is massively enlarged and exceeds the aortic root dimension (Ao) by a ratio of greater than 2:1. An abnormal thickened membrane (bold arrow) is seen within the left atrium superior to the mitral valve (MV). This membrane results in severe supravalvar obstruction to left ventricular filling. The right ventricular outflow tract (RVOT) anterior to the aorta is massively dilated, suggesting pulmonary hypertension.

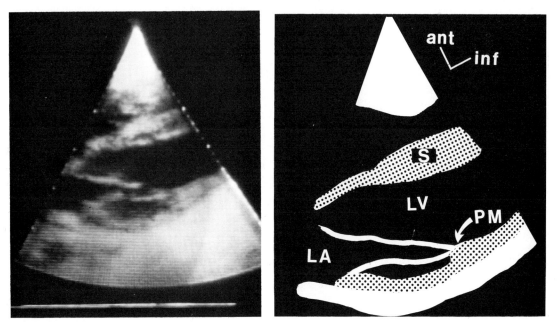

Figure 5–22. "Parachute" mitral valve. Subxiphoidal four-chamber view in a patient with a single papillary muscle (PM) and parachute deformity of the mitral valve. All chordae can be seen to insert into a single hypertrophic posterior papillary muscle. (S = septum; LV = left ventricle; LA = left atrium.)

mitral stenosing ring appears as a thickened structure in close apposition to the mitral valve.[21] The ring differs from the membrane of cor triatriatum in that it is located within the true left atrial cavity, whereas the membrane of cor triatriatum separates the embryologic common pulmonary vein from the true left atrium. The origin of the cor triatriatum membrane, therefore, is above the level of the left atrial appendage. Mitral supravalvar stenosing rings may be associated with more complex intracardiac abnormalities involving obstruction to left ventricular filling at multiple levels as well as obstruction to the left ventricular outflow tract in the form of subvalvar aortic stenosis and aortic coarctation (Shone's syndrome).[22]

The evaluation of the mitral valve as well as left ventricular and left atrial size can best be performed in the long-axis, apical, and subxiphoidal views. *Congenital mitral stenosis,* causing restricted opening of the mitral valve leaflets, also results in left atrial hypertension with bowing of the interatrial septum toward the right atrium (Fig. 5–19). These patients clearly demonstrate thickened, abnormal mitral valve leaflets and, in the most severe form of this entity, the mitral valve orifice may not open at all, resulting in *congenital mitral atresia.* In these cases, there is usually an associated hypoplasia of the left ventricular cavity and the child is dependent upon an interatrial communication in order to survive (Figs. 5–17 and 5–18).

A rare form of subvalvar left ventricular inflow tract obstruction is caused by insertion of both the anterior and posterior mitral chordae tendineae into a single hypertrophic papillary muscle, creating a *parachute mitral valve.* This may be identified in the long-axis, subxiphoidal short axis (coronal) (Fig. 5–22), or apical views. The long-axis echocardiogram shows a single large papillary muscle with insertion of the chordae directly into this muscle. The short-axis view through the apex of the left ventricle, which normally demonstrates an anterior and posterior papillary muscle, shows a single, large, eccentric papillary muscle.

REFERENCES

1. Higgins, C. B., Higgins, S. S., Kelley, M. J., Friedman, W. F.: Heart failure in the neonate due to extreme abnormalities of the heart rate: Clinical and radiographic features. Am J Roentgenol 134:359, 1980.
2. Higgins, C. B.: Radiology of neonatal heart disease. Perinatology-Neonatology 3:24A, 1979.
3. Roberts, W. C., Perry, L. W., Chandra, R. S., Meyers, G. E., Shapiro, S. R., Scott, L. P.: Aortic valve atresia: a new classification based on necropsy study of 73 cases. Am J Cardiol 37:753, 1976.
4. Lakier, J. B., Lewis, A. B., Heymann, M. A., Stanger, P., Hoffman, J. I. E., Rudolph, A. M.: Isolated aortic stenosis in the neonate. Circulation 50:801. 1974.
5. Broderick, T. W., Higgins, C. B., Guthaner, D. F., Friedman, W. F., Stevenson, J. G., French, J. W.: Critical Aortic Stenosis in Neonates. Radiology 129:393, 1978.
6. Gyepes, M. T., Vincent, W. R.: Severe congenital heart disease in the neonatal period. Am J Roentgenol 116:490, 1972.
7. Rudolph, A. M., Heymann, M. A., Spitznas, U.: Hemodynamic considerations in the development of narrowing of the aorta. Am J Cardiol 30:514, 1972.
8. Higgins, C. B., French, J. W., Silverman, J. F., Wexler, L.: Interruption of the aortic arch: Preoperative and postoperative clinical, hemodynamic and angiographic features. Am J Cardiol 39:563, 1977.
9. Moller, J. H., Edwards, J. E.: Interruption of the aortic arch. Anatomic patterns and associated cardiac malformations. J Roentgenol 95:557, 1965.
10. Shone, J. D., Munoz, A. S., Manning, J. A., Keith, J. D.: The mumps antigen skin test and endocardial fibroelastosis. Pediatrics 37:423, 1966.
11. O'Brien, M. S., Schechter, M. M.: Arteriovenous malformations involving the Galenic system. Am J Roentgenol 110:50, 1970.
12. Talner, N. S., Campbell, A. G. M.: Recognition and management of cardiologic problems in the newborn infant. Prog Cardiovasc Dis 15:159 (2), 1972.
13. Hellenbrand, W. E., Kelley, M. J., Berman, M. A.: Heart failure and cyanosis in a newborn: Cerebral arteriovenous malformation involving the vein of Galen. Chest 72:225, 1977.
14. Askenazi, J., Nadas, A. S.: Anomalous left coronary artery originating from the pulmonary artery: Report on 15 cases. Circulation 51:976, 1975.
15. Bookstein, J. J.: Aberrant left coronary artery. Am J Roentgenol 91:515, 1964.
16. Edwards, J. E.: The direction of blood flow in coronary arteries arising from the pulmonary trunk (Editorial). Circulation 29:163, 1964.
17. Talner, N. S., Halloran, K. H., Mahdavy, M., Gardner, T. H., Hipona, F.: Anomalous origin of left coronary artery from the pulmonary artery. A clinical spectrum. Am J Cardiol 15:689, 1965.
18. Liebman, J., Hellerstein, H. K., Ankeney, J. L., Tucker, A.: The problem of the anomalous left coronary artery arising from the pulmonary artery in older children. Report of three cases. N Engl J Med 269:486, 1963.
19. Usman, A., Fernandez, B., Uricchio, J. F., Nichols, H. T.: Aberrant origin of left coronary artery combined with mitral regurgitation in an adult. Am J Cardiol 8:130, 1961.
20. Conley, M. E., Beckwith, J. B., Mancer, J. F. K.,

Tenckhoff, L.: The spectrum of the Di-George Syndrome. J Pediatr 94:883, 1979.

21. Snider, A. R., Roge, C. L., Schiller, N. B., Silverman, N. H.: Congenital left ventricular inflow obstruction evaluated by two-dimensional echocardiography. Circulation 61:848, 1980.

22. Shone, J. D., Sellers, R. D., Anderson, R. C., Adams, P., Jr., Lillehei, C., Edwards, J. E.: The developmental complex of "parachute mitral valve," supravalvar ring of left atrium, subaortic stenosis and coarctation of the aorta. Am J Cardiol 11:714, 1963.

THE ACYANOTIC CHILD WITH NORMAL VASCULARITY OR PULMONARY VENOUS HYPERTENSION

In the older child, obstruction to left ventricular inflow may occur within the left atrium or at the mitral valve level. Obstruction to left ventricular outflow occurs in relation to the aortic valve at the subvalvar, valvar or supravalvar level. These lesions may be acquired (usually on a rheumatic basis) or they may involve specific congenital defects. Depending on the severity of the lesion, the chest radiograph may demonstrate normal vascularity or pulmonary venous hypertension.

RHEUMATIC HEART DISEASE

In the early part of the twentieth century, rheumatic fever was one of the primary causes of morbidity and death in childhood and early adult life. The disease is less prevalent among school children and young adults today, with an estimated incidence of one to two children per thousand.[1] There are an equal number who have had rheumatic fever but who have no residual cardiac involvement. The apparent decline in the prevalence of this disorder may be due to a change in either (or both) the incidence or severity of rheumatic fever.[2]

Acute Rheumatic Fever

Acute rheumatic fever is uncommon in children less than five years of age and is rarely seen under the age of 2.[3] The greatest incidence is between six and 15 years with a peak at age eight years. Carditis is the most important of the major manifestations of acute rheumatic fever, since it is the only one that results in sequelae.[4] The four signs of carditis include (1) significant new heart murmur, (2) cardiomegaly, (3) cardiac decompensation, and (4) pericardial friction rub or effusion.

The mitral valve is the most common site of rheumatic inflammation, being involved three times more frequently than the aortic valve. In the United States, mitral regurgitation is the most common sequela of the acute attack. In this country, mitral stenosis, which takes months or years to develop, is an unusual early manifestation of acute rheumatic fever. It is not unusual, however, in underdeveloped countries. When aortic valvulitis develops, aortic regurgitation may occur early in the course of the disease.

Radiographic Features

From an imaging standpoint, three of the cardinal manifestations of acute rheumatic carditis can be confirmed or initially demonstrated on the chest radiograph. These are cardiomegaly, congestive heart failure, and pericardial effusion. The detection of cardiomegaly is of considerable importance, since it can confirm the impression of carditis in doubtful cases. The methods for obtaining the cardiothoracic ratio outlined in Chapter 2 should be used. In children over age five, this ratio should not exceed 0.56.

During the acute phase of severe rheumatic myocarditis, the heart may have a

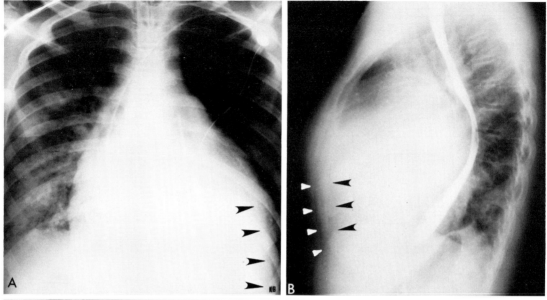

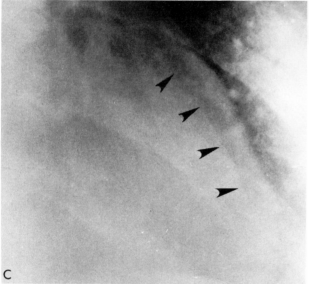

Figure 5–23. *A*, Posteroanterior chest radiograph in a ten-year-old girl with acute rheumatic carditis and congestive failure. There are alveolar infiltrates in the right lung consistent with pulmonary edema. The heart is enlarged and has a globular shape. The acute angle usually present in the right cardiophrenic region is absent. There is a subtle difference in density at the left cardiac margin (arrowheads)—the differential density sign of pericardial effusion.

B, Lateral chest radiograph with barium in the esophagus of the patient shown in *A*. There is marked left atrial enlargement as indicated by posterior deviation of the upper esophagus. A water density separated by substernal and epicardial fat (arrowheads) exceeds 2 mm in width and indicates a substantial pericardial effusion.

C, Close-up of left heart border in a patient with echocardiographic evidence of a moderate pericardial effusion. The differential density sign is well seen (arrowheads).

globular shape. The differentiation between pericardial effusion and generalized cardiac dilatation can readily be solved by obtaining an M-mode echocardiogram (see Fig. 5–27). The plain chest film may also offer clues to the diagnosis of pericardial effusion.

The principal signs are the following:

1. A rapid increase in cardiac size with a decrease in the acuteness of the cardio-diaphragmatic angles (Fig. 5–23A). This is especially suggestive when accompanied by clear lung fields without pulmonary venous hypertensive changes.

2. The presence of a >2 mm water density between substernal and epicardial fat on the lateral chest film (Fig. 5–23B). This sign is seen in less than 15 per cent of adults with echocardiographically proven effusion.[5]

3. The presence of a differential density (lucency) at the outer (usually left) cardiac

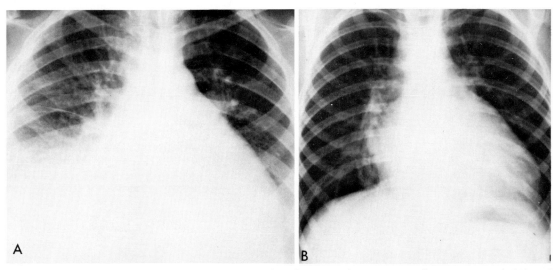

Figure 5–24. Posteroanterior chest radiographs of patient during acute rheumatic attack *(A)* and two months after treatment *(B)*. Severe pulmonary venous hypertension and right pleural effusion have resolved. Cardiomegaly and mild PVH persist in this patient with mitral regurgitation.

margin[5] (Figs. 5–23*A* and *C*). This is due to the difference in attenuation of the fluid-filled pericardial space and the presence of epicardial fat.

The degree of cardiomegaly is a valuable index to severity and to the course of the disease and can be followed by both chest film (Fig. 5–24) and echocardiography. In the majority of patients, heart size returns to normal over a period of weeks to months following the acute attack[6] (Fig. 5–24*B*).

Although it has been stated that acute rheumatic myocarditis does not cause a characteristic cardiac contour,[6] there is invariably fullness of the left heart border (Fig. 5–25). The upper portion of this fullness is due to a dilated left atrial appendage. In fact, the left atrial appendage may add a rather characteristic, if sometimes subtle, bulge to the left upper cardiac contour (Fig. 5–26). Dilatation of the left atrial appendage is more readily apparent after the acute phase of rheumatic fever in children who have residual mitral valve damage (Fig. 5–26). This radiographic marker of rheumatic mitral valve disease has proved useful in distinguishing this lesion from nonrheumatic mitral valve disease as well as from other lesions that result in left atrial enlargement.[7] It also appears to be a sensitive marker for rheumatic mitral disease in adults.[8]

Echocardiographic
Features — Pericardial Effusion

Undoubtedly, the echocardiogram provides the most accurate and sensitive[9] method of detecting pericardial fluid. The echoes generated by the pericardium — usually the strongest source of echoes on an M-mode study — are normally in close apposition to the epicardial echoes. The two structures cannot be distinguished unless fluid intervenes between them. Although a potential pericardial space is present behind the left atrium, the entrance of pulmonary veins in this region generally prevents all but very large effusions from accumulating in this area. Small amounts of pericardial fluid are most easily detected surrounding the apex of the heart. Technical factors such as receiver gain setting are important, and transducer power output must be decreased until only the pericardial echoes are present. Once these have been identified, output is increased until epicardium, endocardium, mitral apparatus, septum, and right ventricular wall are seen. A significant pericardial effusion is indicated by

1. A flat, nonmoving pericardial echo.
2. An echo-free space between the epicardium and the flat pericardium that persists in both systole and diastole (Fig. 5–27).

A large pericardial effusion is present when an echo-free space exists between the

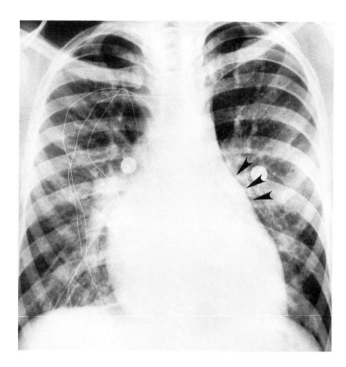

Figure 5–25. Posteroanterior chest radiograph of a child with acute rheumatic carditis. Careful analysis of the fullness along the left upper heart border discloses a subtle bulge of a dilated left atrial appendage (arrowheads).

pericardium and the anterior heart wall. Normally, a small amount of pericardial fluid (< 30 cc) is present in the pericardial space. This may cause a separation between the pericardium and epicardium in systole. This normal separation *should not* persist into diastole nor should the pericardial echo be flat.

The long-axis two-dimensional echocar-diographic view provides a highly reliable means of diagnosing pericardial effusion and is more reliable than the traditional M-mode technique for diagnosing loculated effusions. Separation of the epicardium from the pericardium is easily demonstrated in almost all cases in sections through the body and apex of the left ventricle (Figs. 5–28 to 5–30). The long-axis view provides a

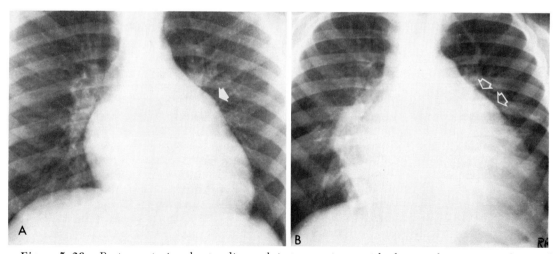

Figure 5–26. Posteroanterior chest radiograph in two patients with chronic rheumatic carditis and mitral regurgitation. The dilated left atrial appendage is readily apparent in *A* (arrow) but more subtle in *B* (arrows).

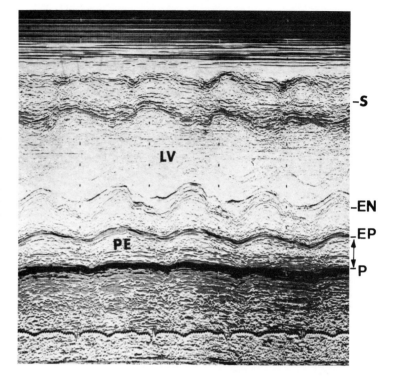

Figure 5–27. M-mode echocardiogram of a 12-year-old with acute rheumatic carditis. There is separation of the epicardium (EP) and pericardium (P) by a moderately large pericardial effusion (PE). The endocardium (EN) and the septum (S) of the left ventricle (LV) are well delineated near the apex.

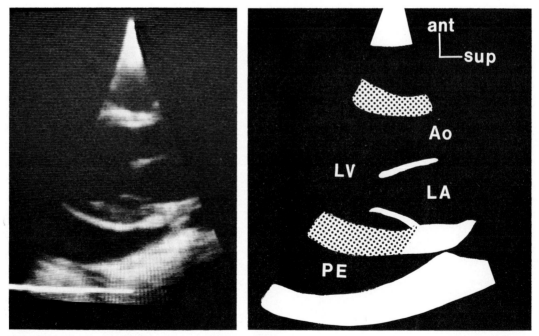

Figure 5–28. Pericardial effusion. Long-axis view of the left ventricle in a patient with a large posterior pericardial effusion (PE). Note the effusion extending to the level of the atrioventricular valve groove, posterior to the left ventricular wall. (LV = left ventricle; LA = left atrium; Ao = aorta.)

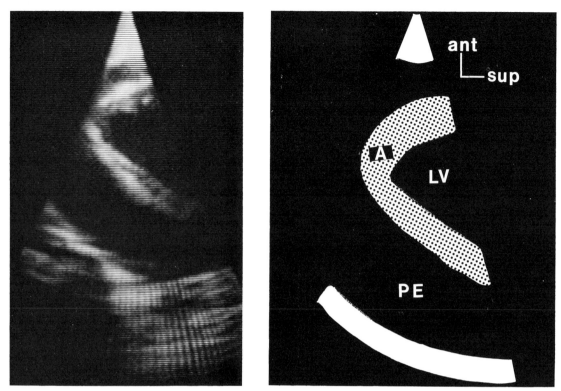

Figure 5–29. Pericardial effusion. Long-axis view at the apex of the ventricle (A) demonstrating a large apical pericardial effusion (PE) that surrounds the apex of the heart both anteriorly and posteriorly. (LV = left ventricle.)

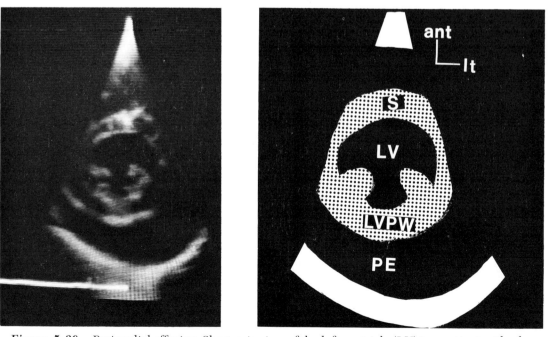

Figure 5–30. Pericardial effusion. Short-axis view of the left ventricle (LV) in a patient with a large posterior pericardial effusion (PE). The pericardial effusion is seen posterior to the left ventricular posterior wall (LVPW). Note the papillary muscles along the lower aspect of the left ventricle. (S = septum.)

gross assessment of the overall quantity of the fluid collection. In massive pericardial effusions, the ventricle shows a chaotic waving motion as it rotates during its contraction within the fluid-filled pericardial sac. Because it provides accurate location of the effusion, two-dimensional echocardiography permits pericardiocentesis to be performed with greater ease and safety[10] and may be of great importance in defining pericardial effusions when they are loculated (for example, following purulent pericarditis or in pericardial effusions that occur after mediastinal irradiation).[11]

Chronic Rheumatic Heart Disease

About one-third of all children with acute rheumatic fever develop chronic heart disease.[12] Autopsy studies of adults show that the mitral valve alone is affected most commonly (80 per cent). Occasionally, both aortic and mitral valves are affected (20 per cent); less frequently, the disease is limited to the aortic valve (7 per cent). Rheumatic carditis involving the right cardiac valves is rare (<5 per cent), but secondary tricuspid regurgitation may occur as a consequence of pulmonary hypertension secondary to the left heart lesion(s). In addition to the valvar lesions, myocardial dysfunction may occur in rheumatic heart disease. This usually results in symptoms of congestive heart failure in the pediatric age group.[13]

Mitral Regurgitation

As healing of the acute process occurs, one or both valve leaflets contract so that they are no longer apposed over the mitral orifice. Fusion and shortening of the chordae further reduce the ability of the valve leaflets to close. As left atrial dilatation occurs, the posterior leaflet of the mitral valve is displaced from the orifice, and this may further aggravate mitral regurgitation. The resulting volume overload of the left ventricle dilates this chamber. This in turn may cause malorientation of the chordae and papillary muscles and further inhibit mitral leaflet closure[14] — in other words, "mitral regurgitation begets mitral regurgitation." Mitral insufficiency is the most common form of rheumatic heart disease in the pediatric age group.

Radiographic Findings

Radiographic findings vary depending on the degree and duration of the regurgitation. Pulmonary vascularity may be normal or there may be mild pulmonary venous hypertension (redistribution of blood flow to the upper lung fields) (Fig. 5–31). The combination of left ventricular and left atrial enlargement is common, since there is volume overload of both chambers (Fig. 5–31). In chronic severe mitral regurgitation both chambers may become huge (Fig. 5–32). In addition, a key radiographic feature is prominence of the left atrial appendage. It has been shown that the radiographic appearance of a dilated left atrial appendage is a unique feature of the chest film in children with rheumatic mitral regurgitation[7] (Fig. 5–31). This sign may separate rheumatic disease from other causes of mitral regurgitation in children. Interestingly, a dilated left atrial appendage rarely occurs in other lesions that cause left atrial enlargement. The explanation for the radiographic appearance of a dilated left atrial appendage may be the unique combination of the inflammatory process that involves the appendage (Aschoff's bodies are commonly found in the appendage),[15] making it more distensible, and the elevated left atrial pressures associated with mitral valve lesions.

Echocardiographic Features

Although mitral regurgitation cannot be directly identified by M-mode echocardiographic techniques, the combination of significant left atrial and left ventricular enlargement should suggest the diagnosis. The mitral valve may be thickened with a decreased closing velocity.

Mitral Stenosis

Mitral stenosis in children is uncommon in this country. It does not occur during the acute attack and may take years to develop. One study that followed 440 children for five years and 347 for ten years reported an incidence of less than 2 per cent in the former and less than 6 per cent in the latter group.[16] In contrast, early mitral stenosis occurring from six months to two years after the acute attack is common in other countries, especially India.[17] The pathologic

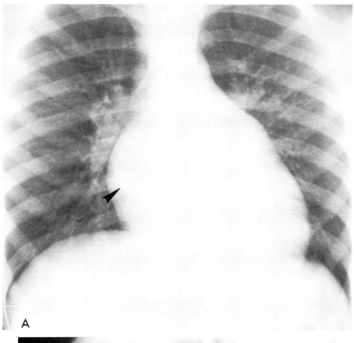

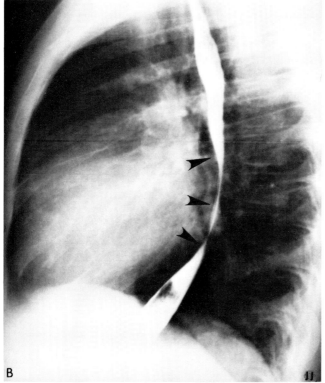

Figure 5–31. Posteroanterior (A) and lateral (B) chest radiographs in a 12-year-old child with chronic rheumatic mitral regurgitation. Mild pulmonary venous hypertension and left ventricular and left atrial enlargement (note double density [arrowhead] and displaced barium esophagram [arrowheads]) indicate volume overload of both left atrium and left ventricle. The left atrial appendage is prominent.

process of mitral stenosis involves fusion of the valve leaflets at the commissures ("fish-mouthing"). In severe cases, the atrioventricular ring, chordae, and even the papillary muscles are involved. Thickening and fusion of the chordae leads to restriction of valve motion and increased stenosis.[18]

Radiographic Features

The pulmonary vascular changes are generally more severe in mitral stenosis than in mitral regurgitation (Fig. 5–33). Even in the face of radiographic evidence of higher levels of pulmonary venous pressure, however,

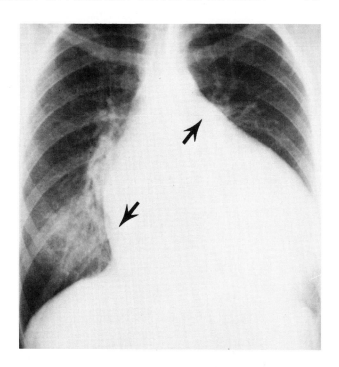

Figure 5–32. Posteroanterior chest radiograph in a child with chronic severe mitral regurgitation. There is massive left ventricular and left atrial enlargement. The left atrial dimension taken between the double density (lower arrow) and the left mainstem bronchus (upper arrow) measured 9.5 cm.

the heart size remains normal and the degree of left atrial enlargement is not as great as in mitral regurgitation (Figs. 5–33 and 5–34). This is due to the nature of the lesion. Basically, mitral stenosis creates pressure overload of the left atrium rather than volume overload of both the atrium and the ventricle as with mitral regurgitation. In more advanced cases associated with increased pulmonary vascular resistance and

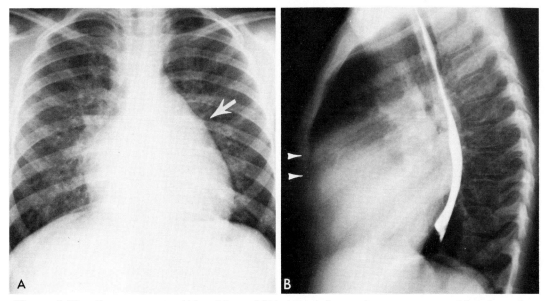

Figure 5–33. Posteroanterior *(A)* and lateral *(B)* chest radiographs in a ten-year-old with predominant rheumatic mitral stenosis. Moderately severe pulmonary venous hypertension is indicated by ill-defined pulmonary vascularity and poorly defined hilar angle. Although the heart appears normal in size on the PA view, right heart enlargement is suggested by the upturned cardiac apex, the prominent right atrial border, and filling in of the retrosternal space on the lateral film (arrowheads). Both the left atrium and the left atrial appendage (arrow) are mildly enlarged.

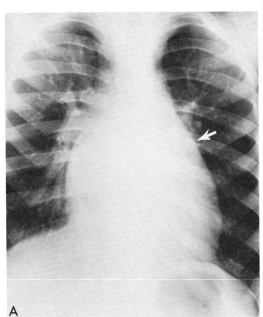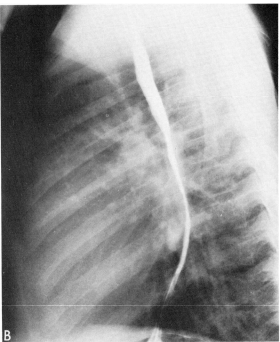

Figure 5–34. Posteroanterior *(A)* and lateral *(B)* chest radiographs in an 11-year-old child with mitral stenosis. The findings are similar to those in Figure 5–33, although the vascularity shows only redistribution. Note the presence of mild left atrial appendage enlargement (arrow).

pulmonary hypertension, right ventricular enlargement may occur. This is manifested on posteroanterior views as an upturned cardiac apex (Fig. 5–33A) and on the lateral view by filling in of a normal clear space between the heart and the sternum (Fig. 5–33B). Calcification of the mitral valve, a common finding in adults with mitral stenosis, is rare in patients under 30 years of age.

Echocardiographic Features

On the two-dimensional examination, the mitral valve can be easily visualized in both the short- and long-axis views. When mitral stenosis is the dominant lesion the valve appears echo-dense owing to fibrosis and/or calcific deposits. The motion of the valve is quite abnormal and is characterized in the long-axis view by doming during diastole with restriction of the orifice primarily at the tips of the valve leaflets (Fig. 5–35A). Left atrial enlargement is reflected as a bowing of the interatrial septum toward the right atrium. In the short-axis view, "fish-mouthing" of the mitral valve may be appreciated (Fig. 5–35B) and the restricted opening may be roughly estimated.[19]

Angiographic Features

Mitral regurgitation can be assessed angiographically and is graded in the following manner:

1+ Evidence of a jet of regurgitant contrast material without opacification of the entire left atrium.

2+ A regurgitant jet with moderate opacification of the left atrium that clears rapidly.

3+ Intense opacification of the left atrium to the same extent as in the left ventricle. Contrast clears slowly from the left atrium. No jet is seen.

4+ Left atrium more densely opacified than left ventricle and remains intensely opacified through the entire film sequence (Fig. 5–36).

The subjective estimate given above may be further compromised when there is decreased left ventricular function or when the left atrium is massively enlarged. When a dilated left ventricle with decreased contractility is demonstrated, the possibility of "rheumatic cardiomyopathy" secondary to pancarditis or myocarditis should be considered.

The angiographic features of mitral steno-

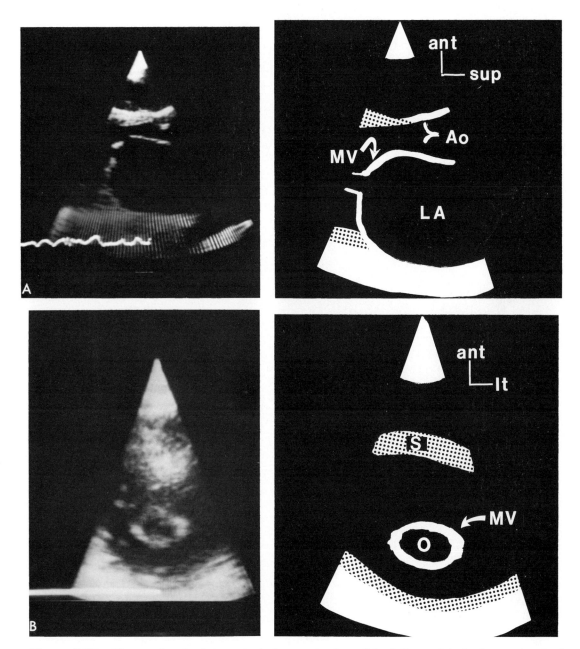

Figure 5–35. Rheumatic mitral stenosis. *A*, Long-axis view of the left ventricle in rheumatic mitral stenosis. There is enlargement of the left atrium (LA) that exceeds the aortic root (Ao) dimension by greater than 3:1. The mitral valve leaflets (MV) are thickened and restrict the orifice. The mitral valve domes during diastole. *B*, Left ventricular short-axis view showing rheumatic mitral stenosis. The left ventricle is moderately dilated due to the presence of mitral insufficiency. The mitral valve orifice (O) is seen in the mid portion of the ventricle below the septum. The valve leaflets (MV) are thickened and the abnormally restricted "fishmouth" motion of the orifice is easily visualized.

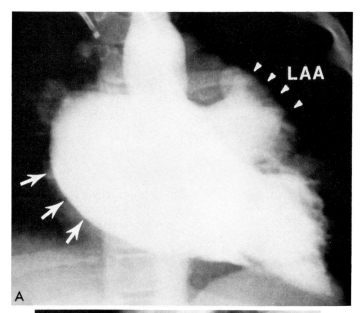

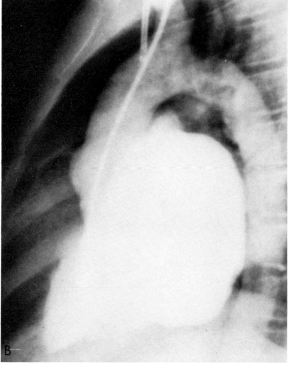

Figure 5–36. Anteroposterior (A) and lateral (B) left ventriculograms in a patient with rheumatic mitral regurgitation. The density of contrast in the markedly dilated left atrium exceeds that in the left ventricle, indicating severe (4+/4+) mitral regurgitation. Note the dilated left atrial appendage (LAA). One can appreciate the origin of the "double density" sign of left atrial enlargement as well (arrows).

sis include a "snapping" forward motion of the mitral valve accompanied by doming in diastole (Fig. 5–37). These features allow one to "see" the abnormal valve, whereas the normal valve rapidly moves forward and disappears into the contrast-containing cavity of the left ventricle. Irregularity at the base of the left ventricle may be secondary to rheumatic scarring, and adherence of

chordal structures in this region may also be noted.

Rheumatic Aortic Valve Disease (Aortic Regurgitation)

Rheumatic involvement of the aortic valve leads to aortic regurgitation in child-

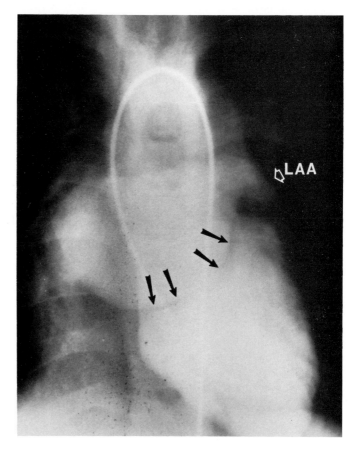

Figure 5-37. Anteroposterior left ventriculogram in a child with combined mitral stenosis and regurgitation. This radiograph, taken in diastole, shows a thickened mitral valve (arrows) "doming" into the left ventricle. The mitral regurgitation was graded as 3+/4+. Note the dilated left atrial appendage (LAA).

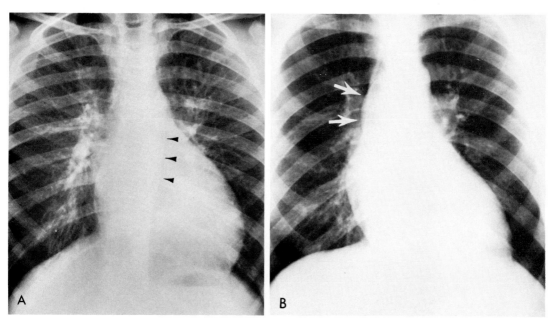

Figure 5-38. Posteroanterior chest radiographs in two teenagers who, following their acute rheumatic fever, developed predominant aortic regurgitation. In both cases, pulmonary vascularity is normal in the face of an enlarged left ventricle. The descending aorta is tortuous in *A* (arrowheads) and the ascending aorta is prominent in *B* (arrows).

hood and adolescence. Predominant aortic stenosis is virtually unheard of in this age group. The aortic valve is usually involved in combination with the mitral valve.

With healing after the acute attack, there is fibrous thickening and contraction of the aortic valve cusps. Fusion of the commissures may occur and, if severe, will gradually lead to aortic stenosis in adulthood.

Radiographic Features

Regurgitant blood flow across the aortic valve in addition to blood arriving from the left atrium increases the volume load on the left ventricle and causes it to dilate. This leads to an enlarged left ventricular configuration on the chest radiograph, usually in the presence of normal pulmonary vascularity (Fig. 5–38). Diastolic blood pressure drops and systolic pressure rises to maintain mean arterial pressure. The vigorous bounding peripheral pulse wave typical of significant aortic regurgitation is reflected in the vigorous pulsation of the thoracic aorta seen fluoroscopically. With time, this leads to prominence of the ascending aorta and aortic knob and to premature tortuosity of the descending thoracic aorta (Fig. 5–38).

Echocardiographic Features

Coarse diastolic fluttering of the anterior leaflet of the mitral valve or septum suggests aortic insufficiency and can usually be seen on the M-mode echocardiographic examination[20] (Fig. 5–39). The aortic root tracing may show increased aortic valve echoes indicative of thickening. Real-time two-dimensional techniques may further substantiate mitral valve diastolic fluttering and occasionally show evidence of abnormal aortic valve anatomy in the form of thickening of or prolapse of aortic valve leaflets (Fig. 5–40).

Angiographic Features

Ascending aortography definitively establishes the presence of aortic regurgitation, and using the assessment below suggests the severity of the valve lesion. Thickening of the leaflets of a *tricuspid* aortic valve is frequently seen in aortic regurgitation secondary to rheumatic carditis. The severity of aortic insufficiency is judged as follows:

1+ Evidence of a jet of regurgitant contrast without opacification of the left ventricle.

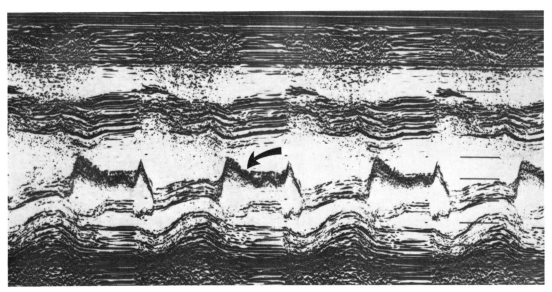

Figure 5–39. Aortic insufficiency. M-mode echocardiogram at the ventricular level in a patient with moderate aortic insufficiency. Note the coarse flutter on the anterior leaflet of the mitral valve during diastole (arrow). This flutter is related to the regurgitant jet of blood striking the anterior leaflet of the mitral valve.

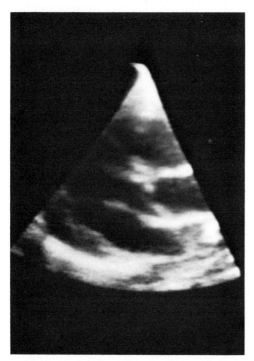
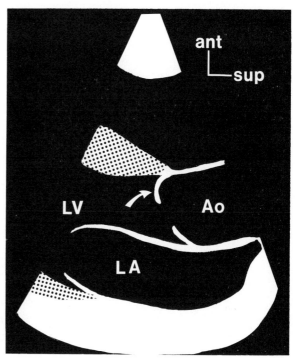

Figure 5-40. Aortic insufficiency. Long-axis view of the left ventricle during diastole. There is a prolapse of both aortic cusps (arrow) inferiorly into the left ventricular cavity, suggesting the presence of aortic insufficiency. Direct evidence of this type for aortic insufficiency is relatively unusual; the diagnosis is most commonly made in the presence of diastolic fluttering on the M-mode echocardiogram (see Fig. 5-39). (Ao = aorta, LA = left atrium, LV = left ventricle.)

2+ Evidence of a jet of regurgitant contrast with faint opacification of the left ventricle.

3+ Dense opacification of the left ventricle with no distinct jet visualized.

4+ Left ventricle is more densely opacified than aorta (Fig. 5-41).

NONRHEUMATIC HEART DISEASE

Aortic Valve Stenosis

Aortic valve stenosis makes up approximately 4 per cent of all congenital heart defects.[21, 22] Approximately 95 per cent of isolated aortic stenosis is due to a congenital abnormality of the aortic valve, and it has been estimated that the frequency of bicuspid valves may approach 2 per cent of the population.[23] The congenitally stenotic aortic valve may be dysplastic, unicuspid, or bicuspid. The more common bicuspid form results from partial failure of the development of the commissures between the three semilunar cusps. The orifice is often eccentrically placed owing to inequality of the size of the cusps. A false raphe representing the underdeveloped third commissure is located in one of the cusps in approximately 50 per cent of patients.[24]

Two basic types of bicuspid valves exist. When the two cusps are located anteriorly and posteriorly (the most common variety), the commissures are right and left, and both coronary arteries arise in front of the anterior cusp (Fig. 5-42B). A false raphe, if present, is located in the right or anterior cusp (Fig. 5-42B). When the cusps are right and left, the commissures are anterior and posterior and the coronary arteries originate above each cusp (Fig. 5-42C). A false raphe, if present, is located in the right cusp (Fig. 5-42C).

Clinical presentation varies with the severity of the stenosis. Critical aortic stenosis in the neonate has been discussed previously. Generally, presentation with isolated aortic stenosis in the first decade of life involves the dysplastic, unicuspid, or (most commonly) the bicuspid valve. Presentation

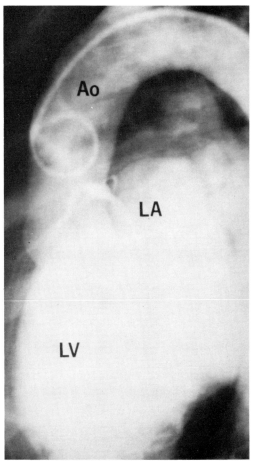

Figure 5–41. Lateral thoracic aortogram showing dense opacification of the left ventricle (LV) greater than that of the aorta (Ao). This represents 4+/4+ aortic regurgitation. There is mitral regurgitation into the left atrium (LA) in this child with rheumatic heart disease.

in the second to seventh decade is usually associated with a bicuspid valve. Calcific aortic stenosis in adults is most commonly related to a congenitally bicuspid aortic valve. Presentation of aortic stenosis after the seventh decade is associated with degeneration of a tricuspid valve.[25] In the latter situation, the basic abnormality arises from acquired degeneration of a normal valve. A congenital bicuspid valve has a progressive tendency to develop calcific aortic stenosis and, less commonly, aortic regurgitation or endocarditis.[23]

Radiographic Features

In the child with aortic stenosis the pulmonary vascularity is usually normal (Fig.

5–43A and B) and the remainder of the chest film is frequently normal. A sign that may suggest the diagnosis is prominence of the ascending aorta (Fig. 5–43). On the frontal film, subtle deviation of the superior vena cava to the right may be the only clue that the ascending aorta is dilated. Occasionally, a prominent ascending aorta will be seen in the child with systemic hypertension, although a common cause for "prominence" is a film that is slightly rotated to the right. Conspicuous dilatation of the ascending aorta suggests that the left ventricular obstruction is at the valve level (rather than at the subvalvar or supravalvar level). A normal ascending aorta may rarely occur with valvar aortic stenosis, and a prominent ascending aorta may occur with discrete subvalvar aortic stenosis, especially when the obstruction is within 1 cm of the aortic valve.[26] A "left ventricular configuration" (a reflection of left ventricular hypertrophy) with a normal heart size is frequent. This is suggested by increased convexity to the apex (Fig. 5–43A) and "sagging" of the lower heart border below the left hemidiaphragm (Fig. 5–43B). In older

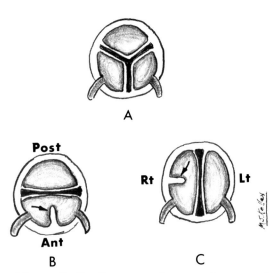

Figure 5–42. Diagram of a normal tricuspid aortic valve (A) and the two types of bicuspid aortic valve (B and C). In the most common bicuspid valve (B), the two cusps are located anteriorly (Ant) and posteriorly (Post), with the commissures right and left. A false raphe (arrow) is located in the anterior cusp. Both coronary arteries arise above the anterior cusp. When the two cusps are right (Rt) and left (Lt) (C), the commissures are anterior and posterior. A false raphe (arrow) is located in the right cusp.

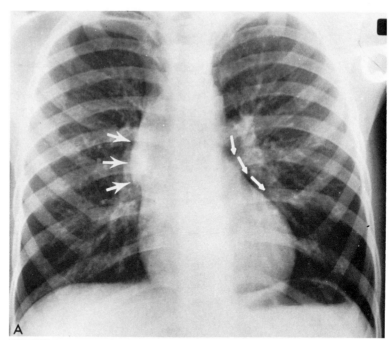

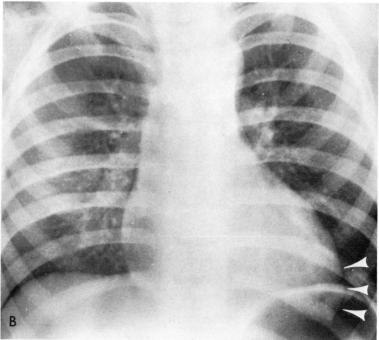

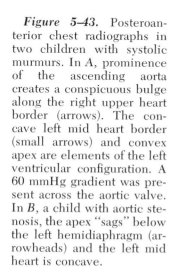

Figure 5–43. Posteroanterior chest radiographs in two children with systolic murmurs. In *A*, prominence of the ascending aorta creates a conspicuous bulge along the right upper heart border (arrows). The concave left mid heart border (small arrows) and convex apex are elements of the left ventricular configuration. A 60 mmHg gradient was present across the aortic valve. In *B*, a child with aortic stenosis, the apex "sags" below the left hemidiaphragm (arrowheads) and the left mid heart is concave.

children and adults this configuration is characterized by a concave left midheart border in the region usually occupied by the pulmonary trunk (Fig. 5–43). Marked enlargement of the left ventricle is seldom noted in children presenting for the first time with aortic valve stenosis. When symptoms of congestive heart failure develop late

in the course of the disease, significant cardiomegaly may be noted.[27]

The most reliable radiographic sign of a congenitally bicuspid aortic valve is the presence of calcium in the valve. However, calcium deposition to the extent that it is visible on the plain chest film is distinctly unusual before the age of 20 years.[24]

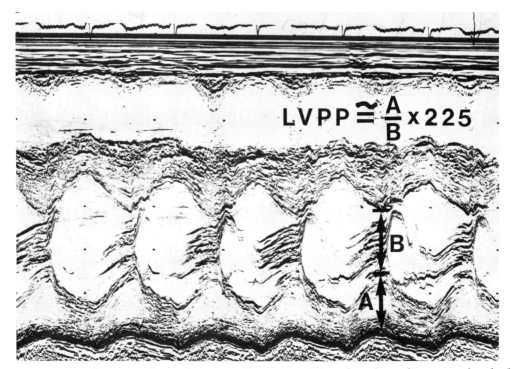

$$LVPP \cong \frac{A}{B} \times 225$$

Figure 5-44. Left ventricular outflow tract obstruction. M-mode echocardiogram at level of the ventricular body. Physiologic normalization of wall stress in the unoperated pediatric patient permits systolic dimensions of the left ventricular cavity and posterior wall to be directly related to intracavity pressure. A simplified formula for estimating cavity pressure is shown in this figure. Left ventricular posterior wall thickness in systole *(A)* is divided by end-systolic cavity dimension *(B)* and this ratio is multiplied by an empirically derived constant (225 torr) to derive an estimate of peak left ventricular cavity pressure. Comparison of this value with clinical measurement of peak systolic blood pressure by cuff correlates well with catheterization measurements of the obstructive gradient of the left ventricular outflow tract in lesions such as membranous subaortic stenosis, valvar aortic stenosis, and coarctation of the aorta.

Echocardiographic Features

Left ventricular outflow tract obstruction, whether at the subvalvar, valvar, or supravalvar level, results in left ventricular hypertension in excess of systolic pressure in the ascending aorta. M-mode echocardiographic evaluation of the dynamic response of the left ventricle to this pressure overload has been successfully used to noninvasively estimate peak systolic pressure within the left ventricular cavity.[28, 29] Previous studies have suggested the inadequacy of physical examination, chest x-ray, and electrocardiography for noninvasive estimation of peak systolic cavity pressure.[30] Recent studies suggest that both end-diastolic and end-systolic left ventricular posterior wall thickness may be related to the left ventricular peak systolic cavity pressure through the use of empirically derived formulae.[28-32]

These formulae appear to have utility only in the preoperative state in the absence of congestive cardiac failure or significant aortic regurgitation.[29] The formula is

Left ventricular peak pressure $\cong$

$$\frac{\text{Left ventricular systolic wall thickness}}{\text{Left ventricular systolic cavity dimension}} \times 225$$

Results indicate an excellent noninvasive estimate of peak left ventricular cavity pressure, which compares well with pressures directly measured at cardiac catheterization (Fig. 5-44).

In aortic stenosis the left ventricular outflow tract is evaluated from the precordial and subxiphoidal short-axis view. In congenital aortic stenosis, the M-mode (Fig. 5-45) and two-dimensional echocardiogram allow visualization of thickened aortic valve

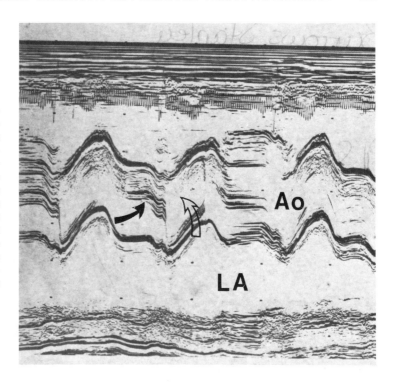

Figure 5–45. Aortic stenosis — bicuspid aortic valve. M-mode echocardiogram of the aortic root (Ao). A stenotic bicuspid aortic valve shows thickening and eccentricity of the leaflets during the diastolic phase (solid arrow). In systole (open arrow), the valve leaflets appear to open fully, but, in fact, the valve leaflets are doming and the portion of the valve that is seen in systole represents only the base of the valve leaflets.

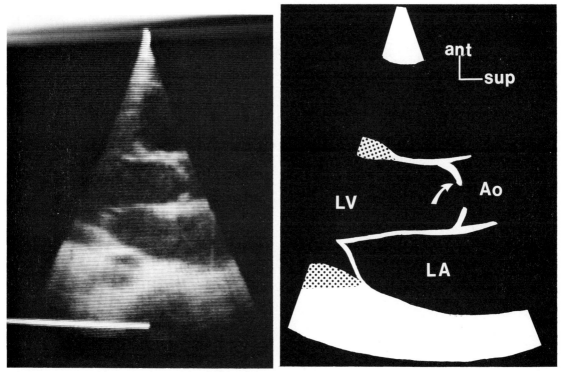

Figure 5–46. Congenital aortic stenosis. End-systolic long-axis view of the left ventricle in the same patient shown in Figure 5–45. Note the incomplete opening with resultant doming of the aortic valve leaflet (curved arrow). (Ao = aortic root; LA = left atrium; LV = left ventricle.)

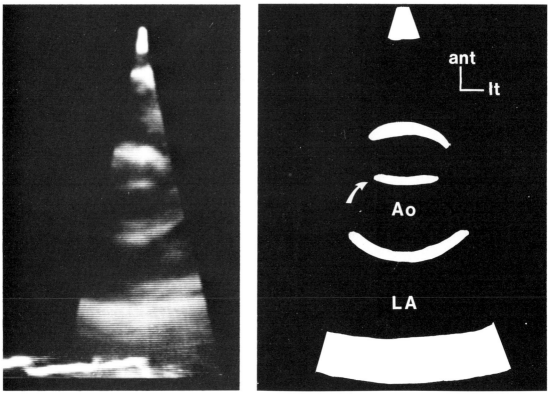

Figure 5–47. Congenital aortic stenosis. Short-axis view of the aortic root in end-diastole, showing eccentric valve closure (arrow) and configuration typical of a bicuspid aortic valve. (Ao = aortic root; LA = left atrium.)

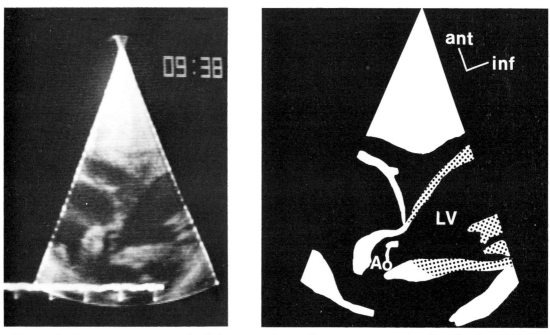

Figure 5–48. Aortic stenosis. The left ventricular outflow tract is visualized in the four-chamber subxiphoidal view. The left ventricular cavity (LV) and aorta (Ao) are well visualized and the aortic valve domes during systole.

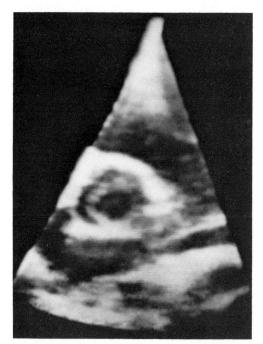
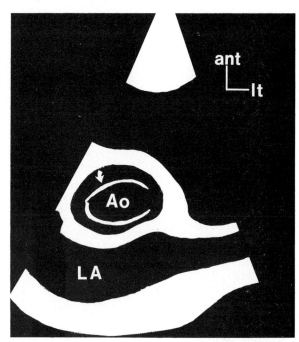

Figure 5–49.   Congenital aortic stenosis. Aortic short-axis view of a bicuspid aortic valve in systole. The bicuspid aortic valve shows an abnormal opening motion. Unlike the triangular opening of the normal tricuspid valve, the bicuspid valve (arrow) forms a "clam shell" configuration as it opens. (Ao = aortic root; LA = left atrium.)

leaflets. There is restricted leaflet motion in systole and doming during left ventricular ejection.[33] This doming of the aortic valve can be seen in the long-axis (Fig. 5–46), short-axis (Fig. 5–47), and subxiphoidal (Fig. 5–48) views. The short-axis view of the aortic valve may be used to identify the "clam shell" bicuspid configuration rather than the normal "Mercedes-Benz" tricuspid valve (Fig. 5–49). The long-axis view of left ventricular outflow tract may also define the presence of a poststenotic dilatation of the ascending aorta.[34]

Angiographic Features

Embryologically, the aortic valve originates from two separate sources. The right and left cusps are derived from the truncal swelling.[35] It is understandable, therefore, that the majority of bicuspid aortic valves have one component represented by the posterior cusp and a second component represented by the fused right and left cusps.

In the child, the characteristic angiographic features of the bicuspid aortic valve are best seen on the ascending aortogram. An eccentric jet of nonopacified blood may be seen above the domed cusps (Fig. 5–50A). Poststenotic dilatation of the ascending aorta (usually the right anterolateral wall) is a fairly constant feature of the significantly stenotic aortic valve (Fig. 5–50A). The most common type of bicuspid valve reveals an enlarged inferior cusp representing the posterior, or noncoronary, cusp (Fig. 5–50B). The smaller fused right and left cusps are superimposed on the dominant posterior cusp in the lateral projection and are often unequal in size (Fig. 5–50B). The false raphe may occasionally be seen as a small radiolucent filling defect separating the right and left cusps. Thickening of the valve cusps is best visualized on the left ventriculogram, where diminished excursion or doming of the leaflets is seen in systole (Fig. 5–51). In the second variety of bicuspid valve, the left cusp is dominant and the right and posterior cusps are fused. This is best appreciated in the frontal projection.

Subaortic Stenosis

Subaortic stenosis is defined as a limited narrowing of the left ventricular outflow tract at or just below the aortic valve. This

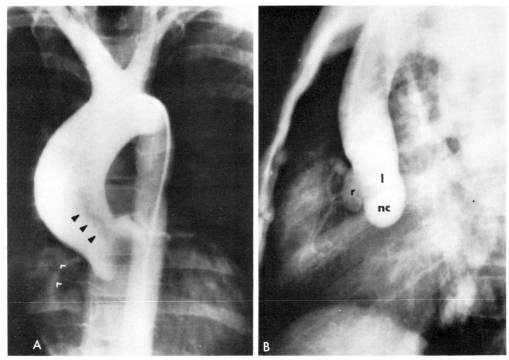

Figure 5–50. A, Posteroanterior ascending aortogram in a child with significant aortic stenosis. The valve is domed, and a jet of nonopacified blood is well visualized (arrowheads). The ascending aorta shows significant poststenotic dilatation. This child's chest film is shown in Figure 5–43A. B, This lateral ascending aortogram was obtained in a patient with aortic coarctation and a bicuspid aortic valve. The noncoronary cusp (NC) is dilated and the right (r) and left (l) cusps are small.

type of left ventricular outflow obstruction is about one-fifth as frequent as valvar aortic stenosis.[36] The lesion is classified into four types, based on angiographic features:[37] Type I, a thin (1 to 2 mm), membranous diaphragmatic stenosis usually located within 2 cm or less of the aortic valve; Type II, a thicker, collar-like stenosis; Type III, a fibromuscular stenosis that is irregular and has additional tissue; and Type IV, a fixed tunnel-like narrowing of the left ventricular outflow tract (so-called "tunnel" aortic stenosis). The aortic valve is usually tricuspid and frequently thickened. Aortic regurgitation occurs in over 50 per cent of patients with subaortic stenosis.[26] The thickening and regurgitation are believed to result from the constant bombardment of the valve by the jet created across the subaortic obstruction.[38] Significant associated defects are present in over 50 per cent of patients and may mask the clinical and catheterization features of subaortic stenosis.[39] The most common associated malformation is a ventricular septal defect.[39]

Another form of subaortic stenosis is dynamic in nature and is found in children with hypertrophic cardiomyopathy who have *functional* subaortic stenosis (hypertrophic subaortic stenosis). Their ventricles demonstrate the following features:[40] (1) greater thickening of the ventricular septum than of the left ventricular free wall (95 per cent); (2) small or normal-sized left and right ventricular cavities (95 per cent); (3) disordered arrangement of myocardial fibers in the ventricular septum (95 per cent); and (4) abnormal intramural coronary arteries (50 per cent). Adults with hypertrophic cardiomyopathy may demonstrate the following additional features:[40] (1) mural endocardial plaque in the left ventricular outflow tract (75 per cent); (2) a thickened mitral valve (75 per cent); and (3) dilated atria.

Most patients with this disorder have some degree of mitral regurgitation. The postulated mechanism for this valvar incompetence in association with a myopathy is thought to relate to an abnormal position

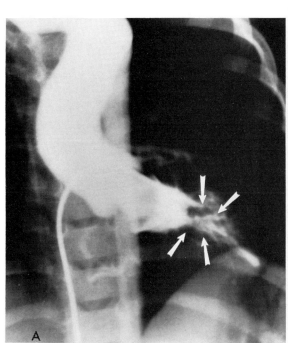
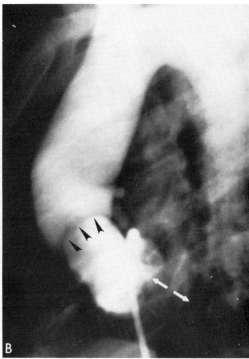

Figure 5–51. Posteroanterior (A) and lateral (B) left ventriculogram in a child with significant aortic stenosis. Left ventricular hypertrophy is indicated by the prominent papillary muscles (arrows) and thickened posterior wall (double arrows) on the lateral view. The domed and thickened aortic valve is best visualized in the lateral view (arrowheads). Significant poststenotic aortic dilatation is present.

of the anterolateral papillary muscle.[41] The hypertrophied septum bulges into the left ventricular cavity, bending the papillary muscles and putting tension on the chordae tendinae, preventing complete closure of the mitral valve in systole.

Radiographic Features

When the gradient across the left ventricular outflow tract leads to significant left ventricular hypertrophy, this may be appreciated on the frontal chest film as a left ventricular configuration (Fig. 5–52). As such it is indistinguishable from the normal-sized left ventricular configuration seen with any left ventricular stress problem (see description under aortic stenosis). Although a normal ascending aorta is the rule with discrete subaortic stenosis (Fig. 5–52), dilatation of the ascending aorta has been described. This is usually mild and associated with a membrane that is 1 cm or less below the aortic valve.[26] With significant volume overload and dilatation of the left ventricle secondary to aortic regurgitation, an en-larged left ventricular configuration may be noted on the chest x-ray (Fig. 5–53).

The radiographic features of the other forms of subaortic obstruction (tunnel aortic stenosis and hypertrophic subaortic stenosis) tend to be rather nonspecific. In the patient with hypertrophic cardiomyopathy (idiopathic hypertrophic subaortic stenosis) the cardiac contour on the chest radiography may reveal an unusually prominent left midheart border (Fig. 5–54A). This is due to hypertrophy of the anterior septal region. Mild left atrial enlargement frequently coexists (Fig. 5–54A), since mitral regurgitation is so common in this lesion. The left ventricle may become considerably enlarged in this entity (Fig. 5–54B).

Echocardiographic Features

Subaortic obstructions can result in characteristic abnormalities of aortic valve motion. M-mode echocardiographic studies of patients with fixed subaortic stenosis may demonstrate early systolic closure of the aortic valve. The jet of blood flowing

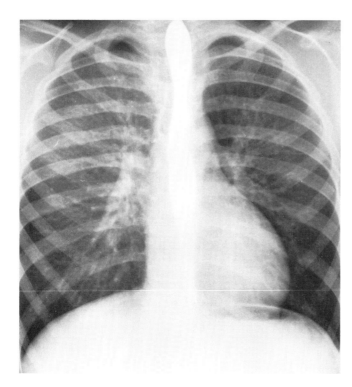

Figure 5–52. Posteroanterior chest radiograph in a 12-year-old boy with a systolic murmur in the aortic position. Pulmonary vascularity is normal. Although the heart is normal in size, there is a left ventricular configuration. Note that the ascending aorta is not dilated. This child had discrete membranous subaortic stenosis.

Figure 5–53. Posteroanterior chest radiograph in a 14-year-old boy with membranous subaortic stenosis and significant aortic regurgitation. There is mild pulmonary venous hypertension (redistribution of flow) and an enlarged left ventricular configuration.

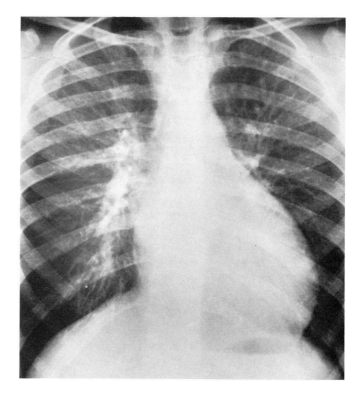

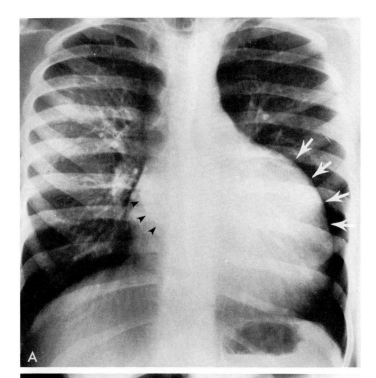

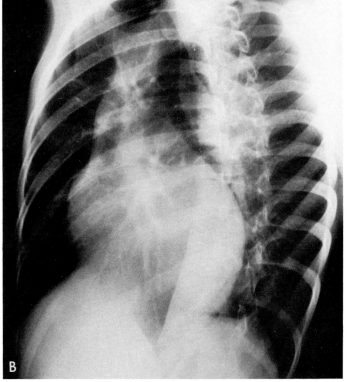

Figure 5-54. Posteroanterior (A) and left anterior oblique (B) chest radiographs in an 18-year-old boy with hypertrophic obstructive cardiomyopathy (idiopathic hypertrophic subaortic stenosis). The unusually prominent left mid heart border (arrows) is due to the hypertrophied anterior septal region. Note the double density along the right heart border (arrowheads), indicating left atrial enlargement. The large left ventricle projects well beyond the spine in the LAO projection, indicating significant left ventricular enlargement.

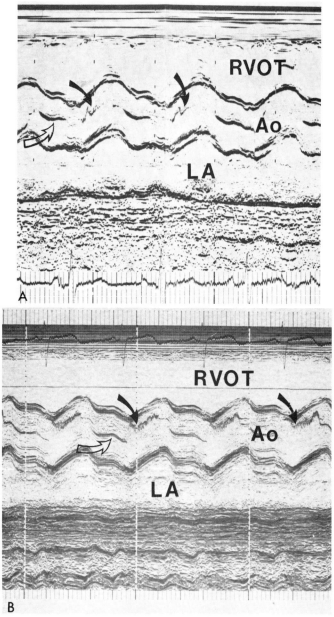

Figure 5–55. Discrete subaortic stenosis. A, In discrete subaortic stenosis, the aortic valve motion is characterized by early systolic closure of the aortic valve secondary to the effect of the jet of blood passing through the center of the aortic valve leaflets. On the M-mode scan, this results in a discrete early systolic notch (closed arrow) with no evidence of aortic valve eccentricity (open arrow). B, Characteristically, the aortic valve is noted to flutter coarsely following the early systolic notch. This is well visualized here (closed arrow). Multiple diastolic echoes may suggest aortic valve leaflet thickening, but the closure line is usually noted in a symmetric position (open arrow).

through the aortic valve in systole creates a Bernoulli effect that partially closes the valve tissue in early systole (Fig. 5–55A). The partially closed leaflets then vibrate coarsely as the jet strikes them during the remainder of systole[42] (Fig. 5–55B). Eventu-

ally, this may damage and thicken the aortic valve and cause subsequent regurgitation. Left ventricular outflow tract obstruction caused by a subaortic membrane is most securely diagnosed by two-dimensional echocardiography (Fig. 5–56).[43] The diag-

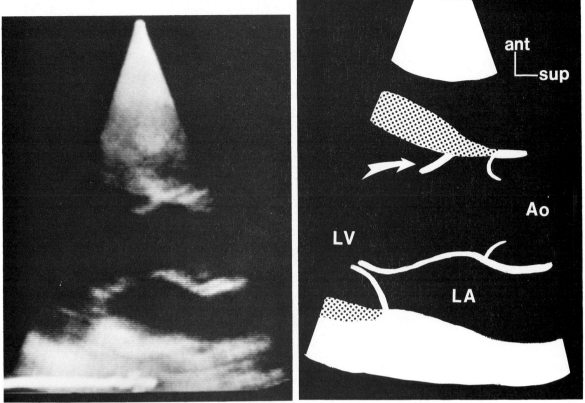

Figure 5–56. Discrete membranous subaortic stenosis. Long-axis view of the left ventricle and outflow tract in a patient with discrete subaortic stenosis. Note the membrane (arrow) arising from the interventricular septum in a position separate from the aortic valve leaflets by approximately 1 cm. (Ao = aortic root; LA = left atrium; LV = left ventricle.)

nostic criteria are highly reliable and specific for this entity, since the membrane produces a directly visible signal on the echocardiogram. The long-axis and sub-xiphoidal left ventricular outflow tract views are preferable for diagnosis of this entity (Fig. 5–56).[43-44] M-mode techniques for prediction of left ventricular peak systolic pressure can be used to estimate the gradient across the subaortic membrane in a manner similar to that of the unoperated patient with valvar aortic stenosis (see Fig. 5–44).

Tunnel subaortic stenosis is best diagnosed on two-dimensional echocardiography using the long-axis or subxiphoidal view (Fig. 5–57). In this entity, the aortic valve leaflets move normally and the valve is composed of three leaflets (demonstrated on the short-axis view). The long-axis view demonstrates excessive thickening of the membranous and upper muscular portion of

the ventricular septum, so much so that it encroaches on the left ventricular outflow tract. The lower portion of the muscular septum, however, is not disproportionately hypertrophied, and there is no evidence of systolic anterior motion of the mitral valve on the M-mode tracing, thus distinguishing this entity from idiopathic hypertrophic subaortic stenosis.

Hypertrophic obstructive cardiomyopathy (idiopathic hypertrophic subaortic stenosis) is best diagnosed from the long-axis view, since the comparative thickness of the interventricular septum and left ventricular posterior wall can be easily compared. Diagnosis can be made with either M-mode (Fig. 5–58) or real-time echocardiography[34, 45] (Fig. 5–59), although the M-mode tracing is useful for documenting the dynamic aspect of the left ventricular outflow tract obstruction by demonstrating abrupt, transient, mid-to-late systolic closure of the

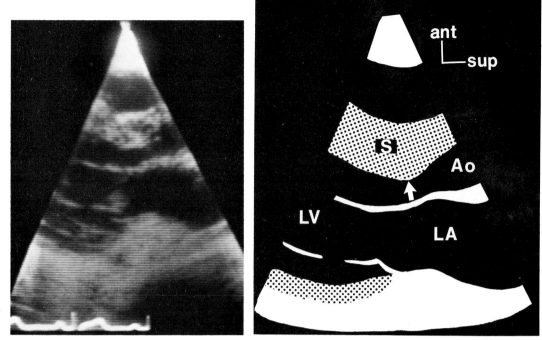

Figure 5–57. Tunnel subaortic stenosis. Left ventricular outflow tract in long-axis of a patient with tunnel subaortic stenosis. The left ventricular outflow tract obstruction is visualized as an elongated area of fixed obstruction below the level of the aortic valve leaflets. Note the area of "heaping up" of excess tissue on the interventricular septum with resulting (arrow) narrowing of the subaortic region. (Ao = aorta; LA = left atrium; LV = left ventricle; S = interventricular septum.)

aortic valve as flow out of the ventricle is interrupted (Fig. 5–58).[46] In this disease, the septum is substantially thicker than the posterior wall and may be triangularly shaped, being thinnest in the upper portion of the ventricular septum. Although systolic anterior motion of the mitral valve ("SAM") can be demonstrated on both the M-mode and real-time tracings, the long-axis two-dimensional view best demonstrates the narrowing of the left ventricular outflow tract resulting from this abnormal mitral motion (Fig. 5–59).

Angiographic Features

Discrete membranous subaortic stenosis may be difficult to diagnose using standard posteroanterior and lateral left ventriculography.[47] This is especially true when the membrane is in its most common location, within 5 mm of the aortic valve[26] or when it is associated with other cardiac defects.[39] When the membrane is well below the aortic valve, standard techniques may be adequate (Fig. 5–60). Left ventriculograms

obtained in the axial projections (long axial oblique and hepatoclavicular views) enhance precision in the diagnosis of subvalvar aortic stenosis. These views may demonstrate the membrane when standard views do not (Fig. 5–61).[48] Discrete membranous subaortic stenosis and hypertrophic subaortic stenosis may have two angiographic features in common. They are both associated with left ventricular hypertrophy and a lucent subaortic filling defect. In the former the defect is the membrane itself (Fig. 5–60), while in the latter it results from the abnormally positioned anterior mitral valve leaflet (Fig. 5–62C). This systolic anterior mitral leaflet position can best be appreciated on the lateral left ventriculogram (see Fig. 5–62B).

The angiographic features of hypertrophic obstructive cardiomyopathy (idiopathic hypertrophic subaortic stenosis) have been well described.[49, 50] In systole, the hypertrophied septum impinges on the left ventricular outflow tract (Fig. 5–62A and B). This is best appreciated in the left anterior oblique or hepatoclavicular projection (Fig.

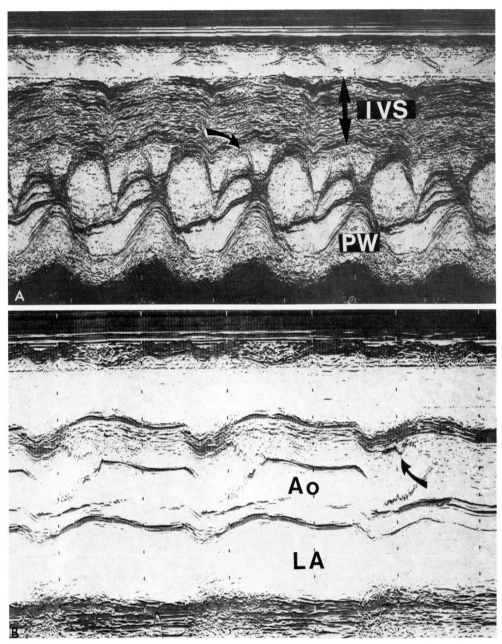

Figure 5–58. Hypertrophic obstructive cardiomyopathy (idiopathic hypertrophic subaortic stenosis). *A,* M-mode echocardiogram shows asymmetric septal hypertrophy with the interventricular septal dimension (IVS) exceeding the thickness of the left ventricular posterior wall (PW) by a ratio of greater than 1.5 in diastole. The anterior mitral valve leaflet shows systolic anterior motion ("SAM"). The leaflet causes dynamic left ventricular outflow tract obstruction by coming into apposition with the interventricular septum in peak systole (curved arrow). *B,* M-mode echocardiogram of the aortic valve in the patient shown in *A.* Note the characteristic mid systolic partial closure of the aortic valve leaflet (arrow). This is due to reduction in aortic flow as a consequence of the dynamic subaortic obstruction. Following the partial closure, the aortic valve leaflet flutters during the remainder of systole. (Ao = aortic root; LA = left atrium.)

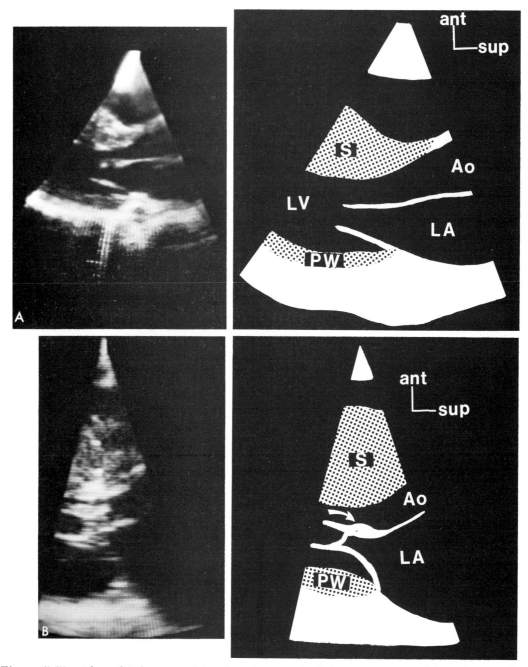

Figure 5–59. Idiopathic hypertrophic subaortic stenosis. *A,* Long-axis view of the left ventricle in diastole. Note the asymmetric thickening of the interventricular septum (S) well in excess of the posterior wall thickness (PW). (LV = left ventricle; Ao = aorta; LA = left atrium.) *B,* Long-axis view of the left ventricle in the same patient during systole. Note the marked thickening of the interventricular septum (S) compared with the thickness of the left ventricular posterior wall (PW). Systolic anterior motion ("SAM") of the mitral valve is seen (curved arrow). The systolic anterior motion of the mitral valve brings it into apposition with the interventricular septum resulting in dynamic subaortic obstruction. (LA = left atrium; Ao = aorta.)

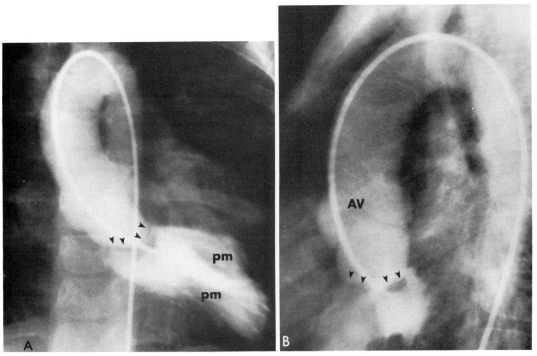

Figure 5-60. Posteroanterior *(A)* and lateral *(B)* left ventriculogram showing a discrete membrane (arrowheads) located well below the aortic valve (AV). Left ventricular hypertrophy is indicated by the large papillary muscles (PM).

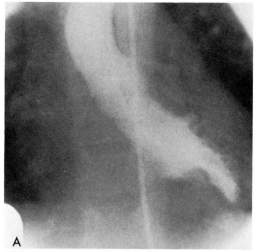

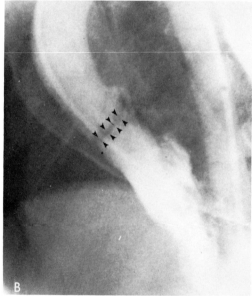

Figure 5–61. *A,* Posteroanterior left ventriculogram. The patient had a 50 mmHg pressure gradient across the aortic valve region. *B,* Repeat left ventriculogram in hepatoclavicular projection clearly shows a thin membrane immediately beneath the aortic valve (arrowheads). This membrane was not appreciated on the standard PA view.

5–62C). The papillary muscles may be extremely hypertrophied (Fig. 5–62A), and mild mitral regurgitation is invariably present (Fig. 5–62A). The LAO view in systole demonstrates the essential deformity of this condition. The anterior (and to a lesser extent, the posterior) mitral leaflet, instead of moving posteriorly to widen the outflow tract, moves anteriorly into the outflow tract to contact the hypertrophied septum (Fig.

5–62C). The line of contact of the anterior leaflet and the septum may be seen as a "V" or "W-shaped" radiolucent line several centimeters below the aortic valve (Fig. 5–62C).

Cardiomyopathy and Myocarditis

Endocardial fibroelastosis and other forms of nonobstructive cardiomyopathy are rare in the older child. When present, they may be of the nonobstructive hypertrophic variety or the dilated, "congestive" type. The latter entity may be idiopathic or associated with previous inflammation of the myocardium (myocarditis). These children usually present with congestive heart failure and cardiomegaly (Fig. 5–63). Frequently, both the left and right ventricles are enlarged (Fig. 5–64).

The rare variety of hypertrophic cardiomyopathy — namely, that associated with *symmetrical* left ventricular hypertrophy — can readily be distinguished from the more common asymmetric variety. Although the left ventriculogram in diastole and systole will show evidence of hypertrophy (Fig. 5–65A–D), the anterior mitral leaflet moves normally in systole (Fig. 5–65B and D) and no lucent line is seen in the subaortic region (Fig. 5–65C and D).

Echocardiographic Features

The long-axis two-dimensional echocardiographic view allows visualization of the contractile pattern of the septum and posterior wall as well as an assessment of left ventricular chamber dimensions in children with left ventricular myopathies (cardiomyopathy and myocarditis) (Fig. 5–66). Some investigators have applied various formulae for evaluation of ventricular volumes to these studies and have claimed accuracy in evaluating ventricular ejection fractions and stroke volumes.[51] Dyskinetic areas as well as areas of aneurysm and hypokinesis can be readily diagnosed.[52, 53] In addition, this technique provides the capacity to follow the progress of a cardiomyopathy without resorting to invasive studies. These clinical problems are frequently found in the adult population and are less often encountered in the pediatric age group. They may, however, be encountered in association with viral myocarditis,

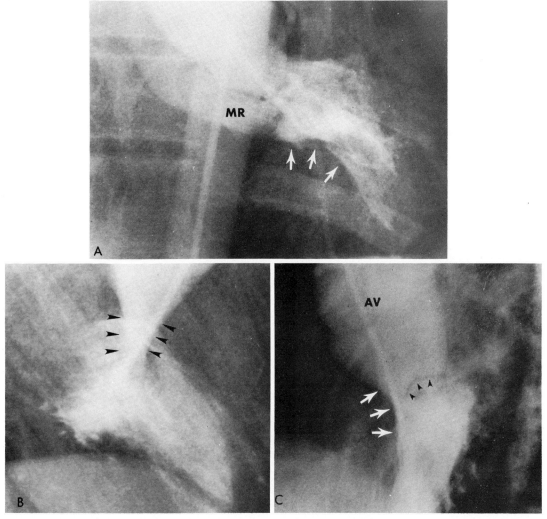

Figure 5-62. Posteroanterior *(A)*, lateral *(B)* and left anterior oblique *(C)* left ventriculograms in a child with hypertrophic obstructive cardiomyopathy. In systole the inferior wall is hypertrophied (arrows) and mitral regurgitation is present (MR). In the lateral view the narrowed outflow tract is seen (arrowheads). In the LAO view obtained in systole, a V-shaped lucency (arrowheads) is well seen beneath the aortic valve (AV). This represents the line of contact between the hypertrophied septum (arrows) and the anterior leaflet of the mitral valve.

congestive cardiomyopathy, and the rare anomalies of coronary artery origin (for example, anomalous left coronary artery from the pulmonary artery)[54] and in patients with coronary aneurysms secondary to the mucocutaneous lymph node syndrome.[55] Echocardiographic studies are of value in the sequential evaluation of left ventricular function in children receiving cardiotoxic medications. These children are seen in increasing numbers in institutions actively involved in chemotherapeutic protocols uti-

lizing drugs such as doxorubicin (Adriamycin)[56] for the treatment of malignant diseases.

Supravalvar Aortic Stenosis

This is the least common form of obstruction to left ventricular outflow. Three distinct types of supravalvar aortic stenosis have been described.[57] The most frequent is a localized, hourglass narrowing just above

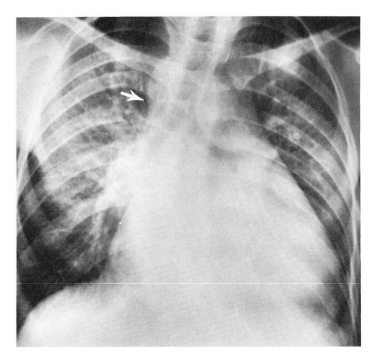

Figure 5–63. Posteroanterior chest radiograph in a seven-year-old child with chronic congestive heart failure. Severe pulmonary venous hypertension is evident as is marked cardiomegaly (both right and left ventricular enlargement). The azygous vein is dilated (arrow), suggesting systemic venous hypertension as well. This child had a history of myocarditis. Two-dimensional echocardiography revealed a dilated, congestive cardiomyopathy (see Fig. 5–66).

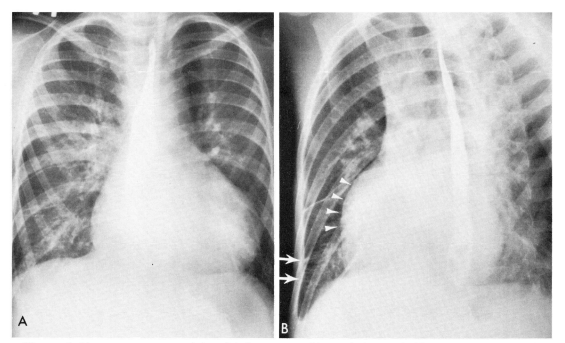

Figure 5–64. Posteroanterior (A) and left anterior oblique (B) in a child with acute myocarditis. There is moderate pulmonary venous hypertension (note the Kerley B lines — arrows) and biventricular enlargement. The enlarged right heart is best appreciated in the LAO view (arrowheads).

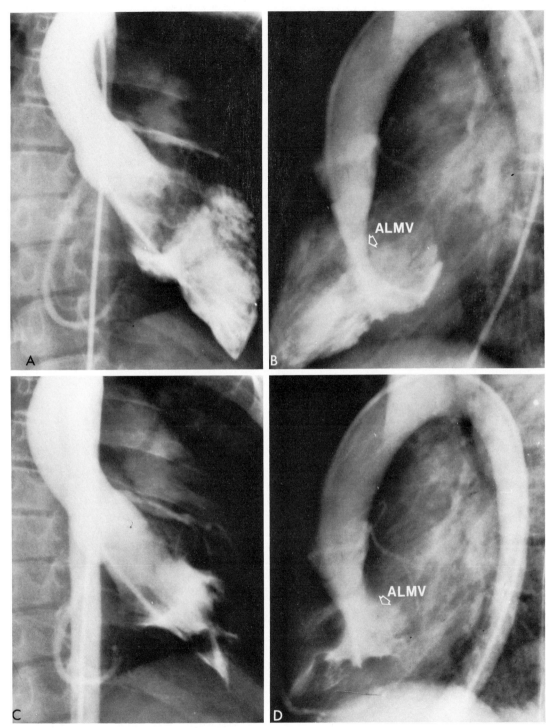

Figure 5–65. Diastolic posteroanterior *(A)* and lateral *(B)* and systolic posteroanterior *(C)*, and lateral *(D)* views of the left ventriculogram in a child with a symmetrical hypertrophic cardiomyopathy. The systolic angiograms show virtual cavity obliteration caused by the hypertrophied myocardium. Note that the anterior leaflet of the mitral valve (ALMV) moves appropriately in diastole and systole and does not cause ventricular outflow tract obstruction.

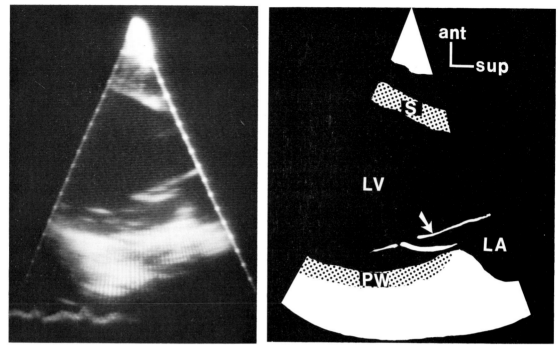

Figure 5-66. Dilated (congestive) cardiomyopathy. Long-axis view of the left ventricle in a patient with severe congestive heart failure. The left ventricle (LV) is massively dilated. The real-time study showed minimal change in left ventricular dimensions between systole and diastole, with a resulting low ventricular ejection fraction. The septum (S) and posterior wall (PW) were poorly contractile. (LA = left atrium, arrow = mitral valve.)

the aortic sinuses. The aortic sinuses are prominent and the ascending aorta above the narrowing is usually normal in caliber. The second type is characterized by a discrete fibrous membrane located in a normal-sized ascending aorta. The third type is associated with tubular hypoplasia of the ascending aorta that begins just above the aortic sinuses and often extends into the aortic arch. The coronary arteries in all three types are often dilated, tortuous, and may undergo early atherosclerotic degeneration.[57] The aortic valve cusps are thickened in almost a third of patients.[58]

Stenosis of the pulmonary artery and its branches,[59] valvar and discrete subvalvar aortic stenosis,[60] coarctation of the aorta,[60] Marfan's syndrome,[61] and rubella syndrome[61] have all been associated with supravalvar aortic stenosis. In addition, a syndrome of supravalvar aortic stenosis, idiopathic hypercalcemia, coexistent pulmonary artery and branch stenosis, physical and mental retardation, and "elfin" facies is well described — the so-called infantile hypercalcemia syndrome.[62, 63]

Radiographic Features

The chest x-ray is indistinguishable from that of aortic stenosis, with one important exception. Since the ascending aorta is small to diminutive in this entity, a prominent ascending aorta is not present. Because of this, the region of the mediastinum usually occupied by the ascending aorta may appear relatively lucent and the right mainstem bronchus may be particularly obvious (Fig. 5–67). We call this the "ascending aortic window."

Echocardiographic Features

In the isolated form of this left ventricular outflow obstruction, the long-axis view of the ascending aorta may demonstrate an area of constriction in the supravalvar aorta consistent with supravalvar aortic stenosis.[34] Associated lesions may be diagnosed when the left ventricular outflow tract is narrowed in the subvalvar area either by a discrete subaortic membrane (Fig. 5–56) or by a

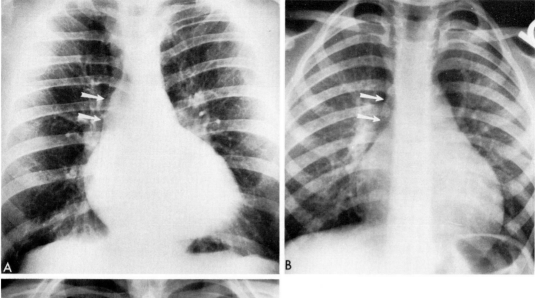

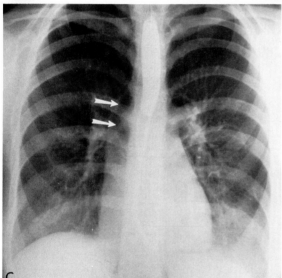

Figure 5-67. Posteroanterior chest radiographs in two children (*A* and *B*) and one teenager (*C*) with supravalvar aortic stenosis. The pulmonary vascularity is normal in all three, and the left ventricle is prominent in the two children. In all three patients, there is a lucent area along the right upper heart border in the region normally occupied by the ascending aorta (arrows). The hypoplastic ascending aorta (see Figs. 5–68 and 5–69) associated with this lesion accounts for this "ascending aortic window."

collar of tissue involving a considerable length of the outflow tract (tunnel subaortic stenosis) (Fig. 5–57).

Angiographic Features

The three anatomic types of supravalvar aortic stenosis can be readily identified using posteroanterior and lateral ascending thoracic aortography. The most frequent type involves a localized "hourglass" constriction immediately above the aortic sinuses of Valsalva (Fig. 5–68). The aorta above the constriction is usually normal or reduced in size. The type associated with uniform hypoplasia begins just above the

sinuses of Valsalva and may extend into the brachiocephalic arteries (Fig. 5–69A). Since the coronary arteries are proximal to the obstruction in this lesion, they are exposed to elevated pressures generated in the noncompliant sinuses of Valsalva. It is not surprising that they become dilated and tortuous (Fig. 5–69C and D) and may undergo premature atherosclerotic changes.[64] The most infrequent variety of supravalvar aortic stenosis is that associated with a discrete membrane above the aortic valve. A pulmonary angiogram should be performed in patients with supravalvar aortic stenosis because of the common association of pulmonary artery branch stenosis (Fig. 5–70).

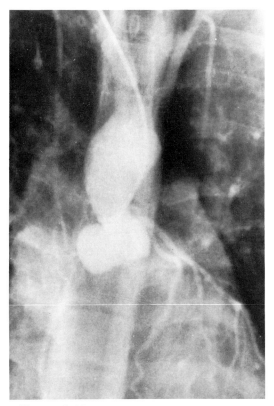

Figure 5–68. Posteroanterior ascending aortogram performed in the teenager whose chest radiograph is illustrated in Figure 5–67C. The constriction immediately above the sinuses of Valsalva gives an "hourglass" appearance to the ascending aorta in this most frequent variety of supravalvar aortic stenosis.

Coarctation of the Aorta

Coarctation refers to a congenital anomaly of the aorta characterized by constriction or obliteration of a section of that vessel. In almost all instances, the constriction is immediately below the origin of the left subclavian artery and the insertion of the ductus arteriosus or ligamentum arteriosum ("juxtaductal" coarctation). Early terminology regarding classification of coarctation of the aorta into "infantile" or diffuse and "adult" or localized forms implied that these anatomic types were characteristic of specific age groups. This terminology should be discarded in light of recent clinical and physiologic data.[65, 66] In a study of 41 infants, 23 had a long segment of diffuse narrowing involving the aortic isthmus (that region distal to the subclavian artery). All 23 infants had other major intracardiac an-

omalies, with VSD being present in 22. In the remaining 18 infants, the aortic obstruction was juxtaductal and usually well localized. Intracardiac anomalies were uncommon in this second group and confined to simple ventricular septal defects.

The basic pathologic lesion in localized aortic coarctation is a juxtaductal indentation, or "shelf," involving the posterior wall of the aorta. It is postulated that during fetal life, when the ductus is patent, there is no aortic obstruction. As the ductus closes after birth, it "removes" its contribution to the narrowed aortic lumen at the site of the posterior shelf, and the result is a local obstruction in the aorta.[66] An obstruction (either functional or organic) to left ventricular flow into the aorta in fetal life would lead to a decrease in flow through the isthmus and increase flow through the pulmonary artery, ductus arteriosus, and descending aorta. This may be the reason for the hypoplasia of the aortic isthmus noted in some infants with coarctation.[67]

Collateral circulation in coarctation of the aorta is well developed and may be extensive even in early life. The major pathways are

1. An anterior pathway through the internal mammary arteries leading to the deep epigastric branches and the external iliac arteries.

2. A posterior system arising from the subclavian arteries and communicating through the costocervical trunk with the highest intercostal arteries and then with the posterior intercostal arteries. Blood flows in a direction opposite the usual into the thoracic aorta below the coarctation.

3. A parascapular anastomosis connecting the subclavian arteries with the descending aorta through the intercostal arteries.

Notching of the ribs occurring in the costal grooves of the posterior ribs results from pulsatile collateral flow through the dilated and tortuous posterior intercostal arteries. The anterior ribs are not involved, since the anterior intercostal arteries do not course in the costal grooves.[68]

Coarctation of the aorta is frequently associated with other cardiac anomalies. Chief among these is a bicuspid aortic valve occurring in 46 per cent of one autopsy series.[69] The valve may be stenotic, incompetent, or functionally normal.[70] Complex intracardiac anomalies are often found

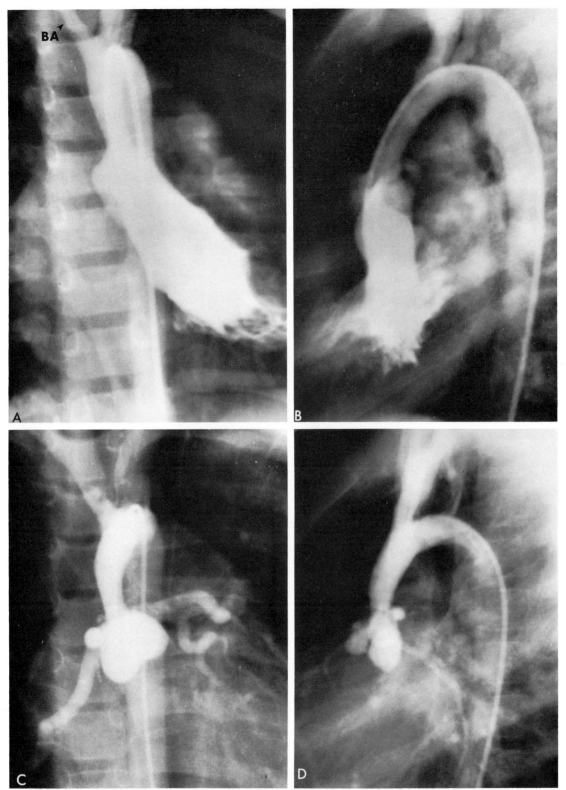

Figure 5–69. Posteroanterior *(A)* and lateral *(B)* left ventriculogram performed in the child whose chest film is shown in Figure 5–67B. The left ventricle is hypertrophied, the ascending aorta is uniformly hypoplastic, and the brachiocephalic artery (BA) is narrowed at its origin. Posteroanterior *(C)* and lateral *(D)* ascending aortograms performed in the same patient show the prominent sinuses of Valsalva and dilated, tortuous coronary arteries.

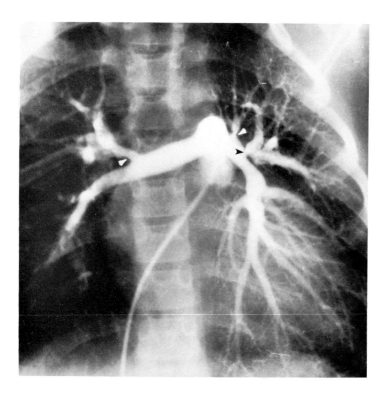

Figure 5–70. Anteroposterior pulmonary angiogram in a child with supravalvar aortic stenosis. Multiple pulmonary artery branch stenoses are present (arrowheads).

when coarctation is associated with aortic isthmus narrowing.[65] There is a close association between aortic coarctation and abnormalities of the mitral apparatus.[71] These consist of leaflet deformities; shortening, lengthening, or fusion of chordae; and single papillary muscle (parachute mitral valve). There also is a well-developed complex consisting of supravalvar mitral stenosis ring, parachute mitral valve, discrete subvalvar aortic stenosis, and coarctation of the aorta.[69]

Congestive heart failure associated with coarctation presents in two well-defined age groups: during early infancy (see first section of this chapter) and after the third decade. Coarctation is one of the most common causes of congestive heart failure in the first months of life.[72]

Radiographic Features

Two diverse chest x-ray appearances manifest themselves depending upon whether coarctation of the aorta presents before or after age two. Radiographic features of coarctation occurring in the infant or young child have been described in the previous section.

Since serious symptoms are uncommon in the child over two years and under 15 years of age with coarctation, the chest film may provide clues that first raise the suspicion of the presence of the lesion. Rib notching occurs in approximately 75 per cent of older children with coarctation,[73] and is more obvious in the older child or adult (Fig. 5–71). This points out the fact that careful evaluation of extracardiac structures can be productive in the evaluation of children with suspected heart disease. Notching is typically confined to the mid or outer undersurfaces of posterior ribs three through eight (Fig. 5–71). Collateral circulation requires patency of the subclavian arteries in the high pressure zone. If notching is confined to the left ribs, one can predict that the right subclavian artery arises anomalously distal to the coarctation. Notching of the right ribs only signifies that the constriction is proximal to the left subclavian artery or involves the orifice of the left subclavian. Another manifestation of collateral circulation is a wavy substernal density seen on the lateral chest film (Fig. 5–71B). This represents the dilated, tortuous internal mammary arteries and is most commonly seen in older children or adults (Fig. 5–71C).

The pulmonary vascularity in the older age group is usually normal (Fig. 5–72A and

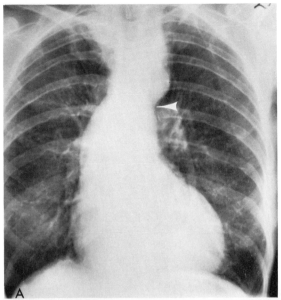

Figure 5–71. Posteroanterior *(A)* and lateral *(B)* chest radiographs and lateral thoracic aortogram *(C)* in an adult with coarctation of the aorta. Rib notching is quite apparent on the undersurfaces of ribs three through nine. There is a left ventricular configuration and prominent ascending aorta. An inward indentation of the proximal descending aorta (arrowhead) marks the point of coarctation. The lateral view shows wavy substernal densities representing dilated internal mammary arterial collaterals (arrows). These are better visualized on the aortogram (arrows). There is heavy calcification of the aortic valve (arrowheads). The angiogram shows a bicuspid aortic valve and the coarctation (arrowheads).

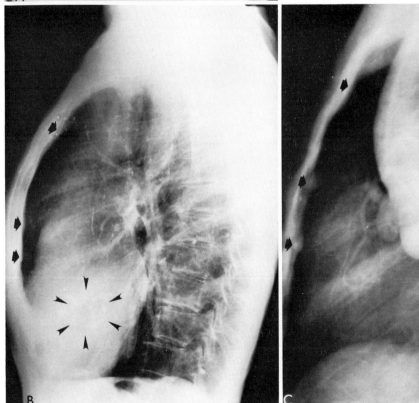

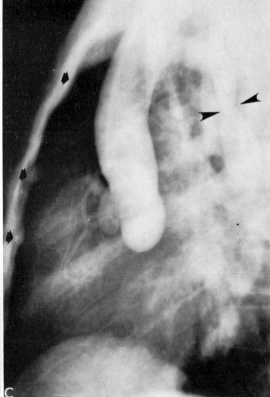

B). The cardiac silhouette may be normal but usually shows a left ventricular configuration and a prominent ascending aorta (Figs. 5–71A and 5–72A). If rib notching is noted the diagnosis is obvious. If not, the findings may be identical to and confused with those of aortic stenosis. An important region to assess in distinguishing these two lesions is the aortic knob. The aortic knob in aortic stenosis is normal or prominent,

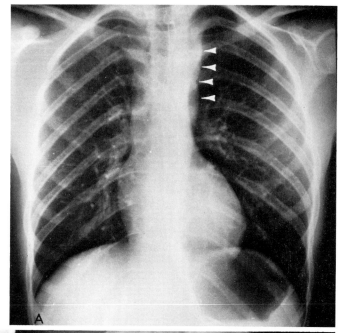

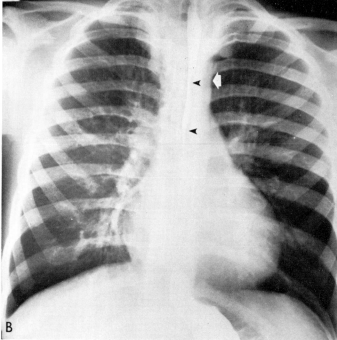

Figure 5–72. Posteroanterior chest radiographs in two children with coarctation of the aorta. Both have normal pulmonary vascularity and normal heart size with a left ventricular configuration. Rib notching is not apparent in either case. The aortic knob region gives valuable clues to the diagnosis in both cases. In *A*, the figure "3" is created by the left subclavian artery and the coarctation (arrowheads). For angiographic correlation see Figure 5–73. In *B*, the aortic knob is indistinct (arrow) owing to hypoplasia of the aortic isthmus. The barium swallow in this case shows the "Ɛ" sign (arrowheads) caused by aortic impressions above and below the coarctation.

while in coarctation it may be flattened or indistinct owing to hypoplasia of the aortic isthmus (Fig. 5–72*B*). The density of the left subclavian artery, which is often inferiorly displaced and dilated in coarctation, may appear in the region normally occupied by the aortic knob (Fig. 5–72*A*). In addition, the region of poststenotic dilatation below the coarctation can often be appreciated (Fig. 5–72*A*), especially if the chest film is overpenetrated. When accompanied by the convex shadow of the left subclavian artery, a figure "3" may be formed (Fig. 5–72*A*). All of these findings can be discerned without the use of barium in the esophagus. With barium, the "Ɛ" sign (mirror image of the

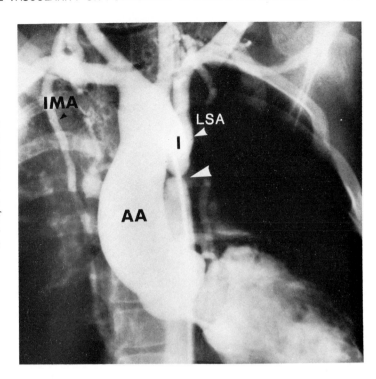

Figure 5–73. Posteroanterior left ventriculogram in the patient whose chest film is illustrated in Figure 5–72A. Note the dilated ascending aorta (AA), the small aortic isthmus (I), inferiorly displaced left subclavian artery (LSA), and the tight coarctation of the aorta (arrowhead). Large internal mammary arteries (IMA) are present.

"3" sign) is created and represents impressions on the esophagus by regions above and below the coarctation (Fig. 5–72B).

Angiographic Findings

Aortic coarctation can be assessed using standard angiographic projections. Care should be taken to visualize the aortic valve (bicuspid or tricuspid?), the aortic isthmus, and origin of the great vessels to the head and extremities (Fig. 5–73). The area of coarctation and the status of the arterial collaterals should also be evaluated (Fig. 5–74). Ischemia to the spinal cord has been associated with injection of contrast into the thoracic aorta in these patients and is thought to be due to high concentrations of contrast material in the anterior spinal artery due to reduction in flow in the low pressure postcoarctation region. Because of this, angiography of coarctation may be carried out as a levophase study following injection of contrast in the pulmonary artery.

Infective Endocarditis

In one series, children with infective endocarditis accounted for 0.5 per 1000 admission to a pediatric hospital center that has an active pediatric cardiology program.[74] The pathogenesis of endocarditis involves a substrate of an abnormal valve or traumatized endocardial surface (due to turbulence or jet effect) that becomes edematous. A sterile platelet-fibrin thrombus forms on the damaged surface and, in the presence of bloodborne clumps of microorganisms (occurring under a wide variety of circumstances), becomes a nidus for the growth of these organisms. Unimpeded by phagocytosis, the organisms become trapped and multiply.[75] Viable organisms may remain during the healing process and fragments of these vegetations may embolize, leading to the formation of an abscess or mycotic aneurysm.

The mitral or aortic valve deformed by rheumatic infections and various congenital cardiac malformations associated with gradients across the defect or valve account for the most common sites of infective endocarditis in childhood.[75] The vegetations occurring in the rheumatic heart tend to form on the atrial surface of the mitral valve and the ventricular surface of the aortic valve.

The sites of vegetations in children with congenital heart disease and their relative incidence is as follows: (These cases make up approximately 10 per cent of pediatric patients with infective endocarditis.[75]) In ventricular septal defects, vegetations occur on the right ventricular rim or on the septal leaflet of the tricuspid valve. Vegetations are found in the right ventricular outflow

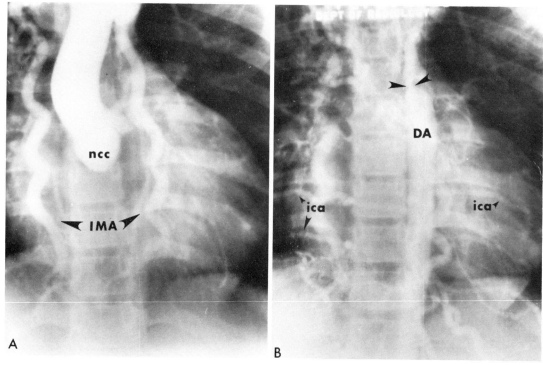

Figure 5–74. Posteroanterior ascending aortogram obtained early *(A)* and late *(B)* following the injection of contrast material. The early film shows a bicuspid aortic valve with a large noncoronary cusp (ncc) and two huge internal mammary arteries (IMA). The descending aorta below the coarctation is not opacified. The late film (B) shows the descending aorta (DA) below the coarctation (arrowhead). It has filled from multiple collaterals, including posterior intercostal arteries (ica) and multiple mediastinal collaterals.

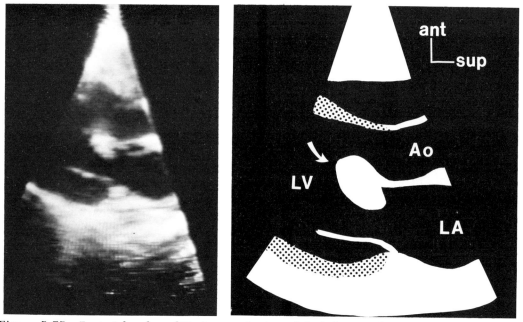

Figure 5–75. Bacterial endocarditis. Long-axis view of the left ventricle in a patient with bacterial endocarditis. A large valvar vegetation (arrow) is seen attached to the anterior leaflet of the mitral valve. This vegetation is seen prolapsing into the left ventricular cavity (LV) during diastole. (Ao = aorta; LA = left atrium.)

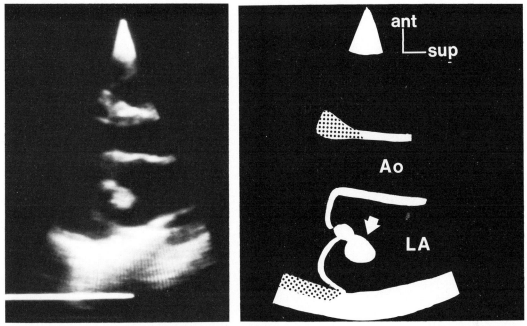

Figure 5–76. Bacterial endocarditis. Long-axis view of the left ventricle in a patient with bacterial endocarditis. A pedunculated valvar vegetation (arrow) is seen attached to the posterior leaflet of the mitral valve, prolapsing into the left atrial cavity (LA) during systole. (Ao = aorta.)

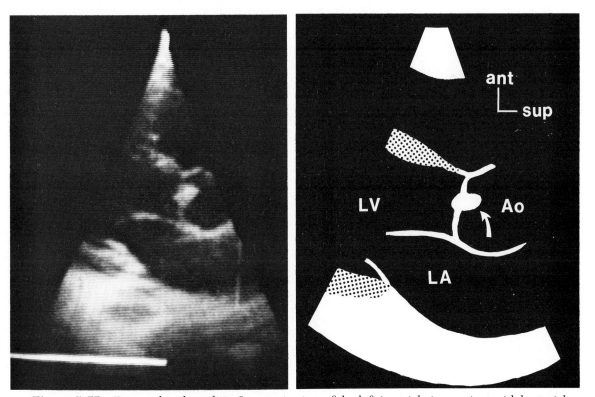

Figure 5–77. Bacterial endocarditis. Long-axis view of the left ventricle in a patient with bacterial endocarditis. A large pedunculated valvar vegetation is seen associated with the aortic valve leaflets (arrow). This patient had bacterial endocarditis superimposed upon a bicuspid aortic valve. (LV = left ventricle; LA = left atrium; Ao = aorta.)

tract or pulmonary valve in tetralogy of Fallot. They occur on a bicuspid aortic valve and on the distal surface of the domed, stenotic pulmonary valve. Vegetations are found on the left pulmonary artery adjacent to the orifice of a patent ductus arteriosus. In coarctation of the aorta, infected material is most commonly located just distal to the coarctation.

In the pediatric population with infective endocarditis, a ventricular septal defect or tetralogy of Fallot is present in approximately 50 per cent of the patients.[75]

Streptococci and staphylococci account for 90 per cent of the cases of childhood infective endocarditis with the most common organism being *Streptococcus viridans*.[76] Unexplained fever is the most common presenting symptom in children with infective endocarditis. A "new" murmur may be difficult to detect in a child who already has organic heart disease. The chest radiograph is of little help in the diagnosis unless unexpected congestive failure is detected in a febrile child with known congenital or rheumatic heart disease.

Echocardiographic Features

Real-time echocardiography can be of value in helping to diagnose the presence of valvar vegetations when the clinical picture suggests infective endocarditis or when positive blood cultures are present.[77] Vegetations may be seen on the mitral (Figs. 5–75 and 5–76) or aortic valve (Fig. 5–77) in the long-axis view and may also be demonstrated in the subxiphoidal view of either the mitral or tricuspid valves. The long-axis view of the right ventricular inflow and outflow tracts is useful for visualizing vegetations on the right-sided valves. The diagnosis of vegetations on echocardiogram may help direct further angiographic studies. The motion of the leaflets may have important implications with regard to the hemodynamic status of the patient, particularly when the complication of ruptured chordae tendineae or prolapsed aortic valve arises. Both these lesions are detectable by two-dimensional echocardiography.

REFERENCES

1. Keith, J. D., Rowe, R. D., Vlad, P.: Heart Disease in Infancy and Childhood. MacMillan Co., New York, 2nd Edition, 1979.
2. Markowitz, M., Gordis, L.: Rheumatic Fever, W. B. Saunders Co., Philadelphia, 1972, p. 1.
3. Ibid., p. 31.
4. Ibid., p. 62.
5. Tehranzadeh, J., Kelley, M. J.: The differential density sign of pericardial effusion. Radiology 133:23–30, 1979.
6. Markowitz and Gordis, op cit, p. 91.
7. Kelley, M. J., Elliott, L. P., Schulman, S. T., Ayoub, E. M., Victorica, B. E., Gessner, I. H.: The significance of left atrial appendage in rheumatic heart disease. Circulation 54:146, 1976.
8. Green, C. E., Kelley, M. J., Higgins, C. B.: Etiologic significance of enlargement of the left atrial appendage in adults. Radiology, In press.
9. Horowitz, M. S., Schultz, C. S., Stinson, E. B., Harrison, D. C., Popp, R. L.: Sensitivity and specificity of echocardiographic diagnosis of pericardial effusion. Circulation 50:239, 1974.
10. Baum, V. C., Hoffman, J. I. E.: Pericardial catheterization. A modification combining two-dimensional echocardiography, an over-the-needle plastic catheter, and a needle-electrode. Pediatr Cardiol 1:159, 1980.
11. Martin, R. P., Bowden, R., Filley, K., Popp, R. L.: Intrapericardial abnormalities in patients with pericardial effusion. Findings by two-dimensional echocardiography. Circulation 61:568, 1980.
12. Markowitz and Gordis, op cit: Chronic rheumatic heart disease, p. 177.
13. Markowitz and Gordis, op cit: Chronic rheumatic heart disease, p. 178.
14. Edwards, J. E., Burchell, H. B.: Pathologic anatomy of mitral insufficiency. Mayo Clin Proc 33:497, 1958.
15. Decker, J. P., Hawn, C., Van, Z., Robbins, S. L.: Rheumatic activity as judged by the presence of Aschoff bodies in auricular appendages of patients with mitral stenosis. Circulation 8:161, 1953.
16. United Kingdom and United States Joint Report: The natural history of rheumatic fever and rheumatic heart disease: Cooperative clinical trial of ACTH, cortisone and aspirin. Circulation 32:457, 1965.
17. Cherian, G., Vytilingam, K. I., Sukumar, I. P., Gopinath, N.: Mitral valvulotomy in young patients. Br Heart J 26:157, 1964.
18. Margarey, F. R.: Pathogenesis of mitral stenosis. Br Med J 1:856, 1951.
19. Henry, W. L., Griffith, J., Michaelis, L. L., McIntosh, C. L., Morrow, A. G., Epstein, S. E.: Measurement of mitral orifice area in patients with mitral valve disease by real-time two-dimensional echocardiography. Circulation 51:827, 1975.
20. Winsberg, F., Gabor, G. E., Hernber, J. C., Weiss, B.: Fluttering of the mitral valve in aortic insufficiency. Circulation 41:225, 1970.
21. Gasul, B. M., Arcilla, R. A., Lev, M.: Heart Disease in Children: Diagnosis and Treatment, Lippincott, Philadelphia, 1966.
22. Krovetz, L. J., Gessner, I. H., Schiebler, G. L.: Handbook of Pediatric Cardiology, Hoeber Harper, New York, 1981.
23. Roberts, W. C.: The congenitally bicuspid aortic valve. A study of 85 autopsy patients. Am J Cardiol 26:72, 1970.

24. Roberts, W. C., Elliott L. P.: Lesions complicating the congenitally bicuspid aortic valve: Anatomic and radiologic features. Radiol Clin North Am 6:410, 1968.

26. Baltaxe, H. A., Moller, J. H., Amplatz, K.: Membranous subaortic stenosis and its associated malformations. Radiology 95:287, 1970.

27. Graham, T. P., Jr., Lewis, B. W., Jarmakani, M. M., et al.: Left heart volume and mass quantification in children with left ventricular pressure overload, Circulation 41:203, Feb., 1970.

28. Bennett, D. H., Evans, D. W., Roy, M. V. J.: Echocardiographic left ventricular dimension pressure and volume overload: Their use in assessing aortic stenosis. Br Heart J 37:971, 1975.

29. Gewitz, M. H., Werner, J. C., Kleinman, C. S., Hellenbrand, W. E., Talner, N. S.: Role of echocardiography in aortic stenosis: Pre- and post-operative studies. Am J Cardiol 43:67, 1979.

30. Glanz, S., Hellenbrand, W. E., Berman, M. A., Talner, N. S.: Echocardiographic assessment of the severity of aortic stenosis in children and adolescents. Am J Cardiol 38:620, 1976.

31. Johnson, G. L., Meyer, R. A., Schwartz, D. C., Korfhagen, J., Kaplan, S.: Echocardiographic evaluation of fixed left ventricular outlet obstruction in children. Circulation 56:299, 1977.

32. Aziz, K. U., van Grondella, A., Paul, M. H., Muster, A. J.: Echocardiographic assessment of the relation between left ventricular wall and cavity dimensions and peak systolic pressure in children with aortic stenosis. Am J Cardiol 40:775, 1977.

33. Weyman, A. E., Feigenbaum, H., Dillon, J. C., Chang, S.: Cross-sectional echocardiography in assessing the severity of valvular aortic stenosis. Circulation 52:828, 1975.

34. Williams, D. E., Sahn, D. J., Friedman, W. F.: Cross-sectional echocardiographic localization of sites of left ventricular outflow tract obstruction. Am J Cardiol 37:250, 1976.

35. Van Mierop, L. H. S.: Ciba Collection: The Heart, Vol. 5.

36. Kelly, D. T., Wulfsberg, E., Rowe, R. D.: Discrete subaortic stenosis. Circulation 46:309, 1972.

37. Deutsch, V., Shem-Tov, A., Yahini, J. H., Neufeld, H. N.: Subaortic stenosis (Discrete form): Classification and angiocardiographic features. Radiology 101:275, 1976.

38. Roberts, W. C.: Congenital Heart Disease in Adults. F. A. Davis Co., Philadelphia, 1979, p. 427.

39. Neufeld, E. A., Muster, A. J., Paul, M. H., Idriss, F. S., Riker, W. L.: Discrete subvalvular aortic stenosis in childhood: Study of 51 patients. Am J Cardiol 38:53, 1976.

40. Roberts, W. C., Ferrans, V. S.: Pathologic anatomy of the cardiomyopathies. Idiopathic dilated and hypertrophic types, infiltrative types, and endomyocardial disease with and without eosinophilia. Hum Pathol 6:287, 1975.

41. Epstein, S. E., Henry, W. L., Clark, C. E., et al.: Asymmetric septal hypertrophy. Ann Intern Med 81:650, 1974.

42. Davis, R. H., Feigenbaum, H., Chang, S., Konecke, L. L., Dillon, J. C.: Echocardiographic manifestations of discrete subaortic stenosis. Am J Cardiol 33:277, 1974.

43. Weyman, A. E., Feigenbaum, H., Hurwitz, R., Girode, D., Dillon, J. C., Chang, S.: Cross-sectional echocardiography in evaluating patients with discrete subaortic stenosis. Am J Cardiol 37:358, 1976.

44. Werner, J. C., Gewitz, M. H., Kleinman, C. S., Hellenbrand, W. E., Talner, N. S.: Real-time echocardiography (RTE) in discrete membranous subaortic stenosis (DMSS). Circulation 58, Suppl. 2:51, 1978 (abstract).

45. Henry, W. L., Clark, C. E., Griffith, J. M., Epstein, S. E.: Mechanism of left ventricular outflow tract obstruction in patients with obstructive asymmetrical hypertrophy. Am J Cardiol 35:330, 1975.

46. Gilbert, B. W., Pollick, C., Adelman, A. G., Wigle, E. D.: Hypertrophic cardiomyopathy: subclassification by M-mode echocardiography. Am J Cardiol 45:861, 1980.

47. Deutsch, V., Shem-Tov, A., Yahini, J. H., et al.: Subaortic stenosis (discrete form): classification and angiographic features. Radiology 101:275, 1971.

48. Kelley, M. J., Higgins, C. B., Kirkpatrick, S. E.: Axial left ventriculography in discrete subaortic stenosis. Radiology 135:77, 1980.

49. Simon, A. L., Ross, J., Jr., Gault, J. H.: Angiographic anatomy of the left ventricle and mitral valve in idiopathic hypertrophic subaortic stenosis. Circulation 36:852, 1967.

50. Simon, A. L.: Angiographic diagnosis of idiopathic hypertrophic subaortic stenosis. Radiol Clin North Am 6:423, 1968.

51. Schiller, N. B., Acquatella, H., Ports, T. A., Drew, D., Goerke, J., Ringertz, H., Silverman, N. H., Brundage, B., Botvinick, E. H., Boswell, R., Carlsson, E., Parmley, W. W.: Left ventricular volume from paried bi-plane two-dimensional echocardiography. Circulation 60:547, 1979.

52. Weyman, A. E., Peskoe, S. M., Williams, E. S., Dillon, J. C., Feigenbaum, H.: Detection of left ventricular aneurysms by cross-sectional echocardiography. Circulation 54:936, 1976.

53. Heger, J. J., Weyman, A. E., Wann, L. S., Dillon, J. C., Feigenbaum, H.: Cross-sectional echocardiography in acute myocardial infarction: detection and localization of regional left ventricular asynergy. Circulation 60:531, 1979.

54. Caldwell, R. L., Weyman, A., Hurwitz, R. A., Girod, D. A., Feigenbaum, H.: Cross-sectional echocardiographic evaluation of coronary artery abnormalities in children. Am J Cardiol 45:467, 1980 (abstract).

55. Yoshikawa, J., Yanagihara, K., Owaki, U., Kato, H., Takagi, Y., Okumachi, F., Furaya, T., Tomita, Y., Baba, K.: Cross-sectional echocardiographic diagnosis of coronary artery aneurysms in patients with the mucocutaneous lymph node syndrome. Circulation 59:133, 1979.

56. Gilladoga, A. C., Manuel, C., Tan, C. C., Wollner, N., Murphy, M. L.: Cardiotoxicity of adriamycin (NSC-123127) in children. Cancer Chemother Rep 6:Suppl 3, 209, 1975.

57. Glieden, L. C., Lucas, R. V., Carter, J. B., Miller, K., Edwards, J. E.: A developmental complex including supravalvular stenosis of the aorta

and pulmonary trunk. Circulation 49:585, 1974.

58. Roberts, W. C.: Valvular, subvalvular, and supravalvular aortic stenosis. Cardiovasc Clinics 5:104, 1973.

59. Folger, G. M.: Further observations on the syndrome of idiopathic infantile hypercalcemia associated with supravalvular aortic stenosis. Am Heart J 93:455, 1977.

60. Keane, J. F., Fellows, K. E., LaFarge, C. G., Nadas, A. S., Bernhard, W. F.: The surgical management of discrete and diffuse supravalvular aortic stenosis. Circulation 54:112, 1976.

61. Cornell, W. P. Elkins, R. C., Criley, J. M., Sabiston, D. C., Jr.: Supravalvular aortic stenosis. J Thorac Cardiovasc Surg 51:484, 1966.

62. Beuren, A. J., Apitz, J., Harmjanz, D.: Supravalvular aortic stenosis, peripheral pulmonary stenosis, mental retardation and similar facial appearance. Am J Cardiol 26:1235, 1962.

63. Garcia, R. E., Friedman, W. F., Kaback, M. M., Rowe, R. D.: Idiopathic hypercalcemia and supravalvular aortic stenosis. N Engl J Med 271:117, 1964.

64. Pansegrau, D. G., Kioshos, J. M., Durnin, R. E., Kroetz, F. W.: Supravalvular aortic stenosis in adults. Am J Cardiol 31:635, 1973.

65. Rudolph, A.: Congenital Diseases of the Heart. Chicago Year Book Med. Publ., 1974.

66. Talner, N. S., Berman, M. A.: Postnatal development of obstruction in coarctation of the aorta: Role of the ductus arteriosus. Pediatrics 56:562, 1975.

67. Cleoria, G. C., Patton, R. B.: Congenital absence of the aortic arch. Am Heart J 58:407, 1959.

68. Boone, M. L., Swenson, B. E., Felson, B.: Rib notching: Its many causes. Am J Roentgenol 91:1075, 1964.

69. Becker, A. E., Becker, M. J., Edwards, J. E.: Anomalies associated with coarctation of the aorta. Circulation 41:1067, 1970.

70. Tarves, R. L., Berry, C. L., Aberdeen, E.: Congenital bicuspid valves associated with coarctation of the aorta in children. Br Heart J 31:127, 1969.

71. Rosenquist, C. G.: Congenital mitral valve disease associated with coarctation of the aorta: A spectrum that includes parachute deformity of the mitral valve. Circulation 49:985, 1974.

72. Coleman, E. N.: Serious congestive heart disease in infancy. Br Heart J 27:42, 1965.

73. Figley, M.: Accessory roentgen signs of coarctation of the aorta. Radiology 62:671, 1954.

74. Littman, D., and Schaaf, R. S.: Therapeutic experiences with subacute bacterial endocarditis. N Engl J Med 243:248, 1950.

75. Blumenthal, S.: Infective Endocarditis. In Heart Disease in Infants, Children, and Adolescents. Moss, A. J., Adams, F. H., Emmanouilides, G. C. (eds.). Williams & Wilkins Co., Baltimore, 1977, p. 552.

76. Lerner, P. I., and Weinstein, I.: Infective endocarditis in the antibiotic era. N Engl J Med 274:199, 1966.

77. Stewart, J. A., Silimperi, D., Harris, P., Wise, N. K., Fraker, T. D., Jr., Kisslo, J. A.: Echocardiographic documentation of vegetative lesions in infective endocarditis: Clinical implications. Circulation 61:374, 1980.

PULMONIC STENOSIS

Isolated obstruction to right ventricular outflow may occur at the subvalvar, valvar or supravalvar level. In the absence of right heart failure and with an intact ventricular septum, pulmonary blood flow is maintained and patients are acyanotic. Critical pulmonary valve stenosis and pulmonary atresia with an intact ventricular septum present in cyanotic infants soon after birth, and these lesions will be discussed in Chapter 7.

Pulmonary Valve Stenosis

This relatively common congenital heart defect (see *Introduction*, Table 1) presents in childhood, and the murmur is frequently heard in the first year of life. The physical examination is characterized by a systolic ejection murmur and an ejection click over the pulmonic area with transmission to the posterior lung fields. The electrocardiogram usually demonstrates right-axis deviation and right ventricular hypertrophy. Survival into adulthood is not uncommon.[1]

The pulmonary valve presents a typical appearance. The unopened valve has the shape of a truncated cone from which three equidistant raphes extend to the wall of the pulmonary artery. Separate leaflets are not present. At the apex of the cone is a small orifice (rarely more than several millimeters in diameter). The pulmonary artery demonstrates poststenotic dilatation, which often extends into the left pulmonary artery but not the right. This is due to the direction of the jet of blood created by the stenotic valve and the direct continuity of the pulmonary trunk with the left pulmonary artery. Calcification of the valve is rare and has been reported only in older individuals.[2] The cardiac output is usually normal due to the high pressure developed in the right ventricle. The development of right ventricular hypertrophy may be reflected in the outflow tract as infundibular stenosis. The so-called "dysplastic" pulmonary valve is a rare form of pulmonary valve stenosis in which there are three distinct cusps without commissural fusion. The cusps in this condition are inordinately thickened and immobile and contain myxomatous tissue.[3]

Classic pulmonary valve stenosis as well

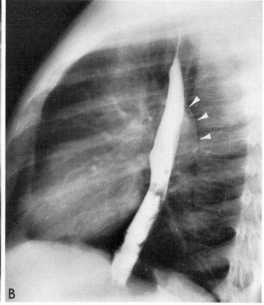

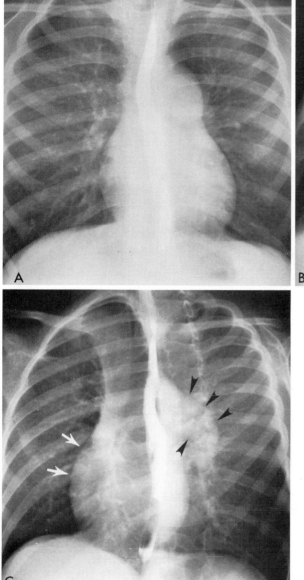

Figure 5–78.   Posteroanterior (*A*), lateral (*B*), and left anterior oblique (*C*) chest radiographs of a child with pulmonary valve stenosis. The pulmonary vascularity and heart size are normal. There is marked dilatation of the pulmonary trunk as well as the left pulmonary artery. The latter is best seen in the lateral and LAO views (arrowheads). Mild right heart enlargement is present in the LAO projection (arrows).

as the dysplastic variety has been associated with noncardiac abnormalities, including small stature, mental retardation, hypertelorism, low-set ears, ptosis, webbed neck, pectus carinatum and excavatum, and undescended testes. This complex, Noonan's syndrome, has also been described as the "male Turner syndrome," although both males and females are affected and karyotypes are normal.[4]

Subvalvar pulmonic stenosis may involve the infundibulum (usually at its inlet) or the subinfundibular region. The latter condition involves hypertrophied anomalous muscle bundles that cross portions of the right ventricle creating a second, subinfundibular chamber.[5] This entity is commonly associated with ventricular septal defects.[6]

Supravalvar pulmonary stenosis may involve narrowing of the pulmonary trunk, its bifurcation, either or both main pulmonary arteries, or lobar and segmental pulmonary arteries. Discrete membranous obstruction is usually localized to the pulmonary trunk and is extremely rare.[7] Pulmonary artery and branch stenosis may be accompanied by poststenotic dilatation or may present as tubular hypoplasia over a long segment of the vessel.

Several types of patients with multiple peripheral pulmonary artery stenoses have been described: (1) Those in whom multiple pulmonary lesions are found as an isolated congenital anomaly. This is often accompanied by some component of central pulmonary artery narrowing. (2) Those in whom the defect occurs in association with pulmonary valve stenosis, supravalvar aortic stenosis, ventricular septal defect, patent ductus arteriosus, and systemic arterial stenosis. (3) Those in whom a familial presentation of multiple peripheral pulmonary stenoses is associated with supravalvar aortic stenosis.[7] (4) Those in whom peripheral pulmonary stenosis occurs following maternal rubella. Central pulmonary artery stenosis, patent ductus arteriosus, and pulmonary valve stenosis are more common in the postrubella syndrome. These infants have a low birth weight, deafness, cataracts, and mental retardation.[8] (5) Finally, a clinical syndrome exists that consists of peculiar facies, abnormal dentition, mental retardation, infantile hypercalcemia, supravalvar aortic stenosis, and bilateral pulmonary artery branch stenosis.[9]

Radiographic Features

Pulmonary vascularity is normal in all of the forms of right heart obstruction previously described, as long as right heart output is adequate (Figs. 5–78 and 5–80). Occasionally, stenosis of the branches of the pulmonary artery is suggested by focal zones of hypovascularity or a fusiform appearance representing poststenotic dilatation (Fig. 5–79).[10]

The key radiographic finding in pulmonary valve stenosis is a dilated pulmonary trunk (Fig. 5–78A). Generally, there is good correlation between the size of the pulmonary trunk and the degree of obstruction: greater degrees of dilatation occur with mild to moderate stenosis, while in severe obstruction the trunk may be unimpressive. Frequently, there is accompanying enlargement of the left main pulmonary artery (Fig. 5–78B and C). This occurs because of the relatively direct posterior extension of the pulmonary trunk, which directs the poststenotic turbulent flow into the left pulmonary artery. This may best be appreciated in the lateral or LAO projection and is in striking contrast to the normal right pulmonary artery (Fig. 5–78B and C). In some patients, the left pulmonary artery will be inordinately dilated and will simulate a left hilar mass (Fig. 5–80).[11] The heart size is

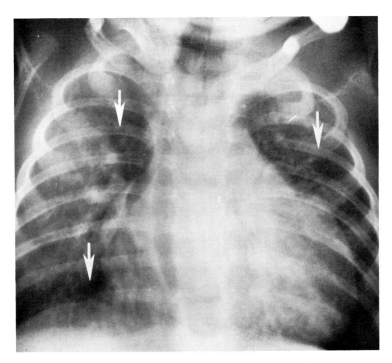

Figure 5–79. Anteroposterior chest radiograph in an infant with pulmonary branch stenoses. Note the focal areas of decreased pulmonary vascularity in both lungs (arrows) (see Fig. 5–86 for angiographic correlation).

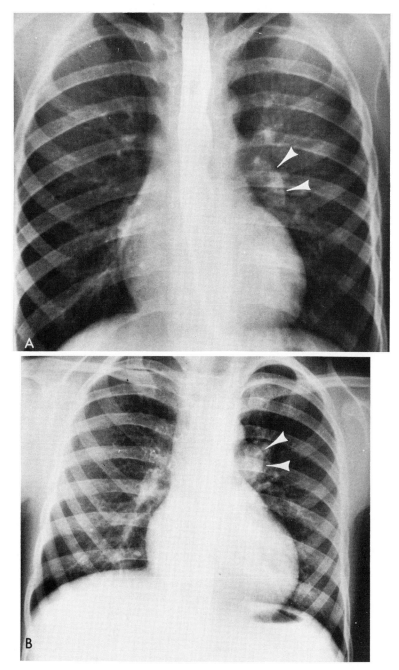

Figure 5–80. Posteroanterior chest radiographs in two children with pulmonary valve stenosis. Pulmonary vascularity and heart size are normal, although both have an upturned cardiac apex. The left pulmonary artery is significantly dilated in both cases (arrows), simulating a left mediastinal mass.

normal, although there may be evidence of right ventricular prominence (Figs. 5–78C and 5–80). A combination of radiographic findings that include normal vascularity, a dilated pulmonary trunk and left pulmonary artery, and a normal-sized heart should

strongly suggest the diagnosis of pulmonary valve stenosis.

When one notes a prominent pulmonary trunk on the chest x-ray, several conditions besides pulmonary valve stenosis should be considered: (1) idiopathic dilatation of the

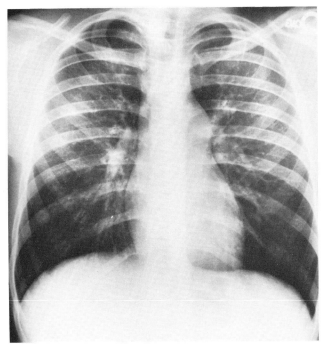

Figure 5-81. Posteroanterior chest radiograph in a teenager with a systolic murmur over the pulmonic area. The pulmonary trunk is prominent but the left pulmonary artery is not dilated. The lack of an ejection click and a normal electrocardiogram led to the diagnosis of idiopathic dilatation of the pulmonary trunk.

pulmonary trunk, (2) partial absence of the left pericardium, (3) thoracic cage abnormalities, (4) normal teenager. Idiopathic dilatation of the pulmonary trunk is an asymptomatic condition associated with a pulmonic ejection murmur (but no ejection click) and dilatation of the pulmonary trunk on the chest x-ray.[12] Although the pulmonary trunk is dilated, the left pulmonary artery generally is not, and this may be a helpful radiographic clue to distinguishing this condition from pulmonary valve stenosis (Fig. 5–81).

With partial absence of the left pericardium, there is herniation of the left pulmonary artery (usually accompanied by the left atrial appendage) through a defect in the upper left pericardium.[13] Again, the left pulmonary artery is not dilated, and the density along the left heart border extends more inferiorly into the region occupied by the left atrial appendage.

Loss of normal thoracic kyphosis ("straight back" syndrome), severe pectus excavatum, or scoliosis may be associated with slight prominence of the pulmonary trunk. This may be due to rotation of the heart to the left (into a slight RAO projection) secondary to these bony deformities.

Normal teenagers (especially girls) may demonstrate a slightly prominent trunk on chest x-ray. Significant pathology can usually be excluded by auscultation.

Echocardiographic Features

In pulmonary valve stenosis, the echocardiogram may show evidence of right ventricular anterior wall thickening and may, more specifically, show evidence of thickening of the pulmonic valve leaflets with systolic doming (Fig. 5–82). There may be, in addition, echocardiographic evidence of poststenotic dilatation of the main and left pulmonary arteries in the long-axis and subxiphoidal views[14] of the right ventricular outflow tract. These latter features are perhaps more consistently demonstrated on the chest film.

The presence of coarctations of the main pulmonary artery branches may be detected by examination of the long-axis view of the right ventricular outflow tract to the level of the bifurcation. The short-axis view of the pulmonary root also permits diagnosis of absent pulmonary valve, coarctation of the origin of the right or left pulmonary arteries, or absence of one of the main branches of the pulmonary artery (Fig. 5–83).

Angiographic Features

Isolated pulmonary valve stenosis is best evaluated with a right ventriculogram (Fig. 5–84). Right ventricular hypertrophy is suggested by increase in trabecular pattern and hypertrophy of the crista supraventricularis (best appreciated in the lateral view) (Fig.

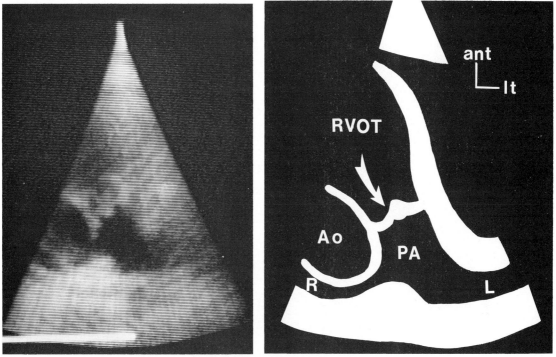

Figure 5–82. Valvar pulmonary stenosis. Short-axis view of the right ventricular outflow tract and pulmonary artery bifurcation. The right ventricular outflow tract (RVOT) is seen anterior to the aorta (Ao). There is marked thickening of the pulmonic valve (arrow), which domes during systole. The main pulmonary artery (PA) and left pulmonary artery (L) have enlarged secondary to poststenotic dilatation. (Note that the left pulmonary artery (L) is larger than the right pulmonary artery (R).)

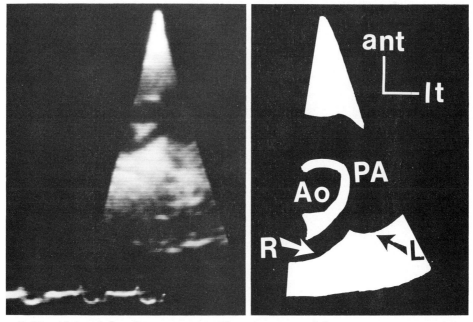

Figure 5–83. Absent left pulmonary artery. Short-axis view of the great arteries in a patient with a normal right and absent left pulmonary artery. Note the pulmonary artery (PA) followed to the point of bifurcation with the identifiable right pulmonary artery (R) and an absent left pulmonary artery (L). (Ao = aorta.)

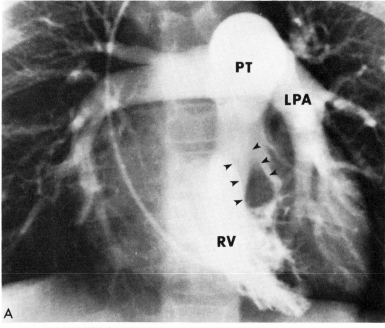

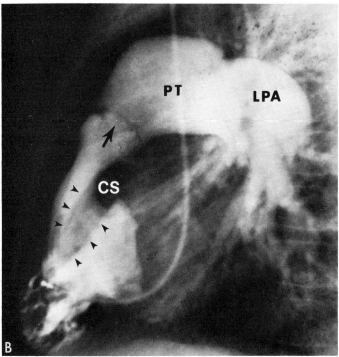

Figure 5–84. Posteroanterior *(A)* and lateral *(B)* views of a right ventriculogram in a child with a 50 mmHg gradient across the pulmonary outflow tract. An anomalous muscle bundle extends from the septal region across the infundibulum (arrowheads). On the lateral view the muscle bundle courses from low anteriorly to high posteriorly (arrowheads). This patient also has significant pulmonary valve stenosis with a thickened pulmonary valve (arrow) and poststenotic dilatation of the pulmonary trunk (PT) and left pulmonary artery (LPA). The crista supraventricularis (CS) is hypertrophied.

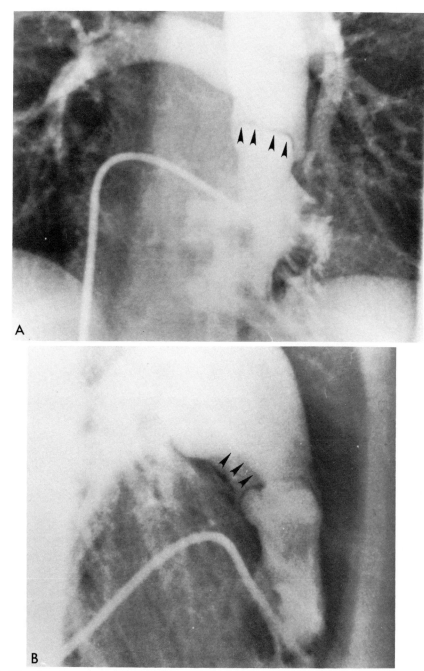

Figure 5–85. Sitting posteroanterior (*A*) and lateral (*B*) projections in a child with a 60 mmHg gradient across the pulmonary valve. The thickened valve (arrowheads) is well seen in the sitting PA view. In the lateral view, a jet of contrast streams (arrowheads) through the valve into the dilated pulmonary trunk.

5–84*B*). The pulmonary valve is domed and thickened (Figs. 5–84 and 5–85) and a jet of contrast may be seen emanating from the apex of the dome (Fig. 5–85*B*). The standard supine posteroanterior view superimposes the valve on the pulmonary trunk (Fig.

5–84*A*). A 30° sitting posteroanterior view is therefore more useful in identifying the abnormal pulmonary valve (Fig. 5–85*A*). Poststenotic dilatation of the pulmonary trunk and left pulmonary artery is usually present (Figs. 5–84*B* and 5–85*B*).

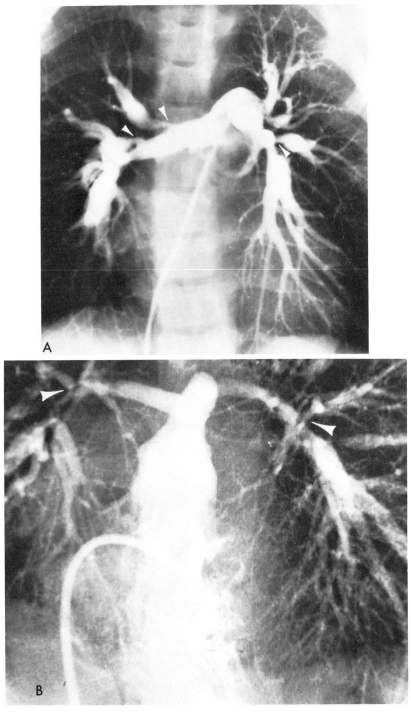

Figure 5–86. Standard posteroanterior *(A)* and sitting posteroanterior *(B)* pulmonary arteriograms showing two types of peripheral pulmonary stenosis. In *(A)*, discrete stenoses are present in the hilar regions (arrowheads). In *B*, there is diffuse hypoplasia of the central pulmonary arteries as well as stenoses of branches in the hilar regions (arrowheads).

The dysplastic pulmonary valve is generally thicker, more immobile, and shows more distortion than the classic domed valve, and poststenotic dilatation is less frequent.

Obstructing muscle bands of the right ventricle may be classified into low and high types, and these can be demonstrated by careful angiographic analysis.[6] In the frontal projection, the low muscle bundle is characterized by a filling defect that extends diagonally from the septal side of the right ventricle to the region of the tricuspid valve and crista supraventricularis (parietal band) (Fig. 5–84). In the lateral view the muscle bundle courses diagonally across the right ventricular sinus from low anteriorly to high posteriorly (Fig. 5–84). In the high obstruction the muscle tissue arises from the septum and encroaches as a horizontal defect on the right ventricular sinus region below the infundibulum. Since ventricular septal defects are commonly associated with this entity (73 to 85 per cent),[6] it becomes important to distinguish this complex from tetralogy of Fallot. The key differentiating point is the presence of a normal (wide), vertical infundibulum with obstructing muscle bands (Fig. 5–84).

Central pulmonary artery stenosis usually exists in association with tetralogy of Fallot or critical pulmonary valve stenosis. The lesion may begin in the distal pulmonary trunk and extend into either main pulmonary artery or may be confined to the origin of either (usually the left) main pulmonary artery. The extent, location, and morphology of peripheral pulmonary artery stenosis (coarctations; branch stenosis) are best appreciated in the posteroanterior pulmonary arteriogram (Fig. 5–86A and B).

REFERENCES

1. Kaplan, D., Adolph, R. J.: Pulmonic Valve Stenosis in Adults. In Congenital Heart Disease in Adults. Roberts, W. C., (ed). F. A. Davis, Philadelphia, 1979, p. 327.
2. Roberts, W. C., Mason, D. T., Morrow, A. G., Braunwald, E.: Calcific pulmonic stenosis. Circulation 37:973, 1968.
3. Koretzky, E. D., Moller, J. H., Korns, M. E., Schwartz, C. J., Edwards, J. E.: Congenital pulmonary stenosis resulting from dysplasia of the valve. Circulation 40:43, 1969.
4. Noonan, J. A. Hypertelorism with Turner phenotype. Am J Dis Child 116:373, 1968.
5. Rowland, T. W., Rosenthal, A. Castaneda, A. R.:

Double chamber right ventricle. Am Heart J 89:455, 1975.
6. Fellows, K. E., Martin, E. C., Rosenthal, A.: Angiography of obstructing muscle bands of the right ventricle. Am J Roentgenol 128:249, 1977.
7. Arvidsson, H., Carlsson, E., Hartman, A., Jr., Tsifutis, A., Crawford, C.: Supravalvular stenosis of the pulmonary arteries. Acta Radiol 56:466, 1961.
8. Venables, A. W.: The syndrome of pulmonary stenosis complicating maternal rubella. Br Heart J 27:49, 1965.
9. Beuren, A. J., Schulze, C., Eberle, P., Harmjang, D., Apitz, J.: The syndrome of supravalvular aortic stenosis, peripheral pulmonary stenosis, mental retardation and similar facial appearances. Am J Cardiol 13:471, 1964.
10. Baum, D., Khoury, G. H., Ongley, P. A., Swan, H. J. C., Kincaid, O. W.: Congenital stenoses of the pulmonary artery branches. Circulation 29:680, 1964.
11. Kelley, M. J., Mannes, E. J., Ravin, C. E.: Mediastinal masses of vascular origin. J Thorac Cardiovasc Surg 76:559, 1978.
12. Deshmukh, M., Guvenc, S., Bentivoglio, L., Goldberg, H.: Idiopathic dilatation of the pulmonary artery. Circulation 21:710, 1960.
13. Nasser, W. K.: Congenital absence of the left pericardium. Am J Cardiol 26:466, 1970.
14. Sahn, D. J., Sobol, R. G., Allen, H. D.: Subxiphoid real-time cross-sectional echocardiography for imaging the right ventricle (RV) and right ventricular outflow tract (RVOT). Am J Cardiol 41:354, 1978 (abstract).

MITRAL VALVE PROLAPSE

Description of a syndrome consisting of clinical and morphologic abnormalities involving the mitral valve were first made in the 1960's.[1-4] A characteristic mid systolic click and late systolic murmur were found to correlate with angiocardiographic findings of billowing of the mitral leaflets into the left atrium and late systolic mitral regurgitation. This condition has variously been termed the prolapsed mitral leaflet syndrome, floppy mitral valve syndrome, Barlow's syndrome, click-murmur syndrome, and billowing mitral valve syndrome. Depending on diagnostic criteria, the syndrome may be quite common, occurring in 6 to 20 per cent of apparently healthy females assessed by echocardiography.[5, 6] Although not generally considered a form of congenital heart disease, mitral valve prolapse has been shown to have a familial occurrence.[1, 3] It also is associated with various syndromes and congenital heart lesions, including ostium secundum atrial septal defect,[7] familial asymmetric hypertrophic car-

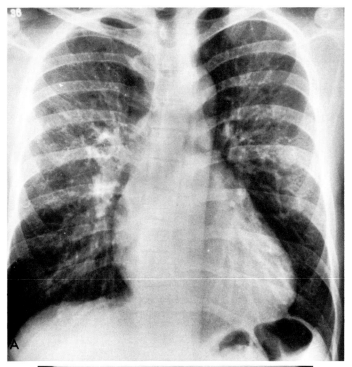

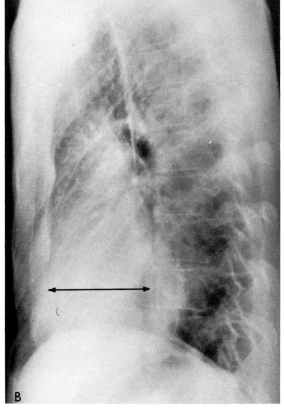

Figure 5–87. Posteroanterior (*A*) and lateral (*B*) chest radiographs in teenage male with mitral valve prolapse. The pulmonary vascularity and the heart appear slightly enlarged. There is mild scoliosis of the thoracic spine. The lateral view shows a decreased anteroposterior dimension (arrows). The AP/transverse thoracic ratio was calculated as 33 per cent—well below the normal mean for males.

diomyopathy,[8] Marfan's and Ehlers-Danlos syndrome,[9] Ebstein's anomaly,[10] Turner's syndrome,[11] and corrected transposition of the great vessels.[12] Although auscultatory manifestations do not usually appear until adulthood, isolated physical findings of the click-murmur syndrome have been described in children.[13] These facts would suggest that this syndrome is a form of congenital heart disease, and its frequency would make it one of the most common congenital heart defects.

With the increased recognition of the mitral valve prolapse syndrome has come documentation of an association of the disorder with certain complications. These include life threatening arrhythmias,[14] significant mitral regurgitation,[15] bacterial endocarditis,[16] embolic episodes,[17] and sudden death.[18]

Pathologically, mitral valve prolapse involves not only the leaflets, but also the chordae tendinae, the mitral annulus, and perhaps the left ventricular wall. Isolated anterior leaflet prolapse is uncommon, and usually the posterior leaflet alone or both leaflets are involved. The involved leaflet(s) is redundant, slightly thickened, wrinkled,

and pale.[19] Myxomatous tissue containing increased acid mucopolysaccharides is present in the redundant leaflets and sometimes in the chordae. The chordae are thinned and elongated. Mitral annulus dilatation is frequently present.[20]

The posterior leaflet of the normal mitral valve has three scallops — a large middle scallop and smaller anterolateral and posteromedial scallops.[21] Mitral prolapse may involve all three, two, or a single scallop. Generally, biscallop prolapse involves the posteromedial and middle scallops.[22]

Abnormal left ventricular systolic contraction patterns seen during angiocardiography have led to the suggestion that there is a myocardial component to the mitral valve prolapse syndrome.[23] Finally, tricuspid valve prolapse has been detected by angiocardiography and echocardiography in approximately 50 per cent of patients with mitral valve prolapse.[24]

Radiographic Features

The pulmonary vascularity, heart size, and configuration are normal unless severe mitral regurgitation is associated with mitral

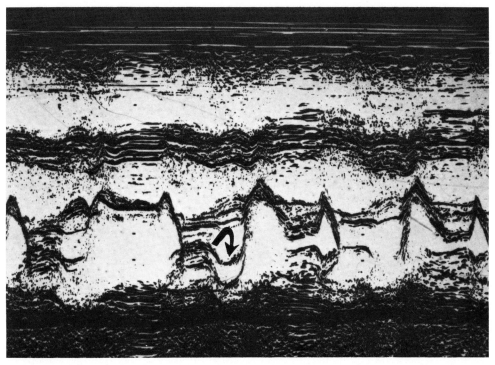

Figure 5–88. Mitral valve prolapse. An M-mode echocardiogram of the ventricle and mitral valve in a patient who has a mid to late systolic prolapse of the posterior and anterior leaflets of the mitral valve (curved arrow).

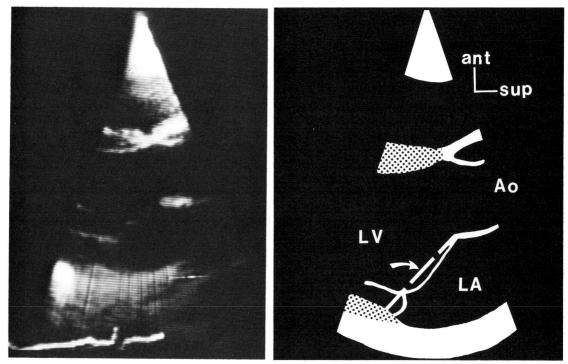

Figure 5–89. Mitral valve prolapse. Long-axis view of the left ventricle (LV) in late systole. Mitral valve prolapse can be diagnosed when either or both the mitral leaflets move posterior to an imaginary line (dashed) connecting the atrioventricular groove with the base of the aortic root (Ao). In this image, both mitral leaflets bow beyond that line (arrow) into the left atrium (LA). (LV = left ventricle.)

valve prolapse. In those cases, signs of left atrial enlargement may be present.

Certain mild abnormalities of the thoracic cage have been described in association with this lesion. These include narrowing of the anteroposterior/transverse thoracic ratio to less than the mean ratio in the normal population — that is, a "flat" chest (Fig. 5–87). This value is a ratio of (1) the perpendicular distance from the anterior surface of the eighth thoracic vertebral body to the posterior cortex of the sternum to (2) the transthoracic distance measured at the level of the diaphragm. In teenagers and adults, the mean value is 45.7 per cent in females and 47 per cent in males.[25] In one study, 64 per cent of patients with systolic click–late systolic murmur syndrome were found to have a "flat" chest.[26] Thirty-nine per cent of these patients had scoliosis (Fig. 5–87); 23 per cent had absence of the normal thoracic kyphosis ("straight back") (Fig. 5–87); and 11 per cent had a pectus excavatum. Sixty-one per cent had at least one abnormality and 12.5 per cent had two. It is well known that individuals with Marfan's syndrome have thoracic cage ab-

normalities, including "straight back," scoliosis, and pectus excavatum. Since mitral prolapse is a relatively frequent finding in this syndrome, it is postulated that individuals with myxomatous changes in the mitral valve are manifesting a forme fruste of the Marfan syndrome — a connective tissue disorder leading not only to myxomatous changes in the mitral valve but to skeletal changes as well.[27]

Echocardiographic Features

Although there is no universal agreement on a specific set of findings for mitral valve prolapse, the M-mode study may be diagnostic, showing abnormal posterior motion of the mitral leaflets in systole (Fig. 5–88). Usually a posterior motion of at least 2 mm is required. The left ventricular inflow tract and mitral valve are best defined in both the long-axis[13] and subxiphoidal short-axis views. The two-dimensional studies show mitral valve leaflets bowing toward the left atrium, extending beyond an imaginary line drawn from the atrioventricular groove to the base of the aortic valve (Fig. 5–89).

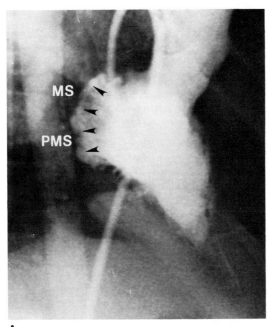
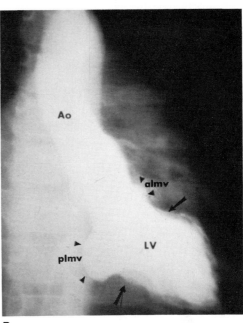

A **B**

Figure 5–90. *A*, Lateral left ventriculogram in a patient with a late systolic click and murmur. In this systolic angiogram there is a convex bulge into the left atrium (arrowheads). The upper portion of the bulge represents the middle scallop (MS) of the posterior leaflet of the mitral valve, while the posteroinferior bulge represents the posteromedial scallop (PMS) of the posterior leaflet. *B*, Postero-anterior left ventriculogram showing prolapse of both the posterior leaflet of the mitral valve (plmv) and the anterior leaflet of the mitral valve (almv). Note the prominent contraction of the midportion of the left ventricle (LV) (arrows). Ao = aorta.

Angiographic Findings

Left ventricular cineangiography in the right anterior oblique or lateral projection allows one to detect both the prolapsed scallops of the posterior mitral leaflet and the presence of mitral regurgitation (Fig. 5–90). Anterior mitral leaflet prolapse is more difficult to detect (Fig. 5–90*B*) and often requires the left anterior oblique projection.

The normal anterior and posterior mitral leaflets overlie each other in the standard (30°) RAO projection, and the atrioventricular ring is often seen as a narrowed ("closed") oval. The normal valve shows little if any systolic bulging beyond the ring. The fornix of the left ventricle is a variably present "pouch" projecting from the inferior base of the ventricle at its junction with the atrioventricular ring. This structure may present a small bulge on the left ventriculogram (see *Normal Ventriculogram*, Chapter 4). It can usually be distinguished from a prolapsing posterior mitral leaflet, since it remains during diastole, while the prolapse occurs during systole.

Prolapse of the posterior leaflet presents angiographically as distinct convex bulges into the left atrium during systole (Fig. 5–90*A* and *B*). A central bulge indicates prolapse of the middle scallop of the posterior leaflet. A posteroinferior bulge occurs with posteromedial scallop prolapse. When isolated, this must be distinguished from a prominent fornix. An anterosuperior bulge is seen when the anterolateral commissural scallop prolapses. Prolapse in this region overlaps the aortic root but may extend anteriorly beyond the root. Prolapse of the middle and posteromedial scallops commonly occur together, while isolated single scallop prolapse most commonly involves the middle scallop. Infrequently, all three bulges may be present ("triscallop" prolapse).

Abnormal patterns of left ventricular contraction have been described in association with mitral valve prolapse. One study reported an 82 per cent incidence of abnormal contraction separated into five contraction patterns:[23]

TYPE I. A "ballerina foot" pattern consisting of a prominent contraction of the diaphragmatic portion of the left ventricle accompanied by convexity of the anterolateral wall (Fig. 5–90A).

TYPE II. An "hourglass" pattern produced by a concentric contraction of the middle portions of the anterior and diaphragmatic walls (Fig. 5–90B).

TYPE III. Inadequate long-axis shortening.

TYPE IV. Posterior basal wall akinesis.

TYPE V. Cavity obliteration.

REFERENCES

1. Barlow, J. B., Pocock, W. A., Marchand, P., Denney, M.: The significance of late systolic murmurs. Am Heart J 66:443, 1963.
2. Barlow, J. B., Bosman, C. K.: Aneurysmal protrusion of the posterior leaflet of the mitral valve: An auscultatory-electrocardiographic syndrome. Am Heart J 71:166, 1965.
3. Criley, M. J., Lewis, K. B., Humphries, J. O., Ross, R. S.: Prolapse of the mitral valve: Clinical and cine-angiocardiographic findings. Br Heart J 28:488, 1966.
4. Stannard, M., Sloman, J. G., Hare, W. S., Goble, A. J.: Prolapse of the posterior leaflet of the mitral valve. A clinical, familial and cineangiographic study. Br Med J 3:71, 1967.
5. Markiewicz, W., Stoner, J., London, E., Hunt, S., Popp, R. L.: Mitral valve prolapse in one hundred presumably healthy young females. Circulation 53:464, 1976.
6. Procacci, P. M., Savran, S. V., Schreiter, S. L., Bryson, A. L.: Prevalence of clinical mitral valve prolapse in 1169 young women. N Engl J Med 294:1086, 1976.
7. Betrui, A., Wigle, E. D., Felderhof, C. H., McLoughlin, M. J.: Prolapse of the posterior leaflet of the mitral valve associated with secundum atrial septal defect. Am J Cardiol 35:363, 1975.
8. Chandraratna, P. A. N., Tolentino, A. O., Mutucumarana, W., Gomez, A. L.: Echocardiographic observations on the association between mitral prolapse and asymmetric septal hypertrophy. Circulation 55:622, 1977.
9. McKusick, V. A.: Heritable Disorders of Connective Tissue, 4th ed. C. V. Mosby, St. Louis, 1972.
10. Roberts, W. C., Glancy, D. L., Seningen, R. P., Maron, B. J., Epstein, S. E.: Prolapse of the mitral valve (floppy valve) associated with Ebstein's anomaly of the tricuspid valve. Am J Cardiol 38:377, 1976.
11. Hancock, W. E., Cohn, K.: The syndrome associated with midsystolic click and late systolic murmur. Am J Med 41:183, 1966.
12. Cowley, M. J., Coghlan, H. C., Mantle, J. A., Soto, B.: Chest pain and bilateral atrioventricular valve prolapse with normal coronary arteries in isolated corrected transposition of the great vessels. Am J Cardiol 40:458, 1977.
13. Sahn, D. J., Allen, H. D., Goldberg, S. J., Friedman, W. F.: Mitral valve prolapse in children:
A problem defined by real-time cross-sectional echocardiography. Circulation 53:651, 1976.
14. Winkle, R. A., Lopes, M. G., Fitzgerald, J. W.: Arrhythmias in patients with mitral valve prolapse. Circulation 52:73, 1975.
15. Hill, D. G., Davies, M. J., Braimbridge, M. V.: The natural history and surgical management of the redundant cusp syndrome (floppy mitral valve). J Thorac Cardiovasc Surg 67:519, 1974.
16. Lachman, A. S., Bramwell-Jones, D. M., Lakier, J. B., Pocock, W. A., Barlow, J. B.: Infective endocarditis in the billowing mitral leaflet syndrome. Br Heart J 37:326, 1975.
17. Barnett, H. J., Jones, M. W., Boughner, D. R., Kostuk, W. J.: Cerebral ischemic events associated with prolapsing mitral valve. Arch Neurol 33:777, 1976.
18. Jeresaty, R. M.: Sudden death in the mitral prolapse click syndrome. Am J Cardiol 37:317, 1976.
19. Devereux, R. B., Perloff, J. K., Reicheck, N., Josephson, M. E.: Mitral valve prolapse. Circulation 54:3, 1976.
20. Roberts, W. C.: Congenital Heart Disease in Adults. F. A. Davis Co., Philadelphia, 1979, p. 427.
21. Ranganathan, N., Lam, J. H. C., Wigle, E. D., Silver, M. D.: Morphology of the human mitral valve II. The valve leaflets. Circulation 41:459, 1970.
22. Ranganathan, N., Silver, M. D., Robinson, T. F., Kostuk, W. J., Felderhof, C. H., Platt, N. L., Wilson, J. K., Wigle, E. D.: Angiographic-morphologic correlation in patients with severe mitral regurgitation due to prolapse of the posterior mitral valve leaflet. Circulation 48:514, 1973.
23. Scampardonis, G., Yang, S. S., Maranhao, V., Goldberg, H., Gooch, A. S.: Left ventricular abnormalities in prolapsed mitral leaflet syndrome. Circulation 48:287, 1973.
24. Gooch, A. S., Maranhao, V., Scampardonis, G., Cha, S. D., Yang, S. S.: Prolapse of mitral and tricuspid valves in systolic murmur click syndrome. N Engl J Med 287:1218, 1972.
25. Twigg, H. L., DeLeon, A. C., Perloff, J. K.: The straight back syndrome: Radiographic manifestations. Radiology 88:274, 1967.
26. BonTempo, C. P., Ronan, J. A., deLeon, A. C., Twigg, H. L.: Radiographic appearance of the thorax in systolic click–late systolic murmur syndrome. Am J Cardiol 36:27, 1975.
27. Read, R. C., Thal, A. P., Wendt, V. E.: Symptomatic valvular myxomatous transformation (the floppy valve syndrome): A possible forme fruste of the Marfan syndrome. Circulation 32:897, 1965.

CONGENITALLY CORRECTED TRANSPOSITION OF THE GREAT ARTERIES

In congenitally corrected transposition of the great arteries, right atrial blood flows across a morphologic mitral valve into a venous ventricle that is morphologically a

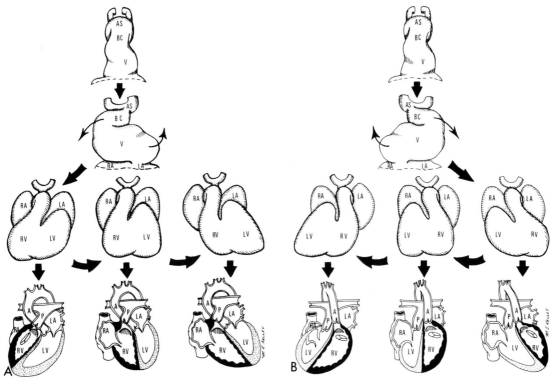

Figure 5–91. Diagrammatic representation of the embryologic ventricular looping process. In *A*, the initially straight cardiac tube bends to the *right* (D [dextro]-loop), and the right ventricle (RV) develops on the right and aligns with the right atrium (RA). The same applies to the development of the left ventricle (LV) and left atrium (LA). The cardiac mass then rotates into the left chest. In *B*, the cardiac tube bends to the *left* (L [levo]-loop). This aligns the left atrium with the right ventricle and the right atrium with the left ventricle. The great arteries (A, P) are shown in the L-transposed position. (A = aorta, AS = aortic sac, B = bulbus cordis, P = pulmonary artery, V = primitive ventricle.) (From Tonkin et al.[5])

left ventricle and then into the pulmonary trunk. Pulmonary venous blood returns to the left atrium, flows across a morphologic tricuspid valve into a systemic ventricle that is morphologically a right ventricle and into the aorta. If one defines transposition of the great arteries as an anatomic arrangement in which both great arteries arise from morphologically inappropriate ventricles, then in this condition the transposition is physiologically corrected, since systemic venous blood (unoxygenated) is transported to the lungs and pulmonary venous blood (oxygenated) is transported to the body. In the presence of situs solitus, this condition involves ventricular discordance (the ventricles and their A-V valves do not relate to their appropriate atria); ventricular inversion (the ventricles and their A-V valves are in positions opposite from normal); and transposition.

In classic corrected transposition, there is both an L-(levo) ventricular loop and L-(levo) transposition. These terms require further definition. During early embryonic development, the initially straight cardiac tube usually bends to the right (D-loop), with the anatomic right ventricle developing on the right (aligned with the right atrium) and the anatomic left ventricle developing on the left (aligned with the left atrium). Subsequently, the cardiac mass rotates into the left chest (Fig. 5–91). In corrected transposition the cardiac tube bends to the left (L-loop). The anatomic right ventricle, therefore, develops on the left and is aligned with the left atrium, and the anatomic left ventricle develops on the right and is aligned with the right atrium (Fig. 5–91). Usually, rotation into the right chest does not occur, so that the cardiac apex remains in the left hemithorax. L-

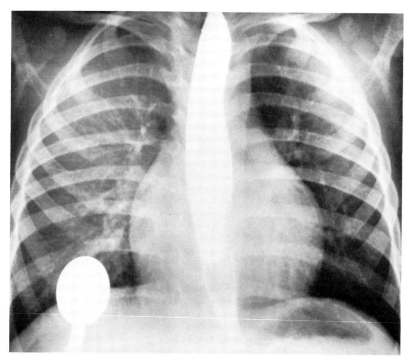

Figure 5–92. Posteroanterior chest radiograph in an asymptomatic child with systolic murmur and a rhythm disturbance. On casual perusal, the film appears normal. However, the normal "triad of densities" (ascending aorta, aortic knob, and pulmonary trunk) is absent and the left mid heart border is slightly prominent. Cardiac catheterization and angiography revealed corrected transposition and a small ventricular septal defect. (See Figure 5–96 for angiographic correlation.)

transposition is a term describing the spatial orientation of the transposed great vessels in which the aorta and its valve are to the left and slightly anterior and superior to the pulmonary trunk. The pulmonary trunk is rightward, posterior, and inferior. These great arteries, therefore, run parallel to each other as they leave their respective ventricles (Fig. 5–91).

In this condition, the importance of internal anatomic landmarks takes on great importance. The left-sided systemic ventricle has anatomic features of a right ventricle; that is, it is heavily trabeculated and has an infundibulum from which the aorta arises. The right-sided venous ventricle has the internal morphology of a left ventricle; that is, it has a fine trabecular pattern and no infundibulum connects the chamber to the pulmonary trunk.

There is a frequent association of corrected transposition with other cardiac defects. Abnormalities of the left A-V valve occur in over 75 per cent of patients. Ebstein's anomaly or dysplasia is the most common anomaly.[1] Ventricular septal defects occur in approximately 75 per cent of patients, while pulmonic stenosis has been described in over 44 per cent of patients with corrected transposition.[2] Abnormalities in position and structure of the atrioventricular conduction system account for the high incidence of conduction disturbances (including complete heart block) in corrected transposition.[3]

Radiographic Features

The plain chest film may first raise the suspicion of corrected transposition in the asymptomatic patient and often provides very useful information when other defects are present. The radiographic features are related to the nature of associated anomalies as well as to the corrected transposition itself.

When corrected transposition occurs as an isolated anomaly with no hemodynamic abnormalities, the pulmonary vasculature and the heart size are normal (Fig. 5–92). In the presence of significant pulmonary stenosis, the vascularity is reduced, while in the

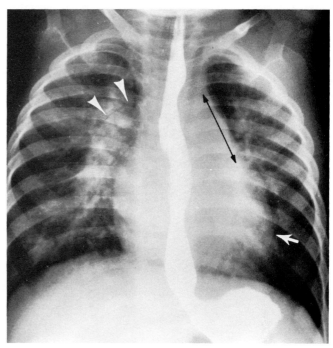

Figure 5-93. Posteroanterior chest radiograph in a child with corrected transposition and a large ventricular septal defect. The pulmonary vascularity is increased and the right main pulmonary artery is elevated (arrowheads). The triad of densities is absent, the left upper heart border is straight (double arrow), and a septal notch can be seen beneath the prominent mid left heart border (arrow).

presence of a moderate to large ventricular septal defect without pulmonary stenosis vascularity of the shunt type is seen. Elevation of the right main pulmonary artery is often a unique feature (Fig. 5–93).[4] Regardless of the intracardiac defects, analysis of the cardiomediastinal silhouette on the chest radiograph often reveals a loss of the normal "triad of densities" (Fig. 5–92). This triad consists of (1) the ascending aorta; (2) the aortic knob–descending aorta continuum; and (3) the pulmonary trunk. In corrected transposition, this triad is absent, since the ascending aorta is on the left and the pulmonary trunk is medial and posterior and therefore no longer border forming. This situation is most apparent when there is an associated large ventricular septal defect and the pulmonary trunk (which one would expect to be prominent when the great vessels are normally related) is not visible on the frontal chest film. The leftward aorta often gives a diagonally straightened or convex border to the left upper cardiac silhouette (Fig. 5–93). Since the proximal descending aorta is medial and rightward rather than lateral and leftward with respect to the ascending aorta, it is superimposed on the spine and the aortic knob may not be seen (Fig. 5–92). The cardiac contour is frequently abnormal. The leftward anatomic right ventricle may cause a prominence to the left midheart border (Fig. 5–92). Occasionally, one may detect a notch below the convex bulge of the systemic ventricle that represents the insertion of the ventricular septum (Fig. 5–93). This has been termed the "septal notch."[5] Left atrial enlargement will be present in those patients with significant left atrioventricular valve regurgitation (suggesting Ebstein's anomaly of the left atrioventricular valve) or a large ventricular septal defect.

Corrected transposition is occasionally associated with situs solitus and right cardiac apex (dextrocardia) (Fig. 5–94). In these cases, the left border of the cardiovascular silhouette presents two convexities: an inferior density formed by the systemic (morphologic right) ventricle and a superior density due to the ascending aorta (Fig. 5–94). The right cardiac border is usually smoothly convex from diaphragm to mediastinum and is formed by the venous (morphologic left) ventricle below and right atrium above (Fig. 5–94). In patients with situs inversus, with the cardiac apex and stomach on the right (a situation often termed "mirror image dextrocardia"), the ascending aorta may form a convexity along the upper right portion of the cardiovascular silhouette with the descending aorta present to the right of the

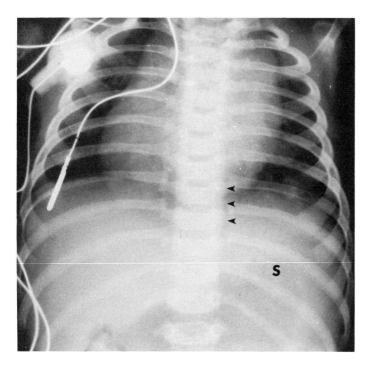

Figure 5–94. Anteroposterior chest radiograph in an infant with heart block. The stomach (S) and descending aorta (arrowheads) are on the left and the cardiac apex on the right. This suggests situs solitus with dextrocardia. This situation is frequently associated with corrected transposition. The convex right cardiac border represents the morphologic left ventricle. (See Fig. 5–97 for angiographic correlation.)

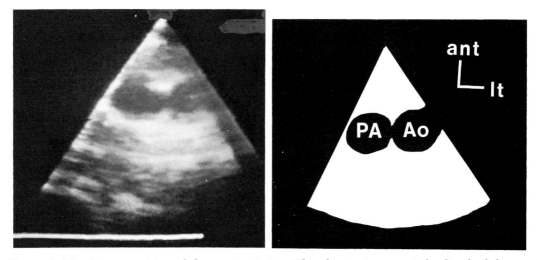

Figure 5–95. L-transposition of the great arteries. The short-axis scan at the level of the great arteries in L-transposition of the arteries demonstrates the side-by-side relationship of the leftward aorta (Ao) and the pulmonary arterial trunk (PA).

thoracic spine. The left heart border no longer shows the superior density of the ascending aorta seen when there is situs solitus and dextrocardia.

Echocardiographic Features

The right atrium is identified by the insertion of the inferior vena cava in the sub-xiphoidal long-axis view. The coarsely trabeculated right ventricular side of the inter-ventricular septum, which identified the anatomic right ventricle, will be found to the left (rather than to the right). This leads to the diagnosis of an L-ventricular loop with atrioventricular discordance.[6] The short-axis view of the great arterial root shows the characteristic "double circle" pattern of transposition with the anterior

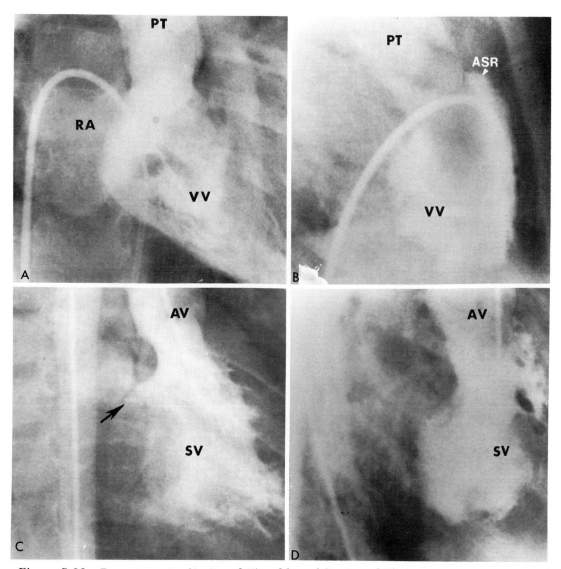

Figure 5–96. Posteroanterior (A, C, and E) and lateral (B, D, and F) angiograms in a patient with corrected transposition and a ventricular septal defect. A and B show the catheter entering a smooth-walled, anteriorly located anatomic left ventricle from the right atrium (RA). This venous ventricle (VV) gives rise to the pulmonary trunk (PT). The lateral view shows the anterosuperior recess (ASR). C and D show the catheter entering the trabeculated, anatomic right ventricle across the aortic valve (AV). A small VSD (arrow) is present in this systemic ventricle (SV).

Illustration continued on following page

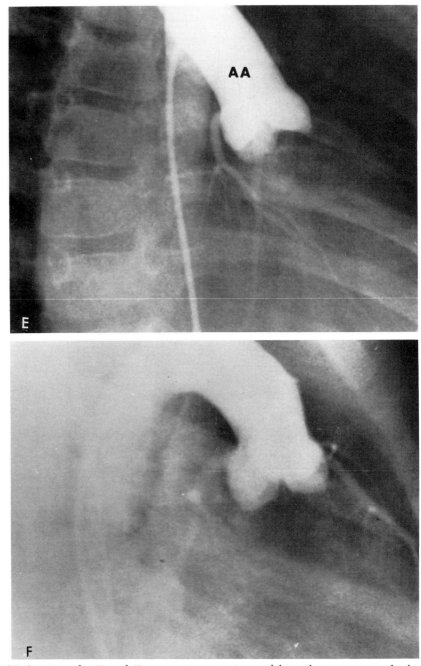

Figure 5–96 *Continued.* *E* and *F* are posteroanterior and lateral aortograms which demonstrate the position of the ascending aorta (AA) above the anatomic right ventricle.

aorta oriented to the left (L-transposition) (Fig. 5–95). Using the segmental approach the echo would define the patient as having situs solitus (S) with an L-ventricular loop (atrioventricular discordance or isolated ventricular inversion) and L-transposition of the great arteries. The lesions frequently associated with L-transposition of the great arteries (interventricular septal defects, pul-

monary stenosis, and left atrioventricular valve dysplasia) can all be diagnosed from the echocardiogram.

Angiographic Features

In the frontal projection in the patient with situs solitus and left cardiac apex, the right-sided venous (morphologic left) ven-

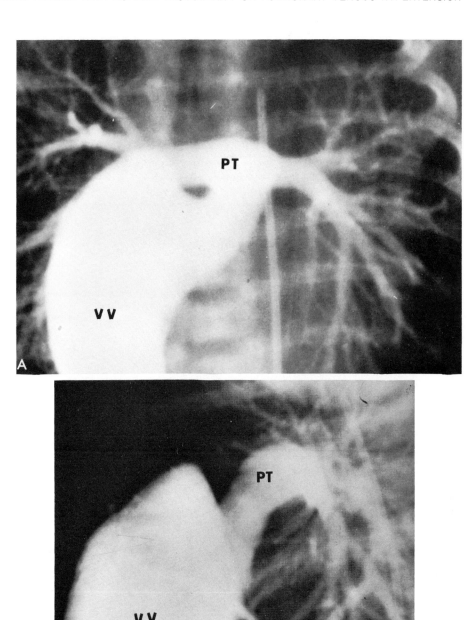

Figure 5–97. Posteroanterior *(A* and *C)* and lateral *(B* and *D)* angiograms in a child with dextrocardia and corrected transposition. The smooth-walled anatomic left ventricle (venous ventricle — VV) is located to the right and gives rise to the pulmonary trunk (PT). The trabeculated anatomic right ventricle (systemic ventricle — SV) is located to the left and gives rise to the aorta (A). Note that the right atrium (RA) connects with the venous ventricle and the left atrium (LA) with the systemic ventricle.

Illustration continued on following page

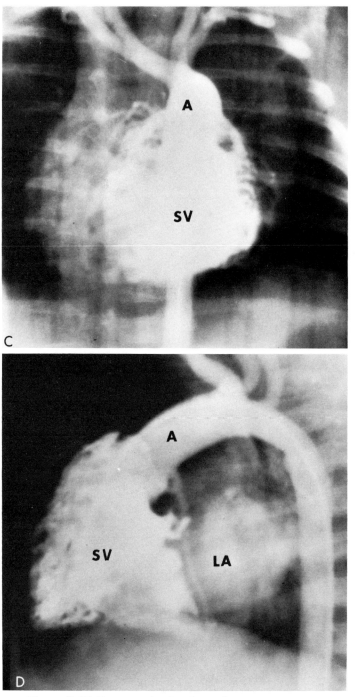

Figure 5–97 Continued. See legend on previous page.

tricle is smooth and triangular in shape and is located inferior and to the right of the left-sided systemic (morphologic right) ventricle (Figs. 5–96A and B). The venous ventricle gives rise to a medial and posterior positioned pulmonary trunk (Figs. 5–96A and B). A blind, anterior, and superior recess (the "anterosuperior recess")[7] is clearly viewed in the lateral angiogram (Fig. 5–96B) and may obscure the outflow tract in the frontal projection. The systemic ventricle is more trabeculated (expected, since it is morphologically a right ventricle) than the venous ventricle (Fig. 5–96C and D). Its rounded left wall forms the left margin of the cardiac silhouette, accounting for one of the characteristic plain chest film features of corrected transposition (see Fig. 5–92). In the lateral view the infundibular outflow tract of this ventricle is either slightly anterior to the venous outflow tract or directly lateral (Figs. 5–96D). The aortic valve plane is more cephalad than the pulmonary valve (Fig. 5–96) and the levo-positioned ascending aorta forms the left superior border of the cardiovascular silhouette (Fig. 5–96E).

When situs solitus with dextrocardia and corrected transposition exists, the morphologic left ventricle (venous ventricle) forms the right heart border and gives rise to the centrally positioned and posterior pulmonary trunk (Fig. 5–97A and B). The morphologic right ventricle (systemic ventricle) fills from the left atrium and forms the left heart border (Fig. 5–97C). It gives rise to the ascending aorta, which is positioned to the left of and anterior to the pulmonary trunk (Fig. 5–97C and D).

REFERENCES

1. Jaffe, R. B.: Systemic atrioventricular valve regurgitation in corrected transposition of the great vessels. Am J Cardiol 37:395, 1976.
2. Allwork, S. P., Bentall, H. H., Becker, A. E., Cameron, H., Gerlis, L. M., Wilkinson, J. L., Anderson, R. H.: Congenitally corrected transposition of the great arteries: Morphologic study of 32 cases. Am J Cardiol 38:910, 1976.
3. Berman, D. A., Aidcoff, A.: Corrected transposition of the great arteries causing complete heart block in an adult. Am J Cardiol 24:125, 1969.
4. Ellis, K., Morgan, B. C., Blumenthal, S., Anderson, D. H.: Congenitally corrected transposition of the great vessels. Radiology 79:35, 1962.
5. Tonkin, I. L., Kelley, M. J., Bream, P. R., Elliott, L. P.: The frontal chest film as a method of suspecting transposition complexes. Circulation 53:1016, 1976.
6. Solinger, R., Elbl, F.: Cardiac malpositions: Deductive echocardiographic analysis. In Echocardiography in Congenital Heart Disease. Lundström, N. R. (ed.). J. B. Lippincott Co., Philadelphia, 1978, p. 293.
7. Carey, L. S., Ruttenberg, H. D.: Roentgenographic features of congenitally corrected transposition of the great vessels. Am J Roentgenol 92:623, 1964.

Chapter 6

ACYANOTIC PATIENT WITH INCREASED PULMONARY FLOW (SHUNT VASCULARITY)

The presence of increased vascularity of the shunt type on the chest film can have several implications, and an appreciation of the clinical setting is necessary to separate the possible pathologic mechanisms involved. The shunt pattern (Fig. 6–1A) is seen whenever there is more than the normal amount of blood flowing to the lungs (approximately 2:1 pulmonary to systemic flow ratio or greater). While this most commonly occurs in the left-to-right shunts discussed in this chapter, it may occasionally be seen in high output states associated with anemia (Fig. 6–1B) or thyrotoxicosis. Once one has determined that the x-ray demonstrates shunt vascularity, it is important to know whether the patient is acyanotic or cyanotic. Certain cyanotic lesions involving preferential flow of excess blood to the lungs and misdirection of venous blood into the aorta with intact septa (for example, complete transposition of the great vessels) or involving excessive pulmonary flow and an obligatory right-to-left shunt (total anomalous venous return above the diaphragm) can have a pulmonary vascular pattern indistinguishable from an uncomplicated left-to-right shunt. Another potential problem involves the infant or child with a substantial left-to-right shunt and mild cyanosis

secondary to congestive heart failure and intrapulmonary right-to-left shunting. Generally, the pattern of shunt vascularity will predominate on the chest x-ray of these patients (Fig. 6–1C). In confusing cases, the clinical and laboratory information will usually be sufficient to indicate whether one is dealing with a case of increased flow and secondary hypoxemia.

Lesions producing increased pulmonary blood flow presenting in an acyanotic, full-term neonate are unusual (the special case of the premature infant with a patent ductus will be discussed later). Isolated ventricular or atrial septal defects or a patent ductus arteriosus rarely produce significant symptomatology in the full-term neonate because the higher pulmonary vascular resistance usually serves to control the volume of left-to-right shunting. Significant shunting may not appear until vascular resistance falls to near adult levels after the first days of life. Once high output states and cyanosis are excluded, the patient can be classified into the clinical-radiographic category of an *Acyanotic Patient with Shunt Vascularity*. Differential diagnosis can then be sought among the lesions listed in Table 6–1 before proceeding to look for clues on the chest radiograph and echocardiogram.

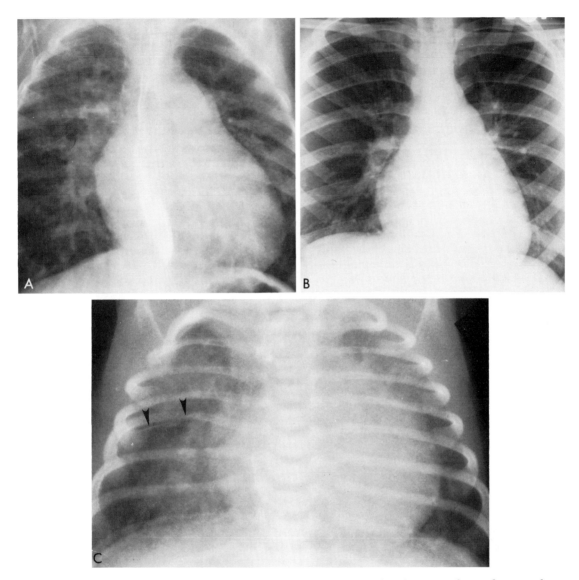

Figure 6–1. *A,* A young acyanotic child with typical radiographic features of a moderate to large left-to-right shunt. There are large hilar vessels and large, distinct peripheral vessels in all areas of the lung. A ventricular septal defect was diagnosed at catheterization, and the calculated pulmonary to systemic flow ratio was 3:1.

B, A teenage female with severe hemolytic anemia and a high output state. Note the prominent central pulmonary vasculature and pulmonary trunk. The chest film simulates a mild to moderate left-to-right shunt.

C, A mildly hypoxic infant with clinical signs of congestive failure. Although the pulmonary vascularity is indistinct and fluid is noted in the minor fissure (arrowheads), large vessels are seen in the lower lung fields and suggest that the predominant lesion is a left-to-right shunt. This pattern is the so-called "flow-failure" pattern. At cardiac catheterization the patient had a large ventricular septal defect and a patent ductus arteriosus.

TABLE 6–1. Lesions Associated with Increased Pulmonary Flow without Hypoxemia

Ventricular Septal Defect
Atrial Septal Defect
Patent Ductus Arteriosus
Endocardial Cushion Defect
Unusual Left-to-Right Shunts
  Left Ventricular to Right Atrial Communication
  Ruptured Sinus of Valsalva Aneurysm
  Coronary Arterial Fistula
  Aorticopulmonary Septal Defect

VENTRICULAR SEPTAL DEFECT

Ventricular septal defects represent the most common lesion among congenitally deformed hearts, accounting for approximately 25 per cent of all congenital cardiac anomalies.[1, 2] The ventricular septal defect (VSD) may be an isolated abnormality or it may be part of a complex malformation involving other cardiac structures (for example, tetralogy of Fallot). A VSD may also be associated with an additional malformation by chance rather than as part of a recognized complex (the association of VSD with coarctation of the aorta). The discussion in this section will be confined to the isolated VSD.

Ventricular septal defects are best classified in relation to anatomic landmarks of the normal right and left ventricle. At the most distal extent of the right ventricular infundibulum is the pulmonary valve. Posterior and inferior to the valve is an inverted U-shaped muscular ridge (the crista supraventricularis) that has a parietal and septal limb (Fig. 6–2). Posterior and inferior to this ridge is the papillary muscle of the conus, which receives chordae from the septal and anterior leaflets of the tricuspid valve. On the left ventricular side, the parietal limb of

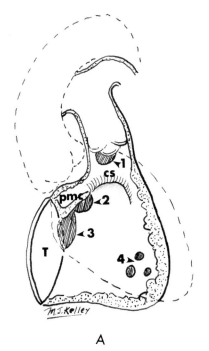
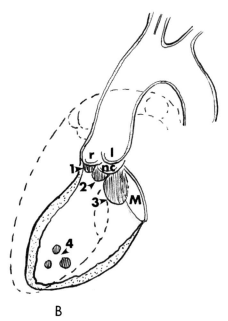

A   B

Figure 6–2. Diagrammatic representation of right ventricular (*A*) and left ventricular (*B*) anatomy illustrating locations of the four types of ventricular septal defect. The supracristal VSD (1) is located just beneath the pulmonary valve in the infundibulum of the right ventricle and just below the commissure between the right (r) and left (l) aortic valve cusps. The membranous VSD (2) is situated inferior and posterior to the crista supraventricularis (cs). This common defect may be located superior or inferior to the papillary muscle of the conus (pmc). On the left ventricular side, membranous defects are centered near the commissure between the right (r) and noncoronary (nc) cusps. Posterior VSDs (3) are adjacent to the septal leaflet of the tricuspid valve (T) and involve the inflow region of the left ventricle near the anterior leaflet of the mitral valve (M). Muscular VSDs (4) are bordered entirely by myocardium and may be located in the central or posterior portion of the muscular septum. They may be multiple.

the crista supraventricularis lies against the right aortic sinus, and the membranous septum lies inferior to the noncoronary aortic leaflet.

Ventricular septal defects are located in a "step ladder" posterior-inferior fashion starting at the pulmonary valve (Fig. 6–2). They may be defined in relation to the crista supraventricularis as follows:[3]

A. VSD Superior to the Crista Supraventricularis (Supracristal VSD)

These defects constitute approximately 8 per cent of isolated VSDs.[4] When viewed from the right ventricle, they are situated immediately beneath the pulmonary valve with the valve forming part of the superior margin of the defect. When viewed from the left ventricle, they are located just below the commissure that joins the right and left aortic valve cusps (Fig. 6–2). Herniation of the right aortic cusp into the defect has been described.[4]

B. VSD Inferior to Crista Supraventricularis (Infracristal VSD)

"MEMBRANOUS" VSD. These defects account for approximately 80 per cent of isolated VSDs. When viewed from the right ventricle, they are situated inferior and posterior to the crista and involve not only the membranous septum but also adjacent muscular septum (Fig. 6–2) (a more appropriate designation might be perimembranous VSD). They may be superior or inferior to the papillary muscle of the conus. In the latter variety, they are hidden by the septal leaflet of the tricuspid valve. When viewed from the left ventricle, these defects are centered near the commissure between the right and noncoronary aortic valve cusps (Fig. 6–2). Defects in the membranous septum may be associated with small aneurysms. These aneurysms are commonly associated with a decrease in size of membranous defects, but their presence does not necessarily predict eventual complete closure.[5]

ENDOCARDIAL CUSHION TYPE VSD (POSTERIOR VSD). This rare, isolated defect is comparable to the VSD seen in endocardial cushion deformities (persistent common atrioventricular canal). When viewed from the right ventricle, it is adjacent to the posterior aspect of the septal leaflet of the tricuspid valve (Fig. 6–2). As viewed from the left ventricle, it involves the inflow region of the ventricle, and the defect runs from the anterior leaflet of the mitral valve to include the membranous septum (Fig. 6–2). It is centered beneath the right and noncoronary aortic valve cusps.

MUSCULAR VSD. These defects are bordered entirely by myocardium. Although they are said to make up less than 5 per cent of VSDs,[6] a recent study suggests that they are more common[7] and that they may occur with other types of VSD. They may be classified into central, posterior, and marginal types.[7] The rare marginal defects are often multiple and have a tortuous, sinusoidal nature.

Aortic regurgitation occurs in 5 to 8 per cent of patients with ventricular septal defects.[8] It is more frequent with the supracristal defect but, since these defects are so uncommon, the association is seen more commonly with infracristal defects. The anatomic basis for the regurgitation appears to be related either to a prolapse of a normal valve that lacks support (with supracristal VSDs) or to an underdevelopment of the right coronary-noncoronary commissure (with infracristal VSDs).[9]

Physiologically, the consequences of a ventricular septal defect depend upon two things — the size of the defect and the pulmonary vascular resistance. The small defect is smaller than the aortic valve orifice and allows relatively little blood to pass into the right ventricle (usually a pulmonary to systemic flow ratio less than 1.5:1). In this situation, pressures in the right heart are normal and the defect acts as an obstructive opening between the two ventricles. Defects approximating the size of the aortic valve orifice are "nonrestrictive" (allowing free access from one ventricle to the other and equalization of pressure between the two chambers). Intermediate situations exist in which a "moderate" defect has physiologic effects between the two extremes.

Three courses are possible in the child with a large VSD and pulmonary hypertension: the defect may decrease in size with a decline in the amount of left-to-right shunt and pulmonary artery pressure; it may remain static and cause continued volume and

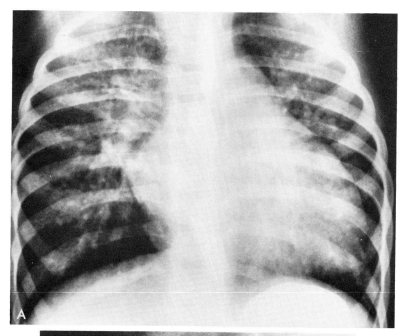

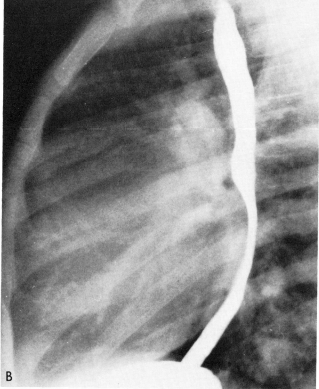

Figure 6–3. Posteroanterior (A) and lateral (B) chest radiographs in an acyanotic patient. There is shunt vascularity with prominent hilar and extrahilar pulmonary vessels, left atrial enlargement (shown by posterior deviation of the barium-filled esophagus on the lateral film), and mild cardiomegaly with a suggestion of left ventricular enlargement. The aorta appears to be normal in size and the findings are typical of a moderate ventricular septal defect.

pressure overload of the left heart and the pulmonary vasculature; or it may be associated with a progressive increase in pulmonary vascular resistance. In the third situation, the elevated pulmonary arterial pressure that accompanies a large VSD may be associated with progressive thickening of the media of the proximal pulmonary arterioles in a manner indistinguishable from the anatomic appearance of the normal fetal pulmonary vascular bed. Persistent increase in pulmonary flow and hypertension may also result in intimal proliferation.[10] These changes lead to an increase in pulmonary vascular resistance (pulmonary vascular obstructive disease). When pulmonary vascular resistance exceeds systemic resistance, the left-to-right shunt ceases and right-to-left shunting may occur (so-called Eisenmenger's physiology). Infants destined to enter this third phase usually do so by the second year of life. This occurs in about 10 per cent of large VSDs[11] and appears to occur earlier in patients with Down's syndrome.[12]

Two factors previously discussed can reduce the volume of the left-to-right shunt through a VSD — namely, a decrease in size or closure of the defect and the development of increasing pulmonary vascular resistance. A third factor may occasionally exist, and that is the development of right ventricular outflow tract obstruction owing to infundibular hypertrophy.

Radiographic Features

The radiologic manifestations of VSD depend on the size of the left-to-right shunt. Small defects (less than 1.5:1 pulmonary to systemic flow ratio) generally result in normal x-rays.

Moderate or large VSDs with low pulmonary vascular resistance have prominent vascularity of the shunt type with prominent hilar and extrahilar pulmonary vessels (Fig. 6–3A and B). In an acyanotic patient with shunt vascularity, the size of the left atrium may suggest the level of the shunt. Since the left atrium is usually normal in atrial septal defects, enlargement of the left atrium suggests a lesion at the ventricular or great vessel level (for example, a patent ductus). Left atrial enlargement (LAE) may be noted on the lateral film of infants as a distinct bulge that elevates the left mainstem bronchus (Fig. 6–4). A double density along the right heart border may suggest LAE, but may also be seen in normal children (Fig. 6–5). Left

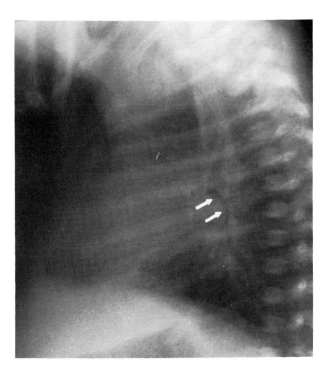

Figure 6–4. Lateral chest radiograph in an infant with moderate-sized ventricular septal defect. Note that the enlarged left atrium elevates the left mainstem bronchus (arrows).

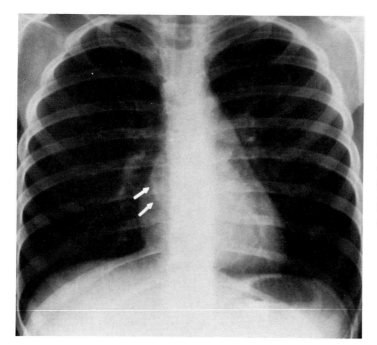

Figure 6–5. A double density (arrows) is noted along the right upper heart margin in this normal child. Although this sign may suggest left atrial enlargement, it may be seen in normal children or in individuals with a prominent right atrium.

atrial enlargement is most accurately assessed on the lateral film as a discrete posterior indentation of the barium-filled esophagus (Fig. 6–3B).

Left ventricular enlargement secondary to volume overload of the left heart is also present with moderate and large VSDs. This is manifested as a downward displacement or "sagging" of the cardiac apex (Figs. 6–1A and 6–3A). When pulmonary hypertension exists, concomitant right ventricular dilatation may exist. The aorta is usually normal or even small, since the increased flow from the shunt does not traverse it (Fig. 6–3). A right aortic arch is seen in approximately 2 per cent of VSDs.[13] Since this is rarely seen with the other common left-to-right shunts listed in Table 6–1, its presence may serve as a valuable clue to the presence of a shunt at the ventricular level.

When pulmonary vascular resistance rises in association with large VSDs, there may be increasing prominence of the pulmonary trunk. As the left-to-right shunt becomes negligible and the volume overload stimulus for cardiac dilatation ceases, the heart may appear normal in size (Fig. 6–6). The only radiographic clue to the development of this high resistance state (Eisenmenger's physiology) is the discrepancy in size between the dilated hilar pulmonary vasculature and pulmonary trunk and the normal-sized heart (Fig. 6–6). A review of serial x-rays may show diminution in size of the left atrium.

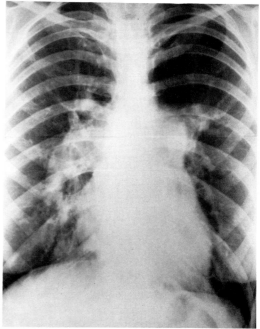

Figure 6–6. Posteroanterior chest radiograph in a cyanotic teenager demonstrating markedly dilated central pulmonary arteries with rapid tapering of vessels in the periphery (especially the left upper lobe). The patient had had a history of a systolic murmur that was no longer audible when this film was taken. Note the normal heart size. At cardiac catheterization the patient was found to have systemic pressures in the pulmonary circulation and markedly elevated pulmonary vascular resistance. Right-to-left shunting through a ventricular septal defect was observed angiographically (Eisenmenger physiology).

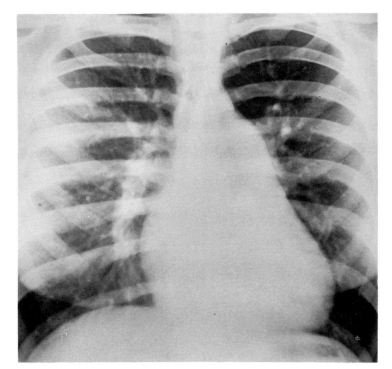

Figure 6–7. Posteroanterior chest radiograph in a young female who at the time of cardiac catheterization had small ventricular septal defect and mild pulmonary valve stenosis. Other than a slightly prominent pulmonary trunk, the chest film is essentially normal.

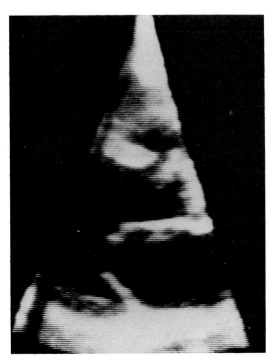 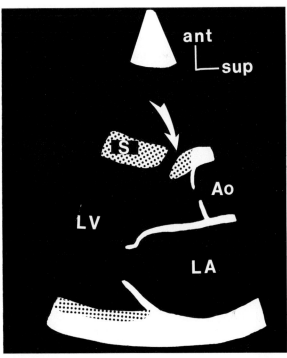

Figure 6–8. Anterior membranous ventricular septal defect. Long-axis view of the left ventricle demonstrating a 3 mm defect in the membranous portion of the interventricular septum (arrow). This defect lies below the aortic valve leaflets. The left-to-right shunt at the ventricular level results in enlargement of the left atrium (LA) compared with the aortic root (Ao). (LV = left ventricle; S = septum.)

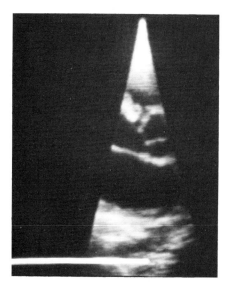
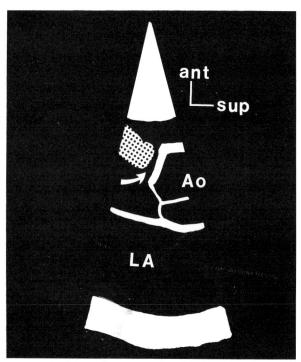

Figure 6–9. Supracristal ventricular septal defect. Long-axis view of the left ventricle. A small interventricular defect (curved arrow) is seen immediately below the noncoronary cusp of the aorta (Ao). This defect is higher than the defect shown in Figure 6–8 and is the result of a malalignment in the region of the conus. This VSD may be associated with aortic insufficiency. The right aortic cusp prolapsed into the defect during the real-time examination. (LA = left atrium.)

Diminished pulmonary vascularity, heart size, and left atrium can occur in patients with VSDs for two reasons: namely, diminished size or spontaneous closure of a VSD, or the development of infundibular pulmonary stenosis. Interestingly, pulmonary vascularity and left atrial size may remain prominent up to a year after successful surgical repair of VSDs.

In patients with aortic insufficiency in association with ventricular septal defect, there may be prominence of the ascending aorta or tortuosity of the descending aorta. This is in contrast to the normal appearance of the aorta in the isolated VSD (Figs. 6–1 and 6–3).

The acyanotic patient with mild pulmonary valve stenosis and a VSD will often have a relatively normal chest film (Fig. 6–7). This is understandable, since the left-to-right shunt is "controlled" by the pulmonary valve stenosis, and the heart size and left atrium are normal. Although this defect is often called an "acyanotic tetralogy of Fallot," in most cases the classic anatomic features of tetralogy are lacking.

Echocardiographic Features

In the presence of shunt vascularity on the chest radiograph, left-to-right shunting at the ventricular or great vessel level may be implied by the presence of left atrial enlargement on the echocardiogram.[14] In addition, the long-axis or apical view of the left ventricle may permit direct identification and measurement of the ventricular septal defect (Fig. 6–8).[15] Defects of the membranous or conal septum have been identified in the long-axis view. Occasionally, the defect is less accessible from this view; although, under ideal circumstances, defects as small as 3 mm in diameter can be visualized (Fig. 6–8). Supracristal interventricular septal defects (conal defects) can be directly seen and may be associated with prolapse of aortic valve leaflets into the defect, resulting in associated aortic insufficiency (Fig. 6–9).[16] Defects of the inflow portion of the interventricular septum (posterior VSD) are best visualized from either the apical or subxiphoidal views (Fig. 6–10). Fenestrations or small muscular defects are

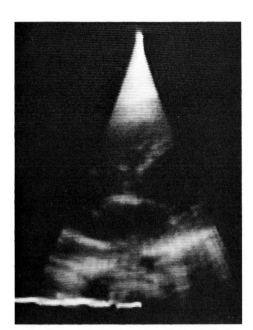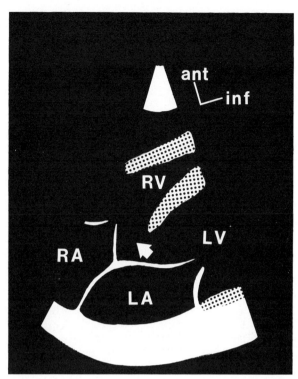

Figure 6–10. Posterior ventricular septal defect. This apical four-chamber view defines the inflow portion of the interventricular septum of a patient with a large posterior or atrioventricular canal type interventricular septal defect (arrow). The interatrial septum was intact. (LV = left ventricle; RV = right ventricle; LA = left atrium; RA = right atrium.)

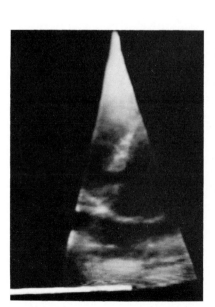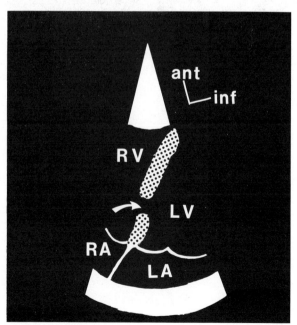

Figure 6–11. Muscular ventricular septal defect. Ventricular septal defects in the trabecular or muscular septum may occasionally be visualized in the apical four-chamber view (arrow). In this patient, the inflow septum and the apical portion of the muscular septum are intact. (LV = left ventricle; RV = right ventricle; RA = right atrium; LA = left atrium.)

more difficult to visualize directly (Fig. 6–11). These defects can be inferred from other evidence of left-to-right shunting, such as an increased left atrial size and previously mentioned radiographic clues.

Angiocardiographic Features

Until recently, left anterior oblique or biplane posteroanterior and lateral left ventriculography had been the standard method of imaging VSDs angiographically (Fig. 6–12A). A more precise way of determining the anatomic type and size of the defect, however, is achieved by axial left ventricular angiocardiography (see Chapter 4). The vertical tube image resulting from the hepatoclavicular (HC) or four-chamber view profiles the *posterior* ventricular septum, while the horizontal tube image from the long-axial oblique view profiles the *anterior* ventricular septum. Left ventriculograms performed in either of these views can localize a defect to the anterior or posterior interventricular septum. If the septum is visualized *through* the defect in the four-chamber view, it must be an anterior perimembranous defect (that is, the defect must be anterior to the profiled posterior septum) (Fig. 6–12B). If the defect allows visualization of the anterior septum through it in the long-axial oblique view, it must be a posterior (Cushion type) defect (that is, the defect must be posterior to the profiled anterior septum). Conversely, if a defect "silhouettes" the septum in the four-chamber view it is a posterior defect (Fig. 6–13), while if it silhouettes the anterior septum in the long-axial oblique (LAXO) view it is an anterior defect. Defects can be localized to the membranous (Fig. 6–12B) or muscular (Fig. 6–13) septum using these projections.

The horizontal tube image of the four-chamber view and the vertical tube image of the long-axial oblique projection provide an angled right anterior oblique left ventriculogram and allows one to (1) relate

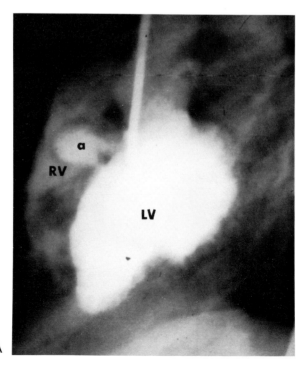

A

Figure 6–12. A, Standard lateral left ventriculogram (LV) shows a large aneurysm (a) in the membranous ventricular septum. Contrast material in the right ventricle (RV) indicates a moderate left-to-right shunt.

Illustration continued on opposite page

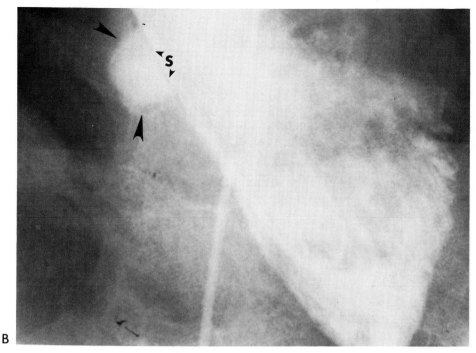

B

Figure 6–12 Continued B, Hepatoclavicular or four-chamber view of a left ventriculogram shows the left ventricle in a caudo-cranial LAO projection. There is an aneurysm of the membranous septum (arrowheads), and a small amount of contrast was seem emanating from this aneurysm during filming. Visualization of the septum (S) through this aneurysm identifies it as an anterior perimembranous defect.

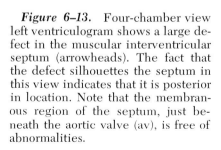

Figure 6–13. Four-chamber view left ventriculogram shows a large defect in the muscular interventricular septum (arrowheads). The fact that the defect silhouettes the septum in this view indicates that it is posterior in location. Note that the membranous region of the septum, just beneath the aortic valve (av), is free of abnormalities.

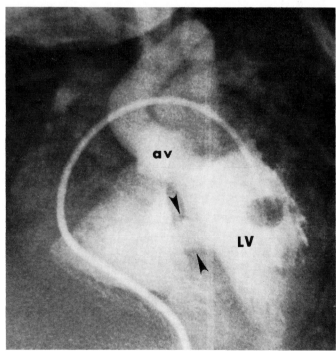

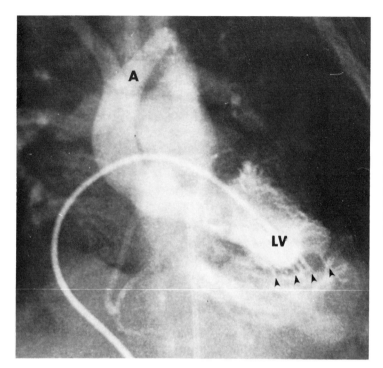

Figure 6–14. Four-chamber view left ventriculogram demonstrates multiple small muscular defects in the interventricular septum (arrowheads). The left ventricle (LV) and the transverse aorta (A) are small.

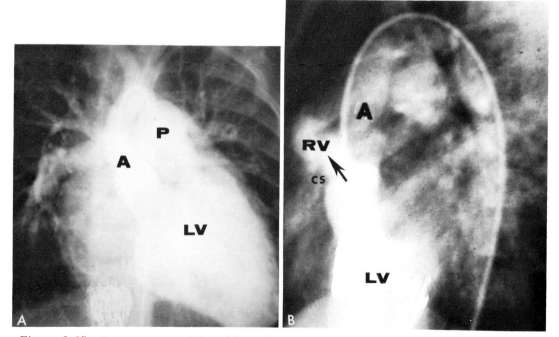

Figure 6–15. Posteroanterior (A) and lateral (B) left ventriculogram shows opacification of the pulmonary artery (P) from the left ventricle (LV). The lateral view (B) indicates that the ventricular septal defect exits beneath the right aortic sinus of Valsalva, passes above the crista supraventricularis (CS), and enters the right ventricular (RV) outflow tract. This is therefore a supracristal VSD.

the defect to the crista supraventricularis and (2) assess the right ventricular infundibulum. Infracristal membranous and infracristal muscular defects are illustrated in Figs. 6–12 and 6–13. Multiple muscular defects are illustrated in Fig. 6–14, and an aneurysm of the membranous septum associated with a left-to-right shunt is illustrated in Fig. 6–12. The four-chamber view may be superior to the long-axial oblique view in locating the posterior (endocardial cushion type) VSD (Fig. 6–13), since it profiles the posterior septum. Otherwise, comparable information is provided by both views.

While the common membranous septal defect can usually be repaired from the right atrial approach, the rare supracristal VSD requires a right ventriculotomy for adequate exposure. It is therefore important to be able to accurately identify the supracristal defect prior to surgery. In the standard frontal and lateral projections, the supracristal VSD will originate between the commissure of the right and left aortic cusps and enter the outflow tract of the right ventricle. In the lateral projection, contrast will enter the right ventricle above the crista supraventricularis or will partially obliterate this structure (Fig. 6–15). It is not reliable to depend on the fact that the supracristal defect opacifies only the outflow tract of the right ventricle while the infracristal defect opacifies the entire right ventricle, since it is not uncommon for flow from a small infracristal defect to be directed upward into the right ventricular outflow tract so that the entire right ventricle will not fill at left ventriculography.[17] The infracristal location of a VSD can best be appreciated in the lateral or RAO projection, since the crista will appear as a round filling defect beneath the contrast column separating the right sinus of Valsalva from the outflow tract of the right ventricle (Fig. 6–15). Since a modified RAO projection makes up one of the views in the four-chamber or long-axial oblique projection in biplane mode, either of these views can be used to locate the VSD with respect to the crista. The additional accuracy available with these views in terms of sizing the VSD, evaluating the left ventricular outflow tract, and ruling out additional muscular defects makes them the projection of choice in patients with suspected VSD.

If significant aortic regurgitation is present in association with a ventricular septal defect, it may be difficult to identify a sinus of Valsalva aneurysm with rupture into the right ventricle through the septal defect. An associated deformity or prolapse of the aortic cusp in such cases (the former seen in membranous VSDs, the latter with supracristal VSDs) makes matters more difficult. Direct catheter placement into the three aortic sinuses usually discloses the source of the shunt.[17]

REFERENCES

1. Keith, J. D., Rowe, R. D., Vald, P.: Heart Disease in Infancy and Childhood. Mac Millan, New York, 1979.
2. Krovetz, L. J., Gessner, I. H., Schiebler, G. L.: Handbook of Pediatric Cardiology. Hoeber-Harper, New York, 1981.
3. Edwards, J. E.: The pathology of ventricular septal defect. Semin Roentgenol 1:2, 1966.
4. Farru, O., Duffan, G., Rodriguez, R.: Auscultatory and phonocardiographic characteristics of supracristal ventricular septal defects. Br Heart J 33:238, 1971.
5. Freedom, R. M., White, R. D., Pieroni, D. R., Varghese, P. J., Krovetz, L. J., Rowe, R. D.: The natural history of the so-called aneurysm of the membranous ventricular septum in children. Circulation 49:375, 1974.
6. Goor, D. A., Lillehei, C. W.: Congenital Malformations of the Heart. Grune and Stratton, New York, 1975, p. 112.
7. Wenink, A. C. G., Oppenheimer-Dekker, A., Moulaert, A. J.: Muscular septal defects: A reappraisal of the anatomy. Am J Cardiol 43:259, 1979.
8. Tatsuno, K., Konno, S., Sakakibara, S.: Ventricular septal defect with aortic insufficiency. Am Heart J 85:13, 1973.
9. Tatsuno, K., Konno, S., Ando, M., Sakakibara, S.: Pathogenetic mechanisms of prolapsing aortic valves and aortic regurgitation associated with ventricular septal defect. Circulation 48:1028, 1973.
10. Wagenvoort, C. A., Neufeld, H. N., DuShane, J. W., Edwards, J. E.: The pulmonary arterial tree in ventricular septal defect: A quantitative study of anatomic features in fetuses, infants, and children. Circulation 23:740, 1961.
11. Collins, G., Calder, L., Rose, V., Kidd, L., Keith, J.: Ventricular septal defect: Clinical and hemodynamic changes in the first five years of life. Am Heart J 84:695, 1972.
12. Chi, T. P., Krovetz, L. J.: The pulmonary vascular bed in children with Down's syndrome. J Pediatr 86:533, 1975.
13. Varghese, P. J., Allen, J. R., Rosenquist, G. C., Rowe, R. D.: Natural history of ventricular septal defect with right sided aortic arch. Br Heart J 32:537, 1970.
14. Lewis, A. B. Takahashi, M.: Echocardiographic assessment of left to right shunt volume in children with ventricular septal defect. Circulation 54:78, 1976.

15. Canales, J. M., Sahn, D. J., Allen, H. D., Goldberg, S. J.: Factors affecting real-time cross-sectional echocardiographic imaging of ventricular septal defects. Am J Cardiol 45:467, 1980 (abstract).
16. Van Praagh, R., McNamara, J. J.: Anatomic types of ventricular septal defect with aortic insufficiency. Am Heart J 75:604, 1968.
17. Baron, M. G., Wolf, B. S., Steinfeld, L., Gordon, A. J.: Left ventricular angiocardiography in the study of ventricular septal defects. Radiology 81:223, 1963.

ATRIAL SEPTAL DEFECTS

The term *atrial septal defect (ASD)* indicates an isolated defect in the atrial septum. Defects in the atrial septum that extend into the atrioventricular canal (ostium primum defects) and that are part of an endocardial cushion malformation will not be included in this discussion. The various types of isolated ASDs and their estimated incidence are listed in Table 6–2.[1] The ASD accounts for approximately 8 per cent of all congenital heart defects.[2]

The *patent foramen ovale* is a small tunnel situated between the superior limbic septum and the septum ovale. Normally, these two septa overlap and, with the higher pressure in the left atrium, the septum ovale is forced against the limbic septum, preventing a left-to-right shunt. If, however, right atrial pressure is higher than left atrial pressure, a right-to-left shunt is possible. This occurs in prenatal life — allowing flow of oxygenated blood from the placenta via the inferior vena cava into the left atrium. Significant elevation of left atrial pressure may lead to a left-to-right shunt. Although the foramen ovale is sealed immediately after birth in most infants, it may remain patent if right atrial pressure remains elevated. It has been found to be probe patent in 25 per cent of normal human hearts.[3]

TABLE 6–2. Classification of Isolated Atrial Septal Defects

Patent Foramen Ovale	25% of normal hearts
Ostium Secundum Defect	70%
Sinus Venous Defect	30%

The *ostium secundum atrial septal defect* (also called septum primum ASD) may involve all or part of the septum ovale and may be singular or multiple. These defects result either from failure of the septum primum to develop or from secondary fenestration of the septum primum.

The *sinus venosus atrial septal defect* (superior or inferior caval ASD) may be located near the entrance of the superior vena cava (high ASD) or in the inferior portion of the septum near the entrance of the inferior vena cava. Both defects are commonly associated with anomalous pulmonary venous connections (from right upper or right lower lobes, respectively) either into the right atrium or into their contiguous caval system.

The altered physiology of the isolated ASD is similar for all varieties of the defect. Generally, a large defect results in free communication between the atria with little or no pressure gradient. The relative distensibility of the two ventricles (the thin-walled right ventricle being more distensible) appears to be the main factor that determines the direction of the shunt. As blood is shunted from the left atrium to the right, it passes through and causes dilatation of the right atrium, right ventricle, pulmonary trunk, and pulmonary arteries and veins. The left atrium does not generally enlarge, since a significant portion of the shunted blood comes from the right pulmonary veins, which deliver it directly into the right atrium. In addition, the right atrium appears to be more distensible than the left.

The ASD is well tolerated in infants and children. Commonly, the defect is suspected for the first time during routine preschool examination. It is also the most common congenital heart defect discovered in adults for the first time.[3] It is more common in females than in males by a ratio of approximately 3:1.[6]

Associated Lesions

Secundum atrial septal defects may be associated with a syndrome consisting of characteristic hand deformities — the Holt-Oram syndrome.[7] Classicially, the thumb is hypoplastic and has an extra phalanx (triphalangeal thumb). Metacarpal and radial hypoplasia may also occur. Children with secundum ASDs are reported to have an incidence of prolapse of the mitral valve of 8 to 37 per cent,[8, 9] and the frequency in adults appears to be even greater.[10] The mitral valve in patients with a long-standing atrial septal defect may be vulnerable to insult, as there is increased occurrence of rheumatic fever with subsequent mitral stenosis (Lutembacher's syndrome).[11]

Radiographic Features

In children and adolescents with an ASD, the chest radiograph findings are characteristic and may provide enough evidence to suggest the presence of a left-to-right shunt at the atrial level. If the left-to-right shunt is 2:1 or greater, the pulmonary vascularity pattern will be of the shunt type. In the typical ASD, the pulmonary vascular resistance is low, and therefore large pulmonary vessels will be seen in the periphery of the lungs (Fig. 6–16A and C). In addition, there will usually be prominence of the pulmonary trunk and a straight or convex left upper heart border due to dilatation of the right ventricular outflow tract (Fig. 6–16A and C). Dilatation of these structures may obliterate the left pulmonary artery and make the right pulmonary artery seem inordinately large (Fig. 6–16A). The right atrium (Fig. 6–17A) and right ventricle are enlarged. The latter can be appreciated as fullness in the retrosternal region in the lateral view (Fig. 6–16B and D) or as a rounded bulge in the LAO view (Fig. 6–17B). The ascending aorta, aortic knob, and superior vena cava are typically inconspicuous (Figs. 6–16A and 6–17A).[12] The key radiographic feature that helps to separate the uncomplicated ASD from the other lesions listed in Table 6–1 is *absence of left atrial enlargement*. In acyanotic patients with moderate or large left-to-right shunts, the absence of left atrial enlargement favors a shunt at the atrial level (Figs. 6–16B and D). The two other common left-to-right shunts in the differential diagnosis (ventricular septal defect and patent ductus arteriosus) are associated with left atrial enlargement. The reason for absence of left atrial enlargement in ASDs has been discussed previously. True left atrial enlargement may occasionally be seen in adults with ASD[13] — apparently because of the long-standing increased flow through the older and presumably more distensible left atrium. "Pseudo" left atrial enlargement may be encountered in patients with large atrial septal defects because of posterior displacement of the left atrium by the dilated right heart.

Although the left ventricle does not enlarge in ASDs, the dilated right ventricle may displace the left ventricle posteriorly, causing it to appear enlarged on the lateral or LAO views (Fig. 6–17B). The shadow of the inferior vena cava on the lateral film can be used to distinguish true left ventricular enlargement in these cases. When the left ventricle is truly dilated, the inferior vena cava will maintain its location midway in the chest between the posterior heart border and the hemidiaphragms. When the left ventricle is pushed posteriorly by a dilated right ventricle (as in ASD), the cava is seen in a more posterior position, although it maintains its position between the posterior cardiac border and the hemidiaphragm.[14]

The previous discussion applies to the radiologic features of all types of ASD (including the ostium primum endocardial cushion defect). Occasionally, the chest film will suggest the type of ASD or a commonly associated anomaly, partial anomalous pulmonary venous connection. In the sinus venosus atrial septal defect, a localized prominence may be seen at the superior vena cava–right atrial junction (Fig. 6–18) (also see Fig. 6–31). This is because of the confluence of an anomalously connected right upper lobe pulmonary vein and the dilated distal superior vena cava. This anomaly is present in 80 to 90 per cent of patients with sinus venosus ASDs.[15] Partial anomalous pulmonary venous connections (pulmonary venous drainage from one lung or lobe into systemic venous structures) involve the right pulmonary veins ten times more commonly than the left lung.[17] The most common variety is partial anomalous pulmonary venous connection to the superior vena cava or right atrium. This type of anomaly invariably coexists with an atrial septal defect.[16]

When the left pulmonary veins drain anomalously or when the inferior vena cava receives anomalous veins from the right lung, an associated ASD is rare.[18] When the left upper lobe pulmonary vein drains to the innominate vein or to a persistent left superior vena cava, the frontal chest film may demonstrate an oblique or vertical density in the left superior mediastinum representing the anomalous vein (Fig. 6–19) (see also Fig. 6–30). The chest film may additionally

Text continues on page 303

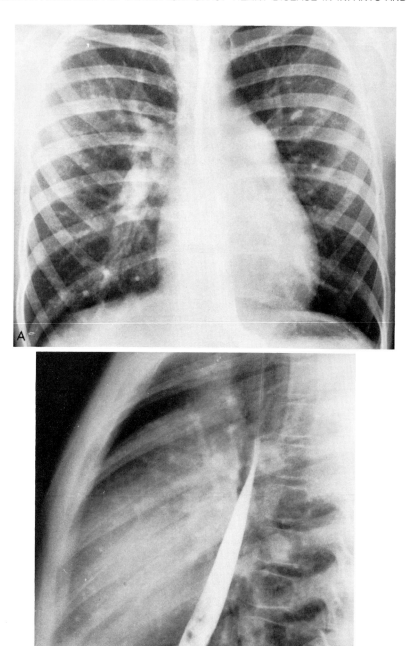

Figure 6–16. Two young children with atrial septal defects. There is shunt vascularity of a moderate degree in both cases. In *A*, the pulmonary trunk is prominent, and in *C* there is fullness along the left heart border due to the dilated right ventricle and right ventricular outflow tract. In both frontal films, the left pulmonary artery is obliterated, making the right pulmonary artery seem inordinately large. The lateral views *B* and *D* show no evidence of left atrial enlargement. There is fullness in the retrosternal region, suggesting right heart enlargement.

Illustration continued on opposite page

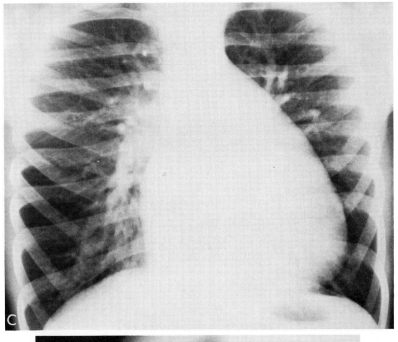

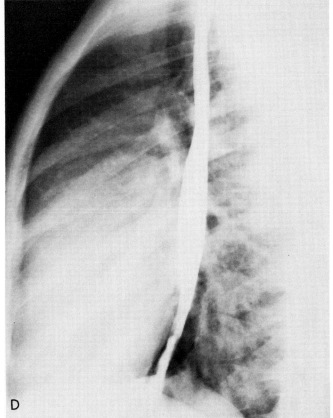

Figure 6–16 Continued

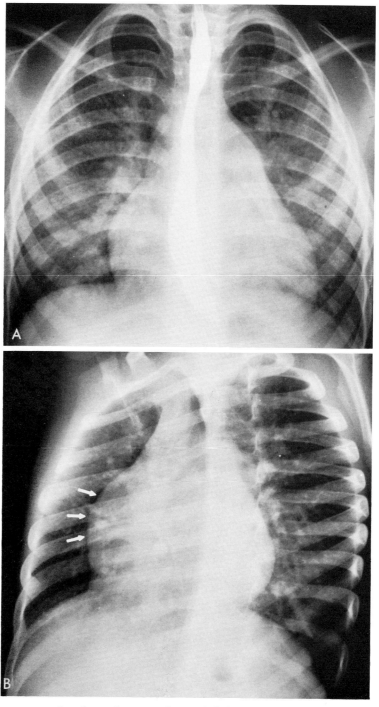

Figure 6–17. A young female with an atrial septal defect. There is prominent, shunt vascularity and the right atrium and pulmonary trunk are dilated on the frontal view (*A*). In the left anterior oblique projection, dilated right heart structures are shown as a distinct bulge (arrows). Note that the left ventricle projects beyond the spine. At angiography the left ventricle was normal in size. This case illustrates that the left ventricle can be pushed posteriorly by the dilated right ventricle. Note in this case and in the cases illustrated in Figure 6–16 that the aortic knob is inconspicuous.

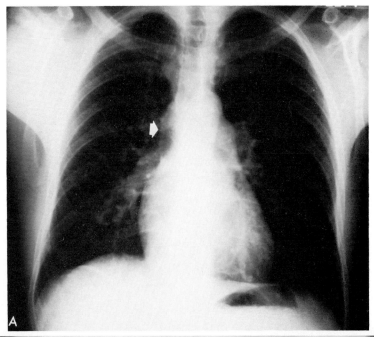

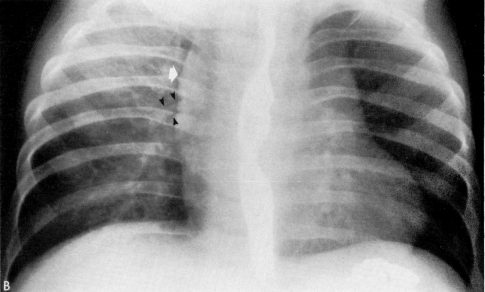

Figure 6–18. An adult (*A*) and an infant (*B*) each with an atrial septal defect. Note the prominence of the superior vena cava in both cases (arrow). In the infant this density may be due to the thymus. However, the density of the right upper lobe pulmonary vein (arrowheads) can be seen entering the superior vena cava. At catheterization and angiography there was partial anomalous pulmonary venous connection from the right upper lobe to the superior vena cava in both cases. (See Fig. 6–31 for the angiogram of case *B*.)

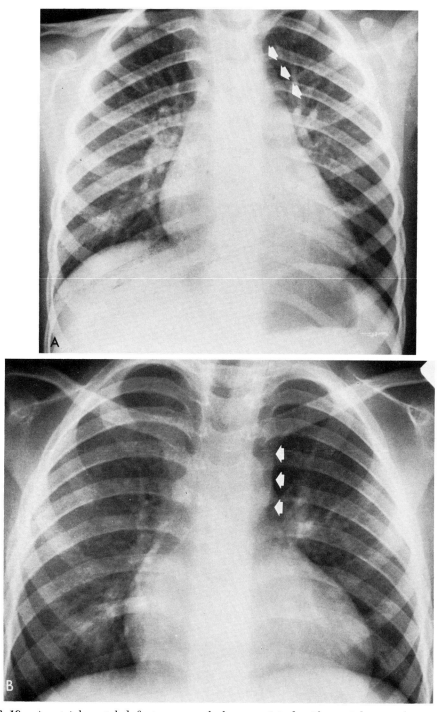

Figure 6–19. An atrial septal defect may rarely be associated with partial anomalous pulmonary venous connection to the innominate vein or persistent left superior vena cava. The frontal chest radiograph in these cases may demonstrate an oblique (A) or vertical (B) density in the left superior mediastinum that represents the anomalous connecting vein (arrows). (See Fig. 6–30 for the angiogram of case A.)

suggest the diagnosis when there is anomalous connection from the right lower lobe or right lung to the inferior vena cava. The anomalous venous structure is crescent shaped and widens as it courses inferiorly (Fig. 6–20). This contour has been likened to a Turkish sword, and the term "scimitar sign" has been applied to it. Commonly, this picture is associated with hypoplasia of one or more lobes of the right lung and a shift of the heart to the right (Fig. 6–20). The term "scimitar syndrome" is applied to this group of findings.[19]

Echocardiographic Features

The M-mode echocardiographic study may provide indirect evidence of the presence of left-to-right shunting at the atrial level. A characteristic pattern of interventricular septal motion termed "paradoxic" is thought to result from posterior displacement of the center of ventricular mass secondary to diastolic volume overload of the right ventricular cavity[20] (Figs. 6–21 and 6–22). The atrial septum is well visualized on two-dimensional studies both from the apical and subxiphoidal approach (Figs. 6–23 through 6–25). The subxiphoidal view may be preferred since it places the septum perpendicular to the interrogating beam axis and thus provides the greatest clarity. Secundum and sinus venosus atrial septal defects are characterized by the absence of reflecting echoes in the mid and upper portions of the interatrial septum (Figs. 6–24 and 6–25). Enlargement of the right atrial and ventricular internal dimensions[22] (Fig. 6–26) and the M-mode echocardiographic documentation of paradoxic interventricular septal motion (Figs. 6–21 and 6–22) along with direct visualization of the defect on two-dimensional scanning (Figs. 6–23 through 6–25) are virtually diagnostic of interatrial septal defects. The use of peripheral vein ultrasonic contrast techniques may be useful in questionable cases to identify transient right-to-left shunting at the atrial level that may be provoked by the Valsalva maneuver.[23, 24] Mitral valve prolapse has been described in 95 per cent of 24 adult patients with atrial septal defect.[10] Predominant involvement of the anterior leaflet has been noted. Paradoxic septal motion was observed in only nine of these 24 patients.[10]

Contrast ultrasonography[25] is a technique that capitalizes on the presence of dissolved microbubbles of air in virtually all injected fluids. The most commonly used fluids are saline or indocyanine-green dye. The microcavitations act as miniature ultrasonic reflecting centers and are visible as a rapidly moving cloud of signals that permit the pattern of blood flow to be visualized on echocardiography. In normals, peripheral vein injection of normal saline will create a

Text continues on page 309

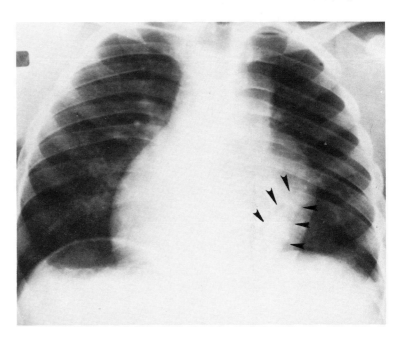

Figure 6–20. Posteroanterior chest radiograph (A) in an acyanotic child with total situs inversus. Note that the "right" lung is smaller than the "left" and that the heart is shifted to the "right." The curvilinear density in the "right" lower lung field ("scimitar sign") (arrowheads) represents the anomalous pulmonary vein that drains into the inferior vena cava. The angiogram of this case is illustrated in Figure 6–29.

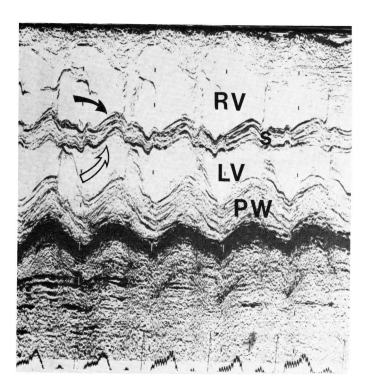

Figure 6–21. Right ventricular volume overload. M-mode echocardiograph of a patient with right ventricular volume overload due to a left-to-right shunt through a secundum atrial septal defect. The septum (S) shows a characteristic motion that has been termed paradoxic septal motion, type "A." The septum is thought to contract toward the center of the ventricular mass during systole. Therefore, because of increased right ventricular volume, both the right side of the septum (closed arrow) and the left side of the septum (open arrow) show an abnormal motion toward the dilated right ventricular cavity (RV). (LV = left ventricle; PW = posterior wall).

Figure 6–22. Right ventricular volume overload. M-mode tracing of a patient with right ventricular volume overload due to a left-to-right shunt through a secundum atrial septal defect. The septum (S) shows a motion that is characterized as paradoxic septal motion, type "B." The right side of the septum (closed arrow) contracts paradoxically toward the right ventricle during systole; however, the left side of the septum (open arrow) has motion that is less clearly abnormal. The diagnostic implications of septal motion showing either paradoxic type "A" or type "B" are the same and imply right ventricular volume overload. The differing patterns of septal motion may be due to the portion of the septum interrogated by the narrow M-mode beam. (RV = right ventricle; LV = left ventricle; PW = posterior wall.)

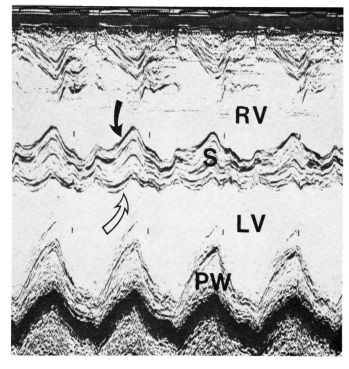

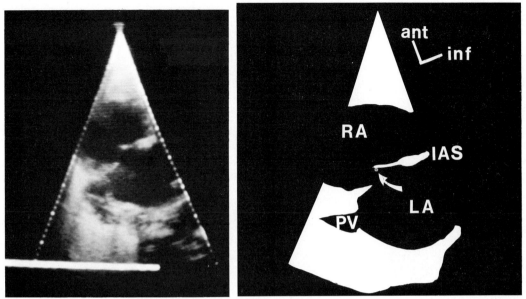

Figure 6–23. Patent foramen ovale. The short-axis view from the subxiphoid position depicts both ventricular inflow tracts. The interatrial septum (IAS) is well seen and appears intact with prolapse of the inferior lip of the foramen ovale (curved arrow) toward the right atrium. (RA = right atrium; LA = left atrium; PV = pulmonary vein.)

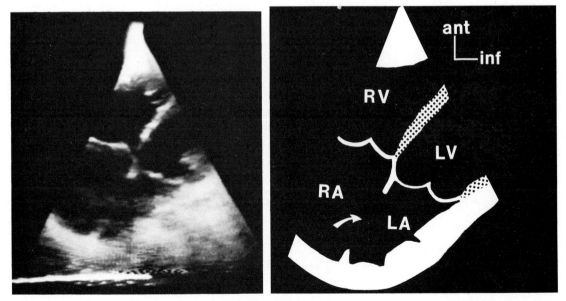

Figure 6–24. Atrial septal defect. Subxiphoidal four-chamber view of an ostium secundum atrial septal defect. The interatrial septum is seen in detail. The upper portion of the atrial septum (septum secundum) is deficient of tissue (curved arrow) and there is a dense echo arising from the intact lower septum (septum primum). The right atrial cavity (RA) is larger than the left atrial cavity (LA). The interventricular septum separating the right and left ventricle (RV and LV) is intact.

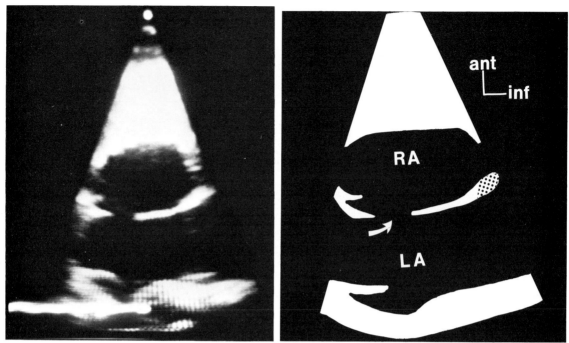

Figure 6–25. Long-axis subxiphoidal view of a secundum atrial septal defect. In this view, the interatrial septum is deficient of tissue in the position of the foramen ovale (arrow). This represents an interatrial septal defect of the secundum type. The lower portion of the septum (septum primum) is intact. (RA = right atrium; LA = left atrium.)

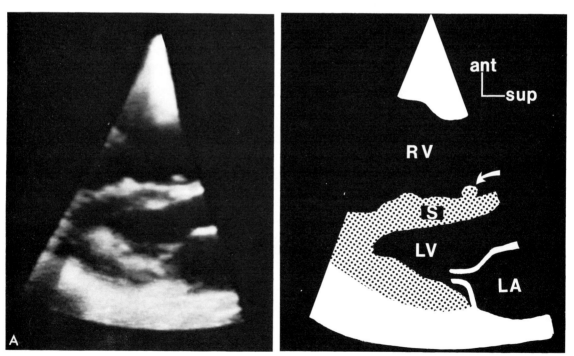

Figure 6–26 See legend on opposite page

Illustration continued on opposite page

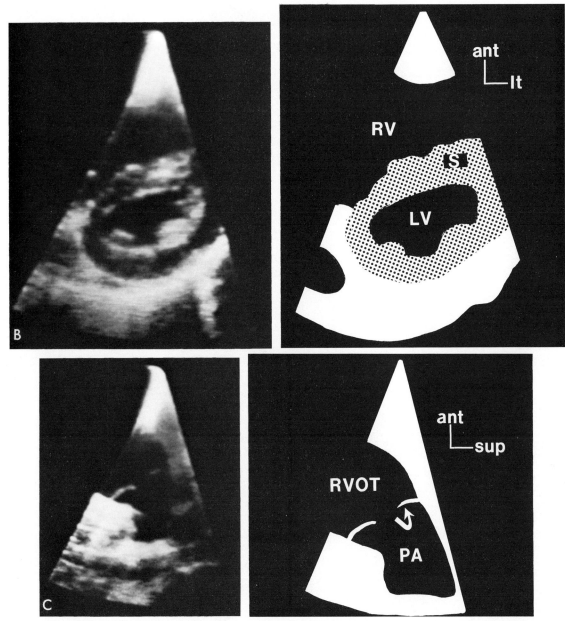

Figure 6–26. Atrial septal defect. *A*, Long-axis view of a patient with secundum atrial septal defect. Right ventricular (RV) cavity enlargement is noted with flattening of the left ventricular cavity (LV). The left atrial cavity (LA) is not enlarged. Prominent right ventricular trabeculations (arrow) can be seen on the right ventricular aspect of the interventricular septum. *B*, Short-axis scan of a patient with a secundum atrial septal defect. The right ventricle is enlarged (RV) with posterior displacement of the septum (S). The left ventricular cavity (LV) has an oval shape rather than the normal circular cross-sectional shape. *C*, Long-axis view showing dilatation of the right ventricular outflow tract (RVOT) in a patient with secundum atrial septal defect. The pulmonary artery (PA) is dilated and the pulmonic valve (arrow) is seen separating the right ventricular outflow tract and the main pulmonary artery.

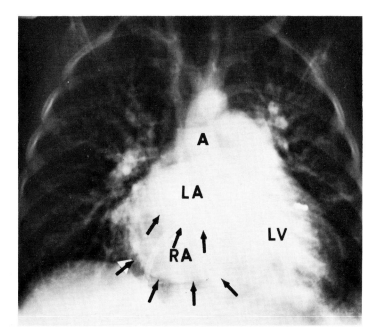

Figure 6–27. Levophase of a standard posteroanterior right ventriculogram showing opacification of the right atrium (RA) shortly after opacification of the left atrium (LA). The floor of the left atrium (upper three arrows) is obliterated by the presence of contrast in the right atrium (lower four arrows). The left ventricle (LV) and aorta (A) are also opacified.

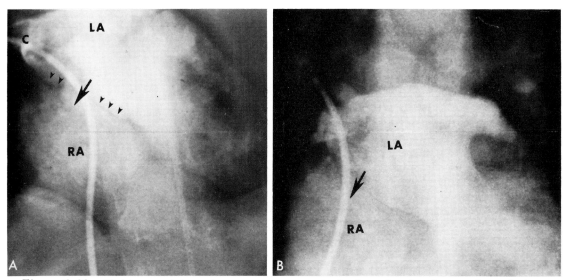

Figure 6–28. Right upper lobe pulmonary venograms in the four-chamber (hepatoclavicular) view showing the angiographic appearances of the various types of ASD.

A, Ostium secundum ASD. Note catheter (*C*) in the right upper lobe pulmonary vein; the lucencies created by the upper and lower portions of the atrial septum (arrowheads); the catheter position and contrast flow across the secundum region of the atrial septum (arrow); and the contrast-filled left atrium (LA) and right atrium (RA).

B, Ostium secundum ASD. Note the break in the lucency of the atrial septum created by flow of contrast (arrow) from the left atrium (LA) to the right atrium (RA).

C, Ostium primum ASD. Note the catheter (*C*) across the foramen ovale (arrowhead) in the right upper pulmonary vein. Contrast crosses the atrial septum in the lower (primum) portion of the septum (arrow). Note also the small left atrium (LA) and large right atrium (RA).

D, Partial anomalous pulmonary venous connection to the right atrium associated with a sinus venous ASD. Note that contrast from the right upper lobe pulmonary vein catheter (*C*) flows directly into the right atrium (RA). Some contrast fills the large right atrial appendage (RAA).

Illustration continued on opposite page

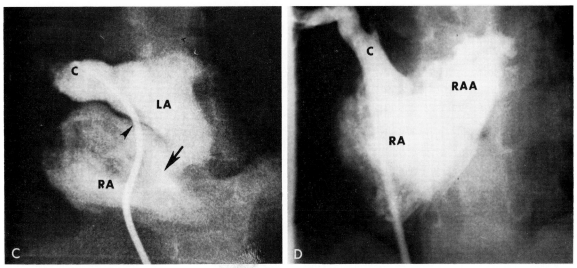

Figure 6–28 Continued

"cloud" of signals that is removed during passage through the lung and that therefore does not appear in the left atrium or ventricle. Patients with atrial septal defect and normal pulmonary vascular resistance will usually shunt blood from left to right atrium and are thus generally undetectable directly by ultrasonic contrast technique. The Valsalva maneuver may result in a transient right-to-left atrial shunt across the defect. With the shunt in this direction, ultrasonic contrast will show the flow of bubbles across the defect and into the left ventricle.

Left-to-right shunts may also be detected by the observation of "negative" contrast in the right atrium following peripheral vein injection of fluid. This is best viewed from the subxiphoidal or apical four-chamber view. The technique is safe and does not result in occlusive arterial gas embolism.

Angiocardiographic Features

In the past, atrial septal defects have been detected indirectly on the levophase of a pulmonary arteriogram or right ventriculo-

Figure 6–29. Selective pulmonary venogram in the child with total situs inversus whose chest film appears in Figure 6–20. The catheter was placed in the "right" lower lobe pulmonary vein (PV) from the inferior vena cava. This illustrates the type of anomalous pulmonary venous connection found in the so-called "scimitar syndrome."

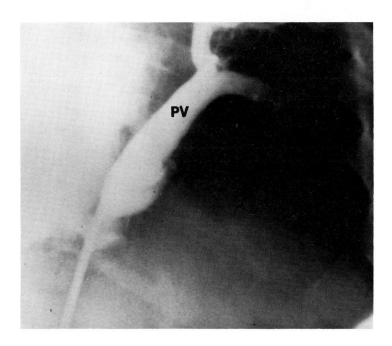

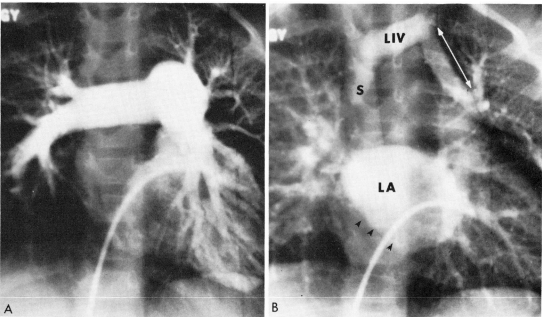

Figure 6–30. A, Angiogram performed in the right ventricular infundibulum showing slightly dilated pulmonary trunk and central pulmonary arteries. On the levophase (B), the left upper lobe pulmonary veins drain into an obliquely oriented venous channel (double arrow) that connects with the left innominate vein (LIV) that in turn drains in the usual fashion into the superior vena cava (S). The left atrium (LA) is opacified from the remainder of the normally draining pulmonary veins and the well-visualized left atrial floor (arrowheads) suggests that there is no ASD. (See Fig. 6–19A for chest film correlation.)

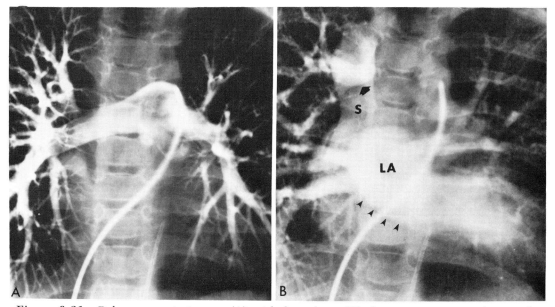

Figure 6–31. Pulmonary arteriogram (A) with levophase (B) demonstrating partial anomalous pulmonary venous connection from the right upper lobe pulmonary vein (arrow) to the superior vena cava (S). The remainder of the pulmonary veins drain normally into the left atrium (LA), and the atrial septum appears to be intact (arrowheads). (See Fig. 6–18B for chest film correlation.)

gram by noting the presence of contrast in the right atrium shortly after the left atrium is opacified (Fig. 6–27). However, angled LAO views with the catheter in the right upper pulmonary vein (hepatoclavicular/four-chamber view) allow detection of the exact location and size of the defect. Ostium secundum defects can be distinguished from ostium primum defects and sinus venous defects (Fig. 6–28). Partial anomalous venous connections from the right upper lobe can readily be evaluated using this view (Fig. 6–28). Anomalous venous return from the right lower lobe to the inferior vena cava can be approached with a direct retrograde injection into the vein (Fig. 6–29). This direct approach can be used to study anomalous venous connections. Pulmonary arteriography with filming carried out into the levophase is also a satisfactory way to evaluate and identify anomalous venous connections either to the left (Fig. 6–30) or to the right (Fig. 6–31) superior vena cava.

Left ventriculography may also be performed to evaluate the mitral valve for prolapse and mitral regurgitation (see Fig. 5–90). The left ventricle in large ASDs may have a concave inferior wall and convex anterior lateral wall that has been termed the "ballerina slipper" appearance. This appearance may be noted in other lesions that cause right ventricular pressure or volume overload.

REFERENCES

1. Goor, D. A., Lillehei, C. W.: Congenital Malformations of the Heart. Grune and Stratton, New York, 1975, p. 104.
2. Krovetz, L. J., Gessner, I. H., Schiebler, G. L.: Handbook of Pediatric Cardiology. Hoeber-Harper, New York, 1969.
3. Taussig, H. B.: Congenital Malformations of the Heart. Commonwealth Fund, New York, 1947.
4. Rowe, G. G., Castillo, C. A., Maxwell, G. M., Clifford, J. E., Crumpton, C. W.: Atrial septal defect and the mechanism of the shunt. Am Heart J 61:369, 1961.
5. Little, R. C.: Volume elastic properties of right and left atrium. Am J Physiol 148:237, 1949.
6. Zaver, A. G., Nada, A. S.: Atrial septal defect — secundum type. Circulation 32 (Suppl. 3):24, 1965.
7. Holt, M., Oram, S.: Familial heart disease with skeletal malformations. Br Heart J 22:236, 1960.
8. Betria, A., Wigle, E. D., Felderholf, C. H., McLaughlin, M. J.: Prolapse of the posterior leaflet of the mitral valve associated with secundum atrial septal defect. Am J Cardiol 35:363, 1975.
9. Devereux, R., Perloff, J. K., Richek, N., Josephson, M.: Mitral valve prolapse. Circulation 54:3, 1976.
10. Lieppe, W., Scallion, R., Behar, V. S., Kisslo, J. A.: Two-dimensional echocardiographic findings in atrial septal defect. Circulation 56:447, 1977.
11. Espino-Vela, J.: Rheumatic heart disease associated with atrial septal defect: Clinical and pathologic study of 12 cases of Lutembacher's syndrome. Am Heart J 47:185, 1959.
12. Chait, A., Zucker, M.: Superior vena cava in the evaluation of atrial septal defect. Am J Roentgenol 103:104, 1968.
13. Kuzman, W. J., Yuskis, A. S.: Atrial septal defects in the older patient simulating acquired valvular heart disease. Am J Cardiol 15:303, 1965.
14. Keats, T. E., Rudhe, U., Foo, G. W.: Inferior vena caval position in the differential diagnosis of atrial and ventricular septal defects. Radiology 83:616, 1964.
15. Davia, J. E., Cheitlin, M. D., Beynek, J. L.: Sinus venosus atrial septal defect. Am Heart J 85:177, 1973.
16. Schumacker, H. B., Jr., Judd, D.: Partial anomalous pulmonary venous return with reference to drainage from inferior vena cava to an intact atrial septum. J Cardiovasc Surg 5:271, 1964.
17. Svellen, H. A., van Ingren, H. C., Hoetsmit, E. C.: Patterns of anomalous pulmonary venous drainage. Circulation 38:45, 1968.
18. Perloff, J. K.: The Clinical Recognition of Congenital Heart Disease. W. B. Saunders Co., Philadelphia, 1978, p. 284.
19. Neil, C. A., Ferencz, C., Sabiston, D. C., Sheldon, H.: The familial occurrence of hypoplastic right lung with systemic arterial supply and venous drainage: "Scimitar syndrome." Bull Johns Hopkins Hosp 107:1, 1960.
20. Pearlman, A. S., Clark, C. E., Henry, W. L.: Determinants of ventricular septal motion: influence of relative right and left ventricular size. Circulation 54:83, 1976.
21. Bierman, F. Z., Williams, R. G.: Subxiphoid two-dimensional imaging of the interatrial septum in infants and neonates with congenital heart disease. Circulation 60:80, 1979.
22. Bommer, W., Weinert, L., Neumann, A., Neef, J., Mason, D. T., DeMaria, A.: Determination of right atrial and right ventricular size two-dimensional echocardiograph. Circulation 60:91, 1979.
23. Kronik, G., Slony, J., Moesslacher, H.: Contrast M-mode echocardiography in diagnosis of atrial septal defect in acyanotic patients. Circulation 59:372, 1979.
24. Fraker, T. D., Jr., Harris, P. J., Behar, V. S., Kisslo, J. A.: Detection and exclusion of interatrial shunts by two-dimensional echocardiography and peripheral venous injection. Circulation 59:379, 1979.
25. Gramiak, R., Shah, P. M., Kramer, D. H.: Ultrasound cardiography: contrast studies in anatomy and function. Radiology 92:939, 1969.

PATENT DUCTUS ARTERIOSUS

In the fetus, the ductus arteriosus provides the normal vascular pathway between the pulmonary trunk and the descending aorta. Its pulmonary end is located near the origin of the left pulmonary artery, while its aortic end is just distal to the origin of the left subclavian artery. Generally, the ductus is largest at its aortic insertion, since it tends to close first on the pulmonary side.[1] In the fetus, most of the output of the right ventricle bypasses the unexpanded lungs via the ductus and enters the descending aorta to reach the fetal organ of oxygenation, the placenta. After birth, continued patency of the ductus may lead to congestive heart failure or may compromise the progress of children being treated for respiratory distress syndrome. On the other hand, ductal patency may be life sustaining in certain complex cardiac lesions associated with diminished systemic blood flow (for example, interrupted aortic arch) or diminished pulmonary blood flow (for example, pulmonary atresia with intact ventricular septum). It may also occur in association with more common lesions such as VSD and coarctation of the aorta.

In the mature infant, functional closure of the ductus due to muscular contraction occurs between 10 and 15 hours after birth. Anatomic closure due to subintimal fibrosis and thrombosis occurs within the first two to three weeks.[2]

The Premature Infant

The premature infant who may be compromised by the respiratory distress syndrome (RDS) frequently has the additional problem of a patent ductus arteriosus.[3] In fact, it has been stated that in very small infants the incidence of patent ductus, whether significant or insignificant, must be considered 100 per cent.[4] Prolonged patency of the ductus and early decline in pulmonary vascular resistance[5] are thought to relate to a relative paucity of pulmonary arteriolar musculature in these preterm infants.[6] The ductal shunt has been implicated in the deterioration of pulmonary function in infants with RDS. Congestive heart failure in this situation is often unrespon-

sive to the usual therapy.[3] It has been shown that the ductus arteriosus in preterm infants with RDS and cardiopulmonary failure can often be constricted and closed by the use of the prostaglandin inhibitor indomethacin.[7, 8]

Radiographic/M-mode Echocardiographic Features

The plain chest film plays an important role in the evaluation of premature infants with suspected patent ductus arteriosus. It has been reported[9] that the appearance of increased vascularity ("pulmonary plethora") on the chest x-ray predates a detectable heart murmur in over half of prematures with a patent ductus (Fig. 6–32A). Most of these infants presented with increased vascularity between the second and sixth days of life with peak pulmonary vascularity being present at the end of the first week or beginning of the second week. Additional pulmonary patterns included the appearance of an alveolar filling process in an infant with resolving RDS, or the appearance of perihilar infiltrates in the presence of shunt vascularity. Although the finding of cardiomegaly (cardiothoracic ratio > 58 per cent) is a relatively unreliable sign of a large volume left-to-right shunt, sequential increase in the cardiothoracic ratio of 0.05 or greater (CT ratio on first day of life divided by maximum CT ratio) is present in over 75 per cent of infants with large shunts (Fig. 6–32B). Prominence of the aortic knob in an infant with respiratory distress syndrome should also suggest a patent ductus (Fig. 6–33).

M-mode echocardiography has been the most widely used method of evaluating the severity of the ductal shunt in premature infants with RDS.[10] This has involved the determination of the left atrial to aortic (LA/Ao) ratio. A ratio in excess of 1.2 indicates a significant left-to-right shunt. Occasionally, patients with large shunts will have LA/Ao ratios on echocardiograms of less than 1.0. Sequential increase in CT ratio of 0.05 or greater is usually present in these patients.[9] Rarely, there may be a "pancaking" phenomena present, involving compression of the left atrium posteriorly by an enlarged left ventricle so that a falsely low value for left atrial size will be recorded

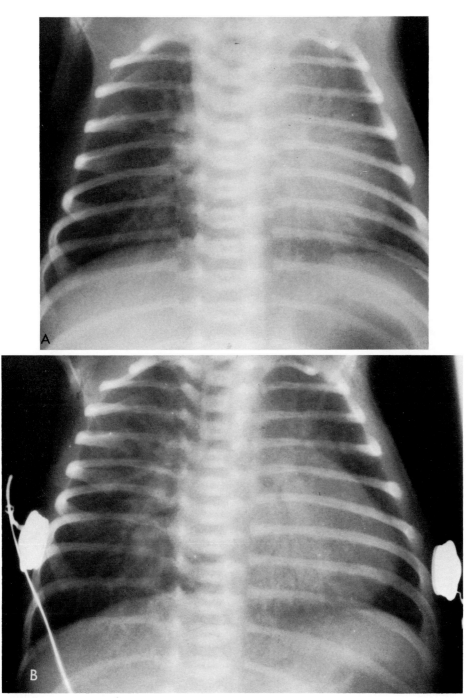

Figure 6–32. Premature infant with mild respiratory distress. In the radiograph taken at birth (A) there is increased vascularity in the perihilar region. There was no detectable heart murmur. A chest radiograph taken six days later (B) shows obvious prominence of the pulmonary vascularity and an increase in the cardiothoracic ratio from 0.52 to 0.58. A large patent ductus was found at catheterization and angiography.

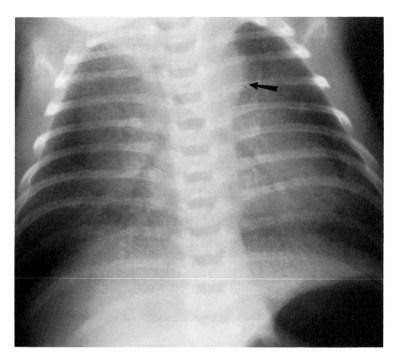

Figure 6–33. Premature infant with moderate RDS (note granular lung fields) and a prominent aortic knob (arrow). A moderate-sized patent ductus arteriosus (PDA) was present at catheterization.

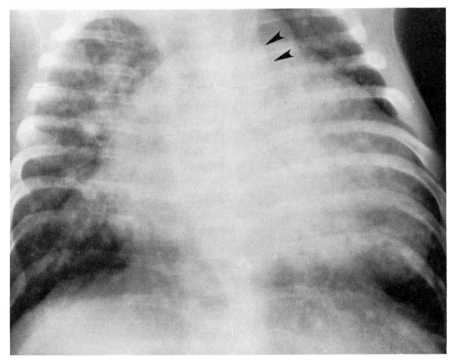

Figure 6–34. A neonate with a large PDA. Marked shunt vascularity (note the large distinct right lower lobe vessels), cardiomegaly, and a prominent thoracic aorta (arrowheads) suggest the diagnosis. When the heart is this size, the M-mode echocardiographic LA/Ao ratio may be falsely low owing to "pancaking" of the left atrium.

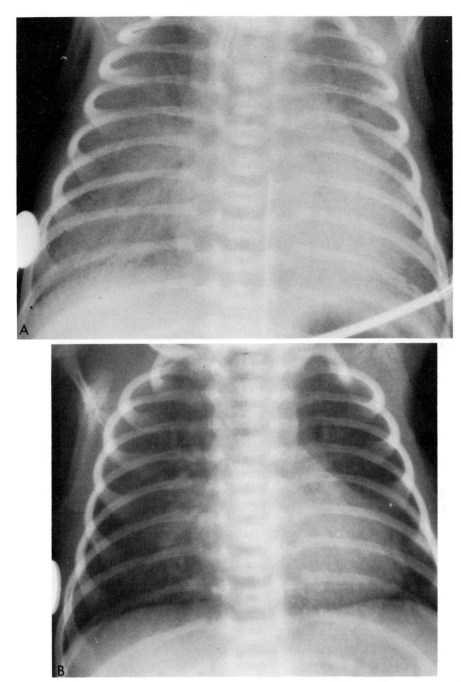

Figure 6–35. A newborn with RDS and PDA. On the initial film (*A*), note the presence of perihilar edema and cardiomegaly. (*B*) After indomethacin therapy there is resolution of the edema, and the heart size has returned to normal.

at echocardiography. The chest film in this situation can also be helpful in suggesting a shunt with cardiomegaly (Fig. 6–34).

Radiographic reduction in shunt vasculature, pulmonary edema, and cardiomegaly tend to precede clinical changes of shunt resolution in newborns treated with indomethacin for patent ductus (Fig. 6–35A and B). Although the exact time of ductus closure is not reliably estimated by the chest radiograph, greater accuracy is attained by using echocardiographic data together with

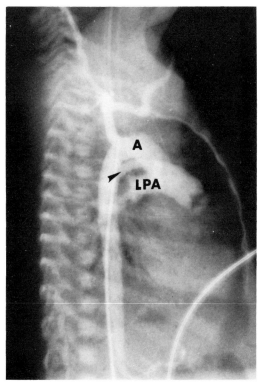

Figure 6–36. Thoracic aortogram performed through an umbilical artery catheter placed at the fifth thoracic level. The infant was placed in a 30° inclined right lateral decubitus position. A moderate-sized patent ductus arteriosus (arrowhead) is clearly seen between the aortic arch (A) and the left pulmonary artery (LPA). (This case courtesy of Dr. Charles B. Higgins.)

the radiographs than by using either method alone.[9]

Angiographic Features

A direct injection of contrast into the umbilical artery catheter placed in the proximal descending aorta may be the only accurate means of assessing ductal patency in cases in which radiographic, echocardiographic, and/or clinical data are unclear with regard to the response of the ductus to indomethacin therapy.[11] Thoracic aortography is performed by advancing the umbilical catheter to the fifth thoracic level. A scout anteroposterior film should be obtained to locate the catheter tip. The infant is placed in a 30° inclined right lateral decubitus position and the mobile x-ray unit is placed above the bed (Fig. 6–36). An alternate method employs a horizontal x-ray beam and supine patient angled 30 to 40° across the bed. Renographin 60 (two parts) diluted with sterile water (one part) is injected in a volume of 1 ml/kg. A single radiograph is obtained near the completion of the injection and will show a patent ductus in the aortopulmonary window (Fig. 6–36).

Radiographic Features in Full-Term Infants and Children

The chest film in the child with a small patent ductus arteriosus is normal. In moderate or large left-to-right shunts pulmonary vascularity of the shunt type will be present (Fig. 6–37). The ascending aorta and aortic knob may be normal in infants but they tend to enlarge in older children

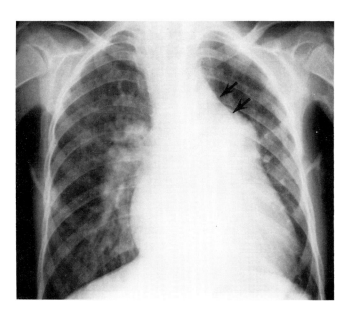

Figure 6–37. A child with a large PDA. There is shunt vascularity, cardiomegaly with a drooping left ventricular apex (suggesting left ventricular enlargement), and filling in of the aortopulmonary window (arrows). Note the presence of calcium in the soft tissues of the thorax. This patient also had myositis ossificans progressiva.

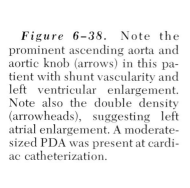

Figure 6-38. Note the prominent ascending aorta and aortic knob (arrows) in this patient with shunt vascularity and left ventricular enlargement. Note also the double density (arrowheads), suggesting left atrial enlargement. A moderate-sized PDA was present at cardiac catheterization.

(Fig. 6–38). This is due to the fact that the entire left ventricular output enters the aorta before reaching the ductal shunt. This may serve as a differentiating point between the ductus and the intracardiac shunts (ASD, VSD). Since increased flow is not directed into the aorta with the intracardiac lesions, the aorta remains normal or small in size (Figs. 6–3 and 6–17). The aortopulmonary window may be filled in by

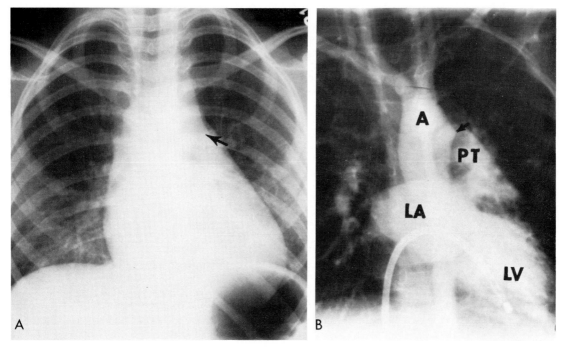

Figure 6–39. A, Note the localized prominence of the descending aorta (arrow) in this patient with a moderate-sized PDA. This bulge in the region of the aortopulmonary window is due to localized dilatation of the descending aorta—the so-called ductus diverticulum ("bump"). The levophase angiogram (B) correlates with the chest film findings and shows the ductus "bump" (arrow) and filling of the pulmonary trunk (PT) from the aorta (A) through the ductus. Both the left atrium (LA) and the left ventricle (LV) are slightly enlarged.

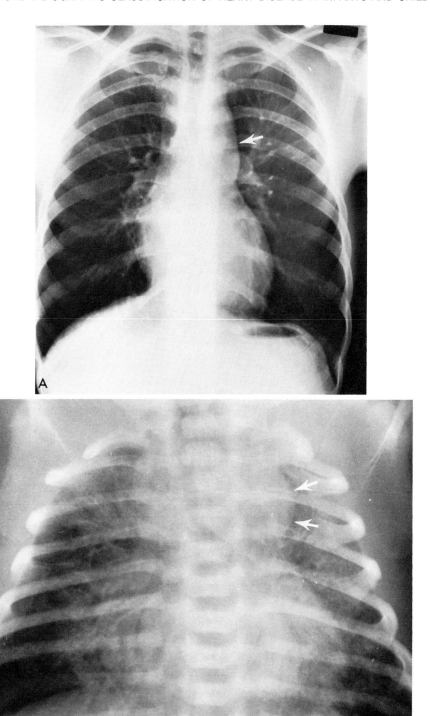

Figure 6–40. *A,* 20-year-old male with a continuous murmur. Although the vascularity and heart size are not impressively abnormal, the aortopulmonary window is obscured (arrow). At fluoroscopy linear calcification was identified in the ductus. There was a small left-to-right shunt at catheterization. *B,* An infant presenting with asphyxia and bounding pulses. Note the prominent mediastinal density on the left (arrows) and the congested lung fields. A large aneurysm of the ductus was found at catheterization and angiography.

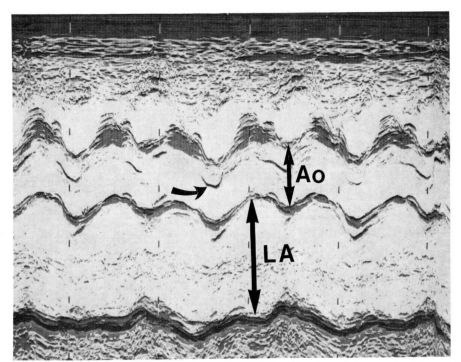

Figure 6–41. Left atrial/aortic root ratio. M-mode echocardiogram at the aortic root. Left-to-right shunting at the ventricular or great vessel level (in the absence of an interatrial communication) creates increased pulmonary arterial flow and results in an increase in pulmonary venous return. The left atrium (LA) enlarges and the LA/Ao ratio increases. This finding may arise from left-to-right shunting due to a ventricular septal defect or a patent ductus arteriosus. The calculated LA/Ao ratio greater than 1.2 in this patient is considered abnormal. Note the aortic leaflets (curved arrow) within the aortic root (Ao).

the ductus (Fig. 6–37). A localized dilatation of the proximal descending aorta (the ductus diverticulum) may be seen in some individuals (Fig. 6–39A). This correlates with angiographic prominence of the descending aorta (Fig. 6–39B). Another point of differentiation between ductal and atrial level shunts is the presence of left atrial enlargement with the former (Figs. 6–38 and 6–39). Volume overload also commonly leads to left ventricular enlargement in patients with a large patent ductus (Figs. 6–37 to 6–39).

In the older child or adult with a patent ductus, the aortopulmonary window may be obscured (Fig. 6–40A) or calcium may be noted in the region of the ductus. Rarely, aneurysms of the ductus will present as a mediastinal mass[12] (Fig. 6–40B). Compression of the airways with resultant asphyxia as well as rupture of the aneurysm and infection has been reported in these infants.[13]

Echocardiographic Features

With associated clinical findings and pulmonary arterial overcirculation on the chest radiograph, the presence of left-to-right shunting through communications at the ventricular and/or great vessel level can be implied by the presence of an enlarged left atrial dimension[10, 14] (Fig. 6–41). In the absence of another explanation for left atrial enlargement (for example, left ventricular inflow tract obstruction),[15] the atrial enlargement is attributed to increased pulmonary venous return secondary to an increase in pulmonary arterial flow from the left-to-right shunt. If there is no interatrial communication allowing "venting" of the increased left atrial return, the left atrial dimension increases both absolutely in size and in relationship to the size of the aortic root. For this reason, measurement of the left atrial to aortic root ratio (LA/Ao ratio)

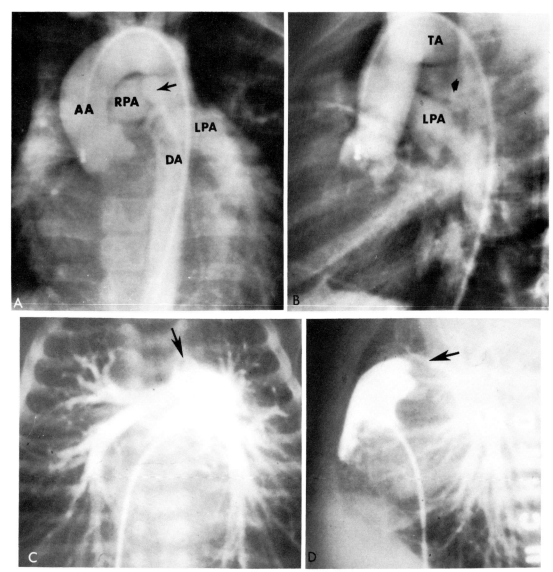

Figure 6-42. *A,* Slight LAO ascending aortogram demonstrating a large ductus diverticulum (arrow) with filling of the right and left pulmonary arteries (RPA, LPA). Note that the ascending aorta (AA) and aortic arch are dilated and larger than the descending aorta (DA). *B,* Lateral ascending aortogram in patient shown in *A* shows a large ductus arteriosus (arrow) beneath the transverse aortic arch (TA) and left pulmonary artery (LPA). Again, note that the aorta proximal to the ductus is dilated. *C,* Posteroanterior, and *D,* lateral pulmonary arteriogram in a young child with a patent ductus arteriosus. Note the negative dilution defect (arrows) in the contrast caused by the ductal left-to-right shunt.

has been used in the presence of clinical and radiographic evidence of increased pulmonary vascularity to imply the presence of a significant left-to-right ventricular and/or ductal shunt.[10, 14] The presence of an LA/Ao ratio in excess of 1.2 is considered consistent with significant left-to-right shunting at these levels but cannot alone distinguish a VSD from a patent ductus.

Direct two-dimensional echocardiographic visualization of the patent ductus is possible,[16] although this cannot be considered a totally reliable diagnostic finding. When the diagnosis of patent ductus arteriosus is considered on clinical grounds, the presence of left atrial enlargement is the best evidence for the presence and size of the shunt.

Angiographic Features

Thoracic aortography is the method of choice for demonstrating a patent ductus in full-term infants and children. A single-plane lateral view, a cross-table lateral view obtained as described in the previous section, or a 45° LAO view is the preferred projection. The ductus originates from the anterior aspect of the aorta just distal to the left subclavian artery and extends in an oblique anterior and cephalad course to connect with the pulmonary trunk where it joins the left pulmonary artery (Figs. 6–39B and 6–42A and B). Indirect evidence of a patent ductus may be indicated by linear dilution of contrast injected into the main pulmonary artery (Fig. 6–42 C and D).

REFERENCES

1. Jager, B. V., Wolenman, O. J., Jr.: An anatomical study of the closure of the ductus arteriosus. Am J Pathol 18:595, 1942.
2. Rudolph, A. M.: The changes in the circulation after birth: their importance in congenital heart disease. Circulation 41:343, 1970.
3. Zachman, R. D., Steinmetz, G. P., Botham, R. J., Graven, S., Ledbetter, M. K.: Incidence and treatment of the patent ductus arteriosus in the ill premature neonate. Am Heart J 87:697, 1974.
4. Merrit, T. A., Gluck, L., Higgins, C. B., Friedman, W., Nyhan, W. L.: Management of premature infants with patent ductus arteriosus. West J Med 128:3, 1978.
5. Danilowicz, D., Rudolph, A. M., Hoffman, J. I. E.: Delayed closure of the ductus arteriosus in premature infants. Pediatrics 37:74, 1966.
6. Wagenvoort, C. A., Neufeld, H. N., Edwards, J. E.: The structure of the pulmonary arterial tree in fetal and early postnatal life. Lab Invest 10:751, 1961.
7. Friedman, W. F., Hirschklau, M. J., Printz, M. P., Pitlick, P. T., Kirkpatrick, S. E.: Pharmacological closure of patent ductus arteriosus in the premature infant. N Engl J Med 295(10):526–9, 1976.
8. Heymann, M. A., Rudolph, A. M., Silverman, N. H.: Closure of the ductus arteriosus in premature infants by inhibition of prostaglandin synthesis. N Engl J Med 295(10):530–3, 1976.
9. Higgins, C. B., Rausch, J., Friedman, W. F., Hirschklau, M. J., Kirkpatrick, S. E., Goergen, T. G., Reinke, R. T.: Patent ductus arteriosus in preterm infants with idiopathic respiratory distress syndrome. Radiographic and echocardiographic evaluation. Radiology 124:189–195, 1977.
10. Silverman, N. H., Lewis, A. B., Heymann, M. A., Rudolph, A. M.: Echocardiographic assessment of ductus arteriosus in premature infants. Circulation 50:821, 1974.
11. Higgins, C. B., DiSessa, T., Kirkpatrick, S. E., Ti, C. C., Edwards, D. K., Friedman, W. F., Kelley, M. J., Kurlinski, J.: Assessment of patent ductus arteriosus in preterm infants by single lateral film aortography. Radiology 135:641–647, 1980.
12. Kelley, M. J., Mannes, E. J., Ravin, C. E.: Mediastinal masses of vascular origin: A review. J Thorac Cardiovasc Surg 76:559, 1978.
13. Falcone, M. W., Perloff, J. K., Roberts, W. C.: Aneurysm of nonpatent ductus. Am J Cardiol 29:422, 1972.
14. Lewis, A. M., Takahashi, M.: Echocardiographic assessment of left to right shunt volume in children with ventricular septal defect. Circulation 54:78, 1976.
15. LaCorte, M., Harada, K., Williams, R. G.: Echocardiographic features of congenital left ventricular inflow obstruction. Circulation 54:562, 1976.
16. Sahn, D. J., Allen, H. D.: Real-time cross-sectional echocardiographic imaging and measurement of the patent ductus arteriosus in infants and children. Circulation 58:343, 1978.

ENDOCARDIAL CUSHION DEFECT

The endocardial cushions are opposing masses of tissue that grow into the common atrioventricular canal of the embryo and complete the formation of the upper ventricular septum, the base of the atrial septum, the anterior leaflet of the mitral valve, and the septal leaflet of the tricuspid valve. Abnormal development of the cushions results in a spectrum of anomalies involving some or all of these structures. The term "endocardial cushion defect" is used in a general way to identify these anomalies. These defects, singly or in combination, involve the atrial septum, the ventricular septum, and one or both atrioventricular valves. The terms "complete endocardial cushion defect" and "partial endocardial cushion defect" will be used to describe the two common varieties of this anomaly. A transitional form exists that shows defects intermediate between the complete and partial forms.

The complete endocardial cushion defect is characterized by

1. A single confluent atrioventricular orifice.

2. A continuous cleft between the anterior leaflet of the mitral valve and septal leaflet of the tricuspid valve.

3. Fusion of the valve segments into a

common atrioventricular valve whose leaflets extend across the atrioventricular orifice on either side of the muscular ventricular septum.

4. A deficient base of the diaphragmatic wall of the ventricles.

Since the atrioventricular septum is absent and the common valve leaflets may have no septal attachments, the consequence of these defects is to allow free communication between the atria above and the ventricles below.

The partial endocardial cushion defect is characterized by

1. A low lying (ostium primum) atrial septal defect.

2. A cleft in the anterior leaflet of the mitral valve.

3. Separate atrioventricular valves that attach to the crest of the defective muscular septum.

4. The tricuspid valve may also be cleft.

In the partial defect, accessory chordae tendinae arise from the cleft anterior leaflet and insert directly onto the ventricular septum. This holds the leaflet close to the septum and helps to create the left ventricular outflow tract deformity typical of the defect.

Endocardial cushion defects may additionally be separated on the basis of chordal attachments, according to the Rastelli classification:[5] Type A — insertion of chordae into the crest of the interventricular septum; Type B — insertion of chordae into a papillary muscle on the *right* ventricular side of the interventricular septum; and Type C — a "free-floating" anterior leaflet with no chordal attachments to the septum.

In both the partial and complete form of this defect, the crest of the muscular septum is deficient and has a concave upper margin. The mitral valve attachment is displaced toward the apex, and the mitral ring shifts its orientation from the usual posterior aspect of the left ventricle so that its orifice is oriented in the sagittal plane.[1] The superior segment of the cleft anterior leaflet maintains its relationship to the aortic annulus but, because the atrioventricular septum is absent, it courses anteriorly along the upper margin of the septum. The inferior segment of the cleft leaflet attaches along the lower margin of the septum. In a frontal view of the normal heart, the right border of the left ventricular outflow tract is formed by the atrioventricular septum. In endocardial cushion defects, because of the

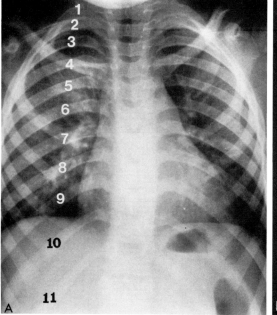 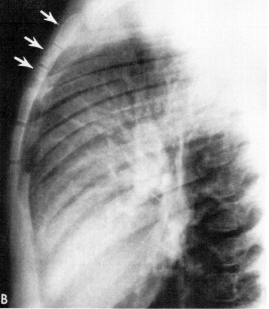

Figure 6–43. Posteroanterior (*A*) and lateral (*B*) chest radiographs in a child with Down's syndrome (trisomy 21, mongolism). There is shunt vascularity, mild cardiomegaly, and a suggestion of right heart enlargement on the lateral film. Note the presence of 11 ribs and a hypersegmental manubrial ossification center (arrows). Although each of these thoracic cage findings may appear in normal individuals, their combined presence on chest radiograph is invariably associated with Down's syndrome.

sagittal orientation of the mitral orifice and the deficient atrioventricular septum, the cleft anterior leaflet forms the right border of the outflow tract of the left ventricle.

Complete endocardial cushion defects generally present in infancy or early childhood with recurrent respiratory infections and congestive heart failure. The prevalence of Down's syndrome is estimated at 40 to 50 per cent in the complete defect.[1] Partial endocardial cushion defects usually present later in childhood. Mitral regurgitation is more common in the partial variety and Down's syndrome is less common.[1] Overall, endocardial cushion defects occur in ~25 per cent of children with Down's syndrome. With rare exceptions, the QRS complex of the electrocardiogram shows left-axis deviation with a counterclockwise loop in the frontal plane.

Radiographic Features

A radiographic clue to the presence of Down's syndrome is the combined presence of a hypersegmented manubrial ossification center and 11 ribs on the chest radiograph (Fig. 6–43). In the complete form of endocardial cushion defects, pulmonary vascularity of the shunt type is invariably present and the left atrium is not enlarged (Fig. 6–44). An element of interstitial edema is not unusual owing to the large volume left-to-right shunt associated with the complete canal deformity (Fig. 6–45). Cardiomegaly is present—especially right heart enlargement (Fig. 6–44 and 6–45). Right atrial appendage enlargement may contribute a characteristic angulated bulge to the right upper margin of the cardiac silhouette (Fig. 6–45). The aorta is usually inconspicuous (Figs. 6–43 to 6–45). Left atrial enlargement is unusual (Fig. 6–46) and should alert one to the presence of a restricted atrial communication and/or significant regurgitation into the left atrium.

The x-ray in partial endocardial cushion defect without mitral regurgitation is indistinguishable from that of a patient with a large secundum or sinus venosus atrial septal defect (Fig. 6–47).

Echocardiographic Features

Primum atrial septal defects occurring as part of a partial or complete endocardial

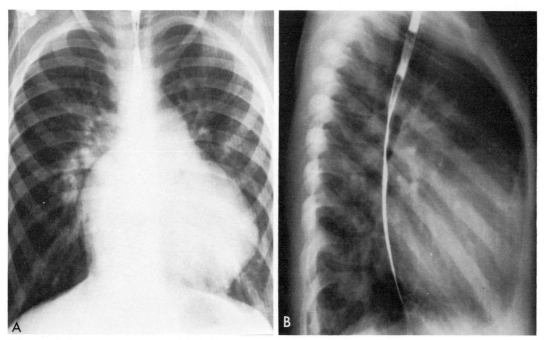

Figure 6–44. This one-year-old child presented with congestive failure. The posteroanterior (A) and lateral (B) chest radiographs demonstrate shunt vascularity, right atrial and right ventricular enlargement, and a normal-sized left atrium. Note the hyperaerated lungs. Although the findings are compatible with an atrial septal defect, a more complex atrial shunt is suggested by the early age of presentation. A complete endocardial cushion defect was present at catheterization and angiography.

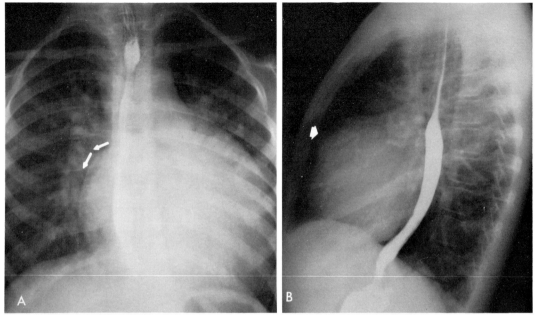

Figure 6–45. In this child with a complete endocardial cushion defect, an element of interstitial edema accompanies the shunt pattern (the lower lobe vessels are indistinct). Note the shelf-like right heart border (arrows) on the posteroanterior film (A). This is due to dilatation of the right atrial appendage and is common in endocardial cushion defects. On the lateral view (B) the right heart is enlarged (arrow) and the left atrium is normal in size.

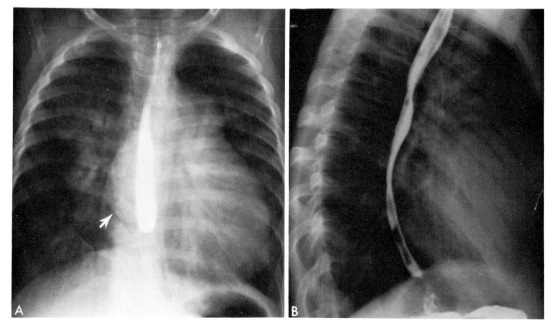

Figure 6–46. A child with a complete form of endocardial cushion defect. Note the presence of a double density (arrows) on the posteroanterior film (A) and left atrial enlargement on the lateral view (B). Significant mitral regurgitation was present in this patient (see Fig. 6–55).

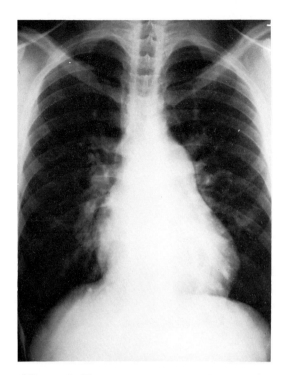

Figure 6–47. Posteroanterior chest radiograph in a young female. The presence of shunt vascularity, mild cardiomegaly, and normal-sized left atrium are all compatible with a moderate or large atrial septal defect. Angiography revealed an ostium primum ASD and a left ventricular contour typical of an endocardial cushion deformity.

cushion defect are identified on two-dimensional echocardiograms using the subxiphoid or apical views (Fig. 6–48). These defects are characterized by the absence of interatrial septal tissue low in the interatrial septum where it comes in contact with the crest of the interventricular septum (Figs. 6–49 and 6–50). In addition, the subxiphoidal and long-axis views of the left ventricular outflow region may show narrowing caused by the abnormal insertion of the anterior leaflet of the mitral valve on the septal outflow portion of the left ventricle. This diastolic deformity is the echocardiographic manifestation of the classic "gooseneck" deformity found at angiography (Fig. 6–51).

Endocardial cushion defects of both the partial and complete variety may be completely evaluated using two-dimensional imaging techniques (Fig. 6–49). With the transducer in the apical or subxiphoidal views, the interatrial septum and central fibrous body are evaluated along with the inflow portion of the ventricular cavities.[6-8] A ventricular septal defect in its typical location (the posterior inflow septum) in addition to a primum atrial septal defect may be detected (Figs. 6–49 and 6–50). The anterior leaflet of the atrioventricular valve is examined, and the site of ventricular insertion of chordae tendinae arising from

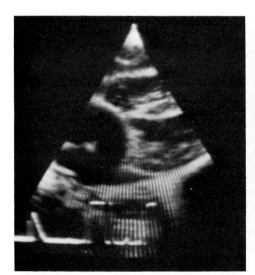

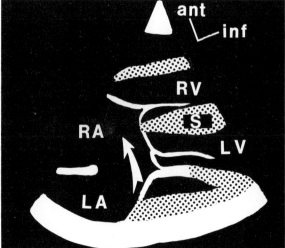

Figure 6–48. Ostium primum atrial septal defect. Subxiphoidal four-chamber view of a primum atrial septal defect. In this view, the right atrium (RA) is larger than the left atrium (LA). There is a large defect in the lower portion of the atrial septum (arrow). The remainder of the septum is intact. The interventricular septum (S) appears intact and there is visualization of both ventricular inflow tracts. (RV = right ventricle; LV = left ventricle.)

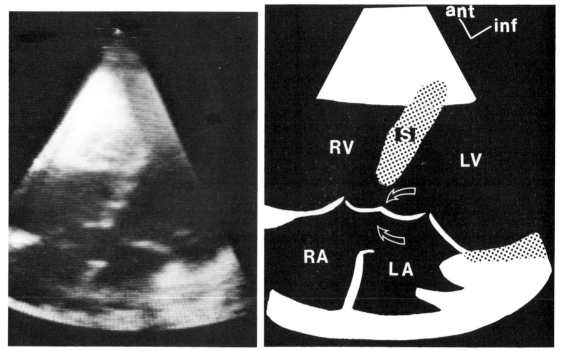

Figure 6–49. Endocardial cushion defect. Apical view of a complete atrioventricular canal defect. In this view, the central fibrous body is absent, resulting in left-to-right communication at both the atrial level in the position of the septum primum (lower arrow) and in the interventricular septum in a position high in the inflow septum (upper arrow). The muscular interventricular septum (S) is intact and both ventricular cavities are visualized (RV = right ventricle; LV = left ventricle; RA = right atrium; LA = left atrium.)

this leaflet can be defined (Fig. 6–50). This allows classification of the defect into Rastelli Types A, B, or C. The typical "gooseneck" deformity of the left ventricular outflow tract is seen both in the subxiphoidal (Fig. 6–51) and in the long-axis view of the left ventricular outflow tract. The presence of right ventricular outflow tract obstruction may be detected on both the long-axis and subxiphoidal view of the right ventricular inflow tract.[6]

Angiographic Features

The frontal projection of the left ventriculogram has proved to be most useful in diagnosing endocardial cushion defects.[3] A review of normal left ventricular anatomy will help to explain the deranged anatomy of this defect (see Chapter 4). During the diastolic phase of a normal left ventriculogram, the attachment of the posterior leaflet of the mitral valve can be visualized by contrast trapped beneath it and the non–contrast-containing left atrial blood. The anterior leaflet attachment is not seen (Fig. 6–52D). The outflow portion of the ventricle extends upward in a smooth, oblique line from the posterior leaflet to the aortic valve (Fig. 6–52D). In systole, as inflow of nonopacified blood from the left atrium ceases, a uniform opacification of the left ventricle occurs and the posterior leaflet attachment is not seen. The smooth, oblique right border of the left ventricle is seen to better advantage in systole and forms a gradually concave curve with the ascending aorta. The papillary muscles may be seen as lucent filling defects arising from the anterior and diaphragmatic surfaces and extending toward the mitral valve.

In the presence of an endocardial cushion deformity the left ventriculogram demonstrates several classic features. In diastole,

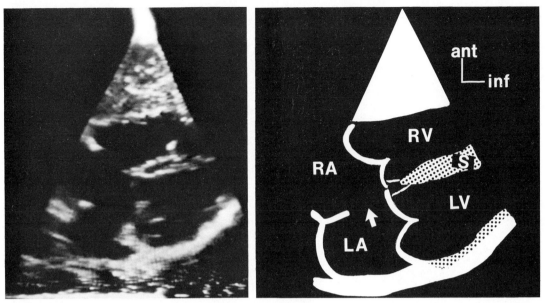

Figure 6–50. Endocardial cushion defect. Subxiphoidal four-chamber view of a complete atrioventricular canal. Both atrial cavities (LA, RA) are separated by a remnant of intact atrial septum secundum. There is a large defect in the septum primium (Ostium primum defect — arrow), and the atrioventricular valves appear to insert into the crest of the interventricular septum (S) (Rastelli Type A). The right and left ventricular cavities appear normal in size. (RV = right ventricle; LV = left ventricle.)

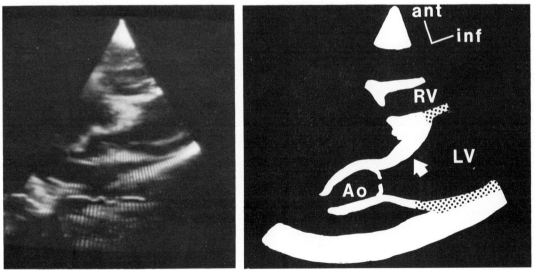

Figure 6–51. Endocardial cushion defect. Subxiphoidal four-chamber view of left ventricular outflow tract in a complete atrioventricular canal. The typical left ventricular outflow tract deformity is demonstrated by this view. The outflow tract is narrowed owing to displacement of the anterior leaflet of the mitral valve (arrow). This diastolic outflow tract narrowing is the echocardiographic manifestation of the configuration identified angiographically as the "gooseneck deformity" (see Fig. 6–52). It is present in both partial and complete forms of atrioventricular canal. (LV = left ventricle; RV = right ventricle; Ao = aortic root.)

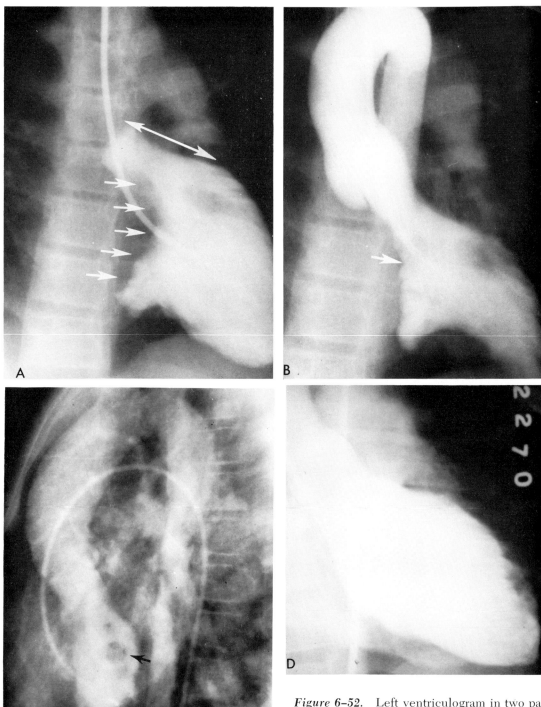

Figure 6–52. Left ventriculogram in two patients with partial endocardial cushion defects. The diastolic frontal projection (*A*) shows the effaced medial border of the left ventricular outflow tract (arrows) and the narrowed, horizontal, elongated outflow region, the "gooseneck deformity" (double arrow). The systolic projection (*B*) demonstrates an irregular, scalloped, slightly concave medial border and a cleft in the anterior leaflet of the mitral valve (arrow). The lateral view (*C*) in a second patient shows the reoriented papillary muscles on end (arrows). Note the catheter passage in this patient: azygous vein → superior vena cava → right atrium → tricuspid valve → atrioventricular canal defect → left ventricle. *D*, Posteroanterior left ventriculogram in diastole in a child with a small VSD. Compare the appearance of this normal left ventricle with the one in Figure 6–52*A*.

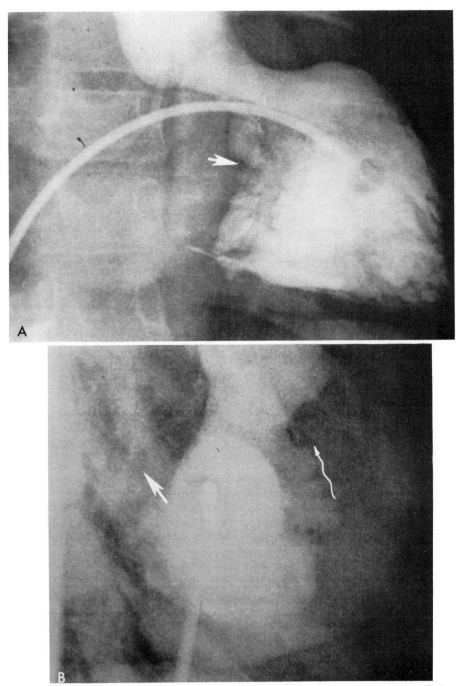

Figure 6–53. Left ventriculogram in a patient with partial endocardial cushion deformity. The posteroanterior view (A) shows the same features as Fig. 6–52A. Note the cleft in the anterior mitral leaflet (arrow) and the narrowed outflow tract. In the lateral view (B) the superior segment of the anterior mitral leaflet projects over the usually smooth outflow tract, giving an irregular appearance to this region (curved arrow). Note the presence of mild mitral regurgitation (arrow).

the inflow of nonopacified blood from the left atrium effaces the medial border of the outflow tract. The superior segment of the anterior leaflet generally moves independently from the inferior segment and is displaced laterally and upward into a horizontal position in the left ventricular outflow tract (Figs. 6–52A and 6–53). The narrowed, elongated outflow tract thus formed has been referred to as the "gooseneck" deformity. When the two anterior leaflet segments are unable to move independently (usually owing to chordal attachments or an incomplete cleft), the superior segment movement into the outflow tract is limited and the "gooseneck" deformity may not be present. Therefore, the absence of this finding does not rule out an endocardial cushion defect.

The left ventricular outflow tract in systole has an irregular, scalloped, slightly concave border (Fig. 6–52B). This is formed by the superior and inferior segments of the anterior mitral leaflets and is an important angiographic sign in this entity. The concave appearance is due to the attachment of the leaflet along the curve of the deficient muscular septum. The scalloping is due to

contrast trapped between the chordal and leaflet margins attached to the septum. The actual cleft between the superior and inferior segments is often visible (Figs. 6–52A and 6–53B). The concavity causes a narrowing of the outflow tract so that it often appears smaller than the ascending aorta (Figs. 6–52B and 6–53B).

In the lateral projection, because of the reorientation of the mitral valve into a sagittal position, the papillary muscles may be seen in cross section (Fig. 6–52C). In addition, the superior segment of the anterior mitral leaflet may project over the usually smooth anterior outflow tract of the left ventricle (Fig. 6–53B). Mitral regurgitation can also be assessed in this projection (Fig. 6–53B). The presence of severe mitral regurgitation may mask the left ventricular features of the endocardial cushion defect in the standard frontal projection (Fig. 6–54).

The partial and complete forms of the endocardial cushion defect generally present the same abnormal left ventricular contour on left ventriculography.[4] The presence of a clear-cut ventricular septal defect favors the complete form of endocardial

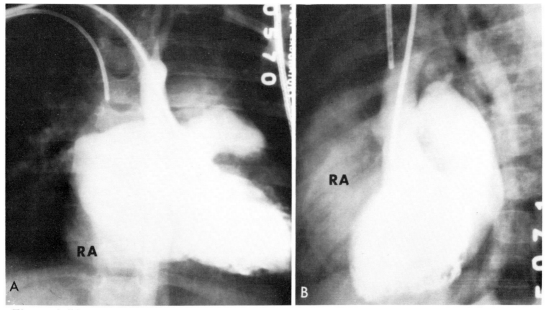

Figure 6–54. Posteroanterior (A) and lateral (B) views of a left ventriculogram in a patient with complete endocardial cushion defect and severe mitral regurgitation. The presence of contrast in the left atrium obscures the left ventricular features of the endocardial cushion deformity. A restrictive ostium primum ASD was present. Note the presence of a small amount of contrast in the right atrium (RA).

cushion defect. This can most readily be appreciated by using the angled four-chamber view, which profiles the inflow portion of the interventricular septum — the usual site of the VSD. This projection is also quite helpful in detecting left ventricular to right atrial communication. An isolated ostium primum defect is best identified by performing a right upper lobe pulmonary venogram with the patient in a hepatoclavicular (four-chamber) view (see Fig. 6–28C).

REFERENCES

1. Feldt, R. H.: Atrioventricular Canal Defects. W. B. Saunders Co. Philadelphia, 1976.
2. MacLeod, C. A.: Endocardial cushion defects with severe mitral insufficiency and small atrial septal defect. Circulation 26:755, 1962.
3. Baron, M. G., Wolf, B. S., Steinfeld, L., Van Mierop, L. H. S.: Endocardial cushion defects. Specific diagnosis by angiocardiography. Am J Cardiol 13:162, 1964.
4. Baron, M. G.: Endocardial Cushion Defects, Radiol Clin North Am 6:3; 343, 1968.
5. Rastelli, G. C., Kirklin, J. W., Titus, J. L.: Anatomic observations of complete form of persistent common atrioventricular canal with special reference to atrioventricular valves. Mayo Clin Proc 41:296, 1966.
6. Lange, L. W., Sahn, D. J., Allen, H. D., Goldberg, S. J.: Subxiphoid cross-sectional echocardiography in infants and children with congenital heart disease. Circulation 59:513, 1979.
7. Bierman, F. Z., Williams, R. G.: Subxiphoid two-dimensional imaging of the interatrial septum in infants and neonates with congenital heart disease. Circulation 60:80, 1979.
8. Hagler, D. J., Tajik, A. J., Seward, J. B., Mair, D. D., Ritter, D. G.: Real-time wide angle sector echocardiography: Atrioventricular canal defects. Circulation 59:140, 1979.

UNUSUAL LEFT-TO-RIGHT SHUNTS

In the group of conditions presented here, the plain chest film shows features similar to those previously described in the sections dealing with the more common left-to-right shunts. The echocardiographic findings may also be nonspecific, and hemodynamic findings may not specify the anatomic source of the shunt. In the left ventricular to right atrial communication the patient presents with a systolic murmur, while in the remaining three defects involving systemic to right heart run off, the murmur is usually continuous. In the presence of shunt vascularity on the chest film, the latter should suggest some form of communication between the aorta and a lower pressure right heart structure. Thus, the thoracic aortogram becomes an essential factor in the diagnostic work-up of these patients.

Left Ventricular to Right Atrial Communication

This is a relatively uncommon form of ventricular septal defect. The defect originates in the membranous septum below the crista. It opens either through a cleft or fenestration in the septal leaflet of the tricuspid valve[1] or as an opening just above the insertion of the septal leaflet of the tricuspid valve.[2]

Radiographic Features

At first glance, the x-ray resembles that of an ordinary atrial or ventricular septal defect with increased flow, prominent pulmonary trunk, small aorta, and cardiomegaly. The left atrium is enlarged in approximately one-third of cases.[1] The most helpful radiographic finding is an inappropriately enlarged right atrium (which is unusual in ventricular septal defects). Selective dilatation of the right atrial appendage may give a conspicuous bulge to the right heart margin (Fig. 6–55A). The findings of right atrial enlargement in conjunction with left atrial enlargement (Fig. 6–55B) should raise the question of a left ventricular–right atrial communication. The only other lesion that results in biatrial enlargement is an endocardial cushion defect with significant mitral regurgitation.

Angiocardiographic Features

Left ventriculography reveals immediate opacification of the right atrium (Fig. 6–56). Ideally, this should be performed in the four-chamber (hepatoclavicular) view. Right atrial opacification from a left ventriculogram can occur in three other conditions that must be distinguished from left ventricular to right atrial communication:

1. A ventricular septal defect in association with tricuspid regurgitation may present a similar picture. In this situation, right

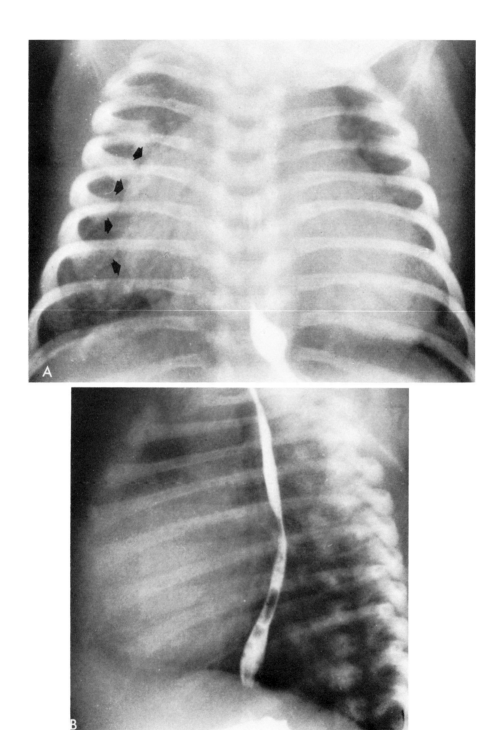

Figure 6–55. Posteroanterior (A) and lateral (B) chest radiographs in an infant who presented with congestive heart failure. There is evidence of increased pulmonary blood flow with large vessels at the right lung base. There is obvious cardiomegaly and the right atrium is quite large (arrows). The lateral view shows esophageal displacement by an enlarged left atrium. Biatrial enlargement should raise the question of a left ventricular to right atrial communication (see Fig. 6–56).

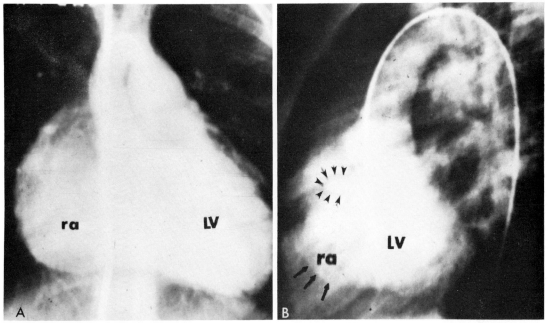

Figure 6–56. Left ventriculogram in posteroanterior (A) and lateral (B) projections performed in the child shown in Fig. 6–55. Note that contrast fills the right atrium (ra and arrows) directly through the ventricular septal defect (arrowheads). The left ventricle (LV) is displaced posteriorly by the dilated right heart structures.

ventricular opacification occurs before right atrial opacification, and right atrial opacification tends to be less than that seen with left ventricular to right atrial communication.

2. Endocardial cushion defects may be associated with left ventricular to right atrial shunting. Left ventriculography should reveal the typical distortion of the outflow tract and the displaced anterior leaflet of the mitral valve (see Figs. 6–52 and 6–53).

3. On left ventriculography, a ruptured sinus of Valsalva aneurysm into the right atrium may give an appearance similar to left ventricular–right atrial communication. Thoracic aortograms should distinguish the two (see Fig. 6–58).

Aneurysms of the Sinuses of Valsalva

The sinuses of Valsalva are the three dilatations above the aortic cusps and are named according to their relationship with the coronary arteries — the left coronary sinus, the right coronary sinus, and the noncoronary sinus. This congenital defect appears to involve a deficiency between the aortic media and the annulus fibrosis of the aortic valve. It is postulated that hydrostatic pressure from the aorta causes distention of the tissue and eventual aneurysm formation.[3] Since the aortic sinuses are essentially intracardiac in location, their relationship to other cardiac structures determines the site of aneurysm rupture. Over 90 per cent of these aneurysms originate in the right or noncoronary sinus, with the right being the most frequent site.[4] Aneurysms of the right coronary sinus generally rupture into the right ventricle (occasionally the right atrium), while aneurysms of the noncoronary sinus almost always rupture into the right atrium. The congenital nature of an aneurysm of the left coronary sinus that ruptures into the left heart is debatable.[4] Aneurysms that enter the right ventricle may be associated with a ventricular septal defect, with both lesions having a similar congenital origin.[4]

The clinical presentation relates to the acuteness and size of the rupture. The majority of patients present after puberty but

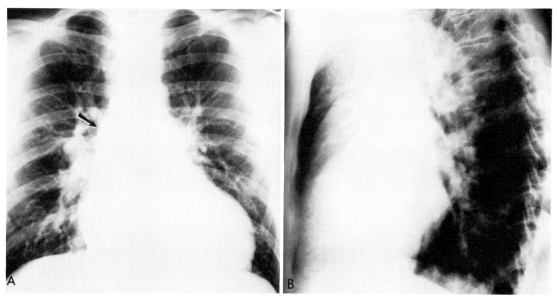

Figure 6–57. An 18-year-old male with sudden onset of chest pain and dyspnea. A continuous murmur was heard over the right parasternal region. There is shunt vascularity, cardiomegaly, and a prominent ascending aorta (arrow) on the posteroanterior chest radiograph (A). The lateral view (B) shows prominence of right heart structures in the retrosternal region. Ascending aortography revealed a large sinus of Valsalva aneurysm that had ruptured into the right ventricle.

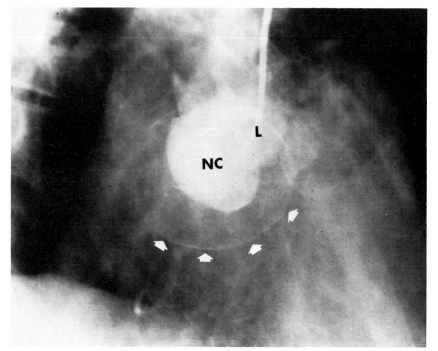

Figure 6–58. Lateral view ascending aortogram demonstrates normal noncoronary (NC) and left (L) sinuses of Valsalva. Note the fine crescent of calcium (arrows) beneath the normal sinuses. This represents calcium in a large right sinus of Valsalva aneurysm.

before age 30.[5] The classic presentation of a large, acute rupture is that of a young person who suddenly develops retrosternal chest pain, dyspnea, and a continuous murmur.

Radiographic Features

Chest film findings depend on the volume of the shunt and the presence or absence of associated congestive heart failure. When the rupture involves the right coronary sinus with communication into the right ventricle, the radiographic appearance is that of a ventricular septal defect. When the rupture is into the right atrium, this chamber may show enlargement. The ascending aorta is often prominent, since this defect represents an aortic runoff lesion much like a patent ductus arteriosus (Fig. 6–57). Direct visualization of the aneurysm is rare, but a crescent-shaped calcification has been reported in association with an unruptured sinus of Valsalva aneurysm (Fig. 6–58).[6]

Angiocardiographic Features

Thoracic aortography will usually demonstrate the position, size, and extent of the aneurysm as well as the chamber with which it communicates. Usually the entire sinus is not dilated, but instead the aneurysm projects as a narrow extension of the sinus with the perforation at its tip.

Coronary Arterial Fistula

In this generally isolated lesion, one of the coronary arteries arises normally from the aorta to communicate with a cardiac chamber, the pulmonary trunk, coronary sinus, vena cava, or pulmonary vein. The right coronary artery is more commonly involved than the left coronary artery.[7] Over 90 per cent of coronary arterial fistulae empty into right heart structures[7] in the following order of frequency: the right ventricle, the right atrium, the pulmonary trunk,[8] and rarely the coronary sinus or superior vena cava.

The hemodynamic consequences of the fistula relate to the amount of blood flowing through the communication, the volume overload of the site of drainage, and myocardial ischemia, which may result as the fistula diverts flow from other coronary arteries.[8] Generally, coronary arterial fistulae result in relatively small left-to-right shunts (less than 1.5:1 pulmonary to systemic flow ratio).[9]

Radiographic Features

The chest x-rays in this entity are usually nonspecific. They are either normal with the smaller shunts[9] or show cardiomegaly (chamber dilatation depending on the site of drainage) with prominence of the pulmonary vasculature when the shunt is larger (Fig. 6–59).

Angiocardiographic Features

Thoracic aortography or selective coronary arteriography demonstrates the dilated tortuous coronary artery that forms the fistula and opacifies the chamber or vessel with which it communicates (Fig. 6–59). Saccular aneurysms as well as calcification of the wall of this vessel have been reported.[10]

Aorticopulmonary Septal Defect (Aorticopulmonary Window)

This rare anomaly is characterized by the presence of a relatively large round or oval communication between the left wall of the ascending aorta and the right wall of the pulmonary trunk. It results from a defect in the septation process of the primitive truncus arteriosus. Clinically the lesion resembles a large patent ductus arteriosus. Occasionally, the two lesions coexist.[11]

Radiographic Features

The chest film findings are not diagnostic and cannot usually be distinguished from those of a large patent ductus, since they demonstrate shunt vascularity and left ventricular and left atrial enlargement (Fig. 6–60). The aortic knob may be less prominent and the pulmonary trunk more prominent[12] than in patent ductus. A right aortic arch has been described with the defect (Fig. 6–60).[13]

Angiocardiographic Features

Ascending thoracic aortography or left ventriculography in the posteroanterior pro-

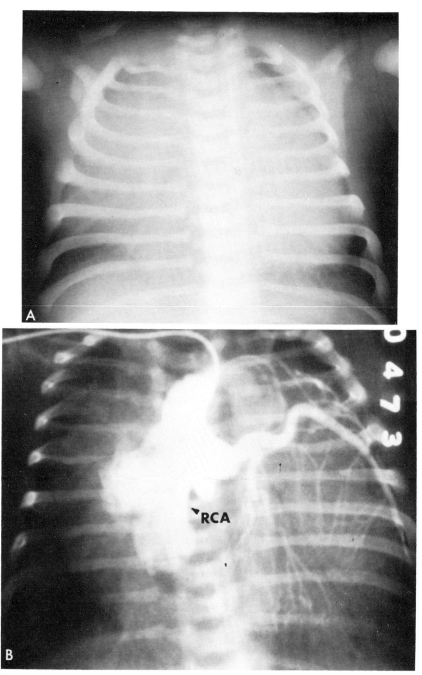

Figure 6–59. A, Anteroposterior chest radiograph in an infant with congestive heart failure and a continuous murmur over the right precordium. The pulmonary vascularity is difficult to evaluate because of the massive dilatation of the right atrium. Ascending aortograms in posteroanterior (*B* and *D*) and lateral (*C* and *E*) projections demonstrate a dilated, tortuous right coronary artery (RCA) that drains into the dilated right atrium (RA). The positions of the left anterior descending (LAD) and circumflex (CX) coronary arteries indicate that the left ventricle is displaced posteriorly by the dilated right heart structures. Ascending aortogram (Ao) performed in an older child in posteroanterior (*F*) and lateral (*G*) projections shows a smaller left coronary artery (lca) to right ventricular (RV) fistula (arrowheads).

Illustration continued on opposite page

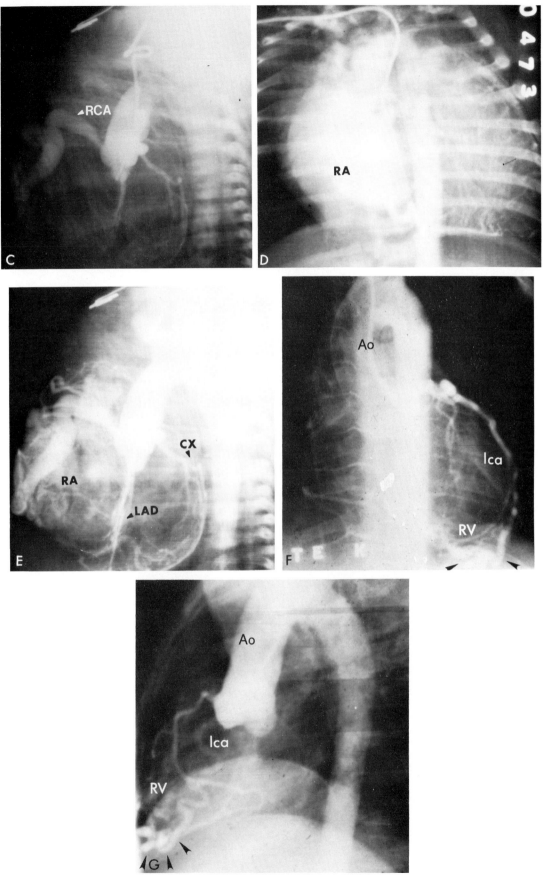

Figure 6-59 Continued

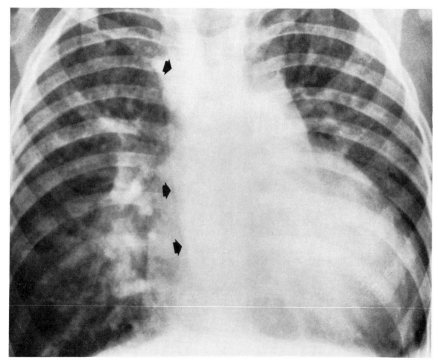

Figure 6–60. This one-year-old child presented with congestive heart failure, bounding pulses, and a continuous murmur over the aortic area. A patent ductus arteriosus was suspected. The posteroanterior chest radiograph shows shunt vascularity, cardiomegaly, and a prominent left ventricle and pulmonary trunk. The aortic knob and descending aorta are relatively inconspicuous and are located on the right (arrowheads). Cardiac catheterization demonstrated a left-to-right shunt at the great vessel level. Angiography is illustrated in Fig. 6–61.

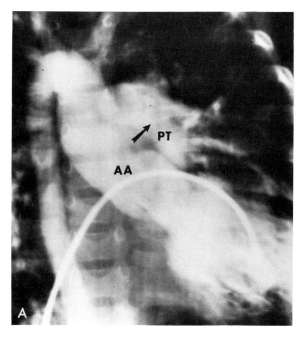

Figure 6–61. Posteroanterior left ventriculogram (A) and lateral ascending aortogram (B) in patient shown in Fig. 6–60. The pulmonary trunk (PT) fills with contrast on both injections and there is a mirror image right aortic arch. Note the linear lucency (arrows) between the ascending aorta (AA) and the pulmonary trunk below the aorticopulmonary septal defect (arrow). The posteroanterior right ventriculogram (C) shows that the pulmonary trunk (PT) arises from the right ventricle (RV). This distinguishes the aorticopulmonary window from persistent truncus arteriosus (see Chapter 8).

Illustration continued on opposite page

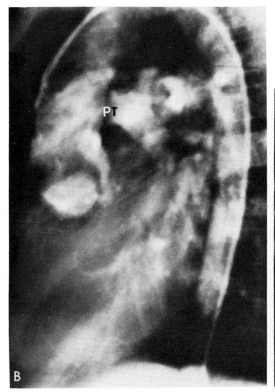

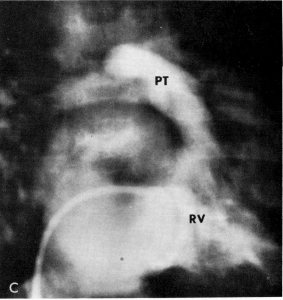

Figure 6–61 Continued

jection should demonstrate the window-like defect connecting the aorta with the pulmonary trunk (Fig. 6–61). The defect occurs several millimeters above the aortic valve. A linear negative filling defect representing the residual truncus septum should be visualized above and below the defect (Fig. 6–61A). It is important to identify the pulmonary valve as well in order to distinguish this entity from persistent truncus arteriosus (Fig. 6–61C). The latter defect is characterized by the presence of a *single* semilunar valve and trunk from which the pulmonary arteries arise (see Chapter 8). A large patent ductus arteriosus will often allow reflux into the pulmonary trunk from the aortic injection. However, the descending, rather than the ascending, aorta is shown to be the source of the shunt.

REFERENCES

1. Elliott, L. P., Gedgandus, E., Levy, M. J., Edwards, J. E.: The roentgenologic findings in left ventricular–right atrial communication. Am J Roentgenol 93:304, 1965.
2. Kramer, R. A., Abrams, H. L.: Radiologic aspects of operable heart disease: VII. Left Ventricular–Right Atrial Shunts. Radiology 78:171, 1962.
3. Edwards, J. E., Burchell, H. B.: Specimen exhibiting the essential lesion in aneurysms of the aortic sinus. Proc Staff Meet Mayo Clin 31:407, 1956.
4. Sakakibara, S., Konno, S.: Congenital aneurysm of the sinus of Valsalva: Anatomy and classification. Am Heart J 63:405, 1962.
5. Winfield, M. E.: Rupture of an aneurysm of the posterior sinus of Valsalva into the right atrium. Am J Cardiol 3:688, 1969.
6. Reinke, R. T., Coel, M. N., Higgins, C. B.: Calcified, nonsyphilitic aneurysms of the sinuses of Valsalva. Am J Roentgenol 122:783, 1974.
7. McNamara, J. J., Gross, R. E.: Congenital coronary fistula. Surgery 65:59, 1969.
8. Edis, A. J., Schattenberg, T. T., Feldt, R. H., Danielson, G. K.: Congenital coronary artery fistula. Mayo Clinic Proc 47:567, 1972.
9. Jaffe, R. B., Glancy, D. L., Epstein, S. E., Brown, B. G., Morrow, A. G.: Coronary arterial right heart fistulae. Circulation 47:133, 1973.
10. Bjork, V. O., Bjork, L.: Coronary artery fistula. J Thorac Cardiovasc Surg 49:921, 1965.
11. Neufeld, H. N., Lester, R. G., Adams, P., Jr., Anderson, R. C., Lillehei, C. W., Edwards, J. E.: Aorticopulmonary septal defect. Am J Cardiol 9:12, 1962.
12. Cooley, D. A., McNamara, D. G., Latson, J. R.: Aorticopulmonary septal defect: Diagnosis and surgical treatment. Surgery 42:101, 1957.
13. Blieden, L. C., Moller, J. H.: Aorticopulmonary septal defect. Br Heart J 36:630, 1974.

Chapter 7

CYANOTIC PATIENT WITH NORMAL OR DIMINISHED VASCULARITY

Previous studies have emphasized a stepwise diagnostic approach to the cyanotic infant or child and have emphasized clinical, radiographic, and electrocardiographic findings associated with the various defects.[1, 2] With the advent of M-mode and cross-sectional echocardiography, the physician involved in the evaluation of the cyanotic child has been given an invaluable tool that noninvasively provides specific information about *internal* cardiac antomy. One can arrive at a specific diagnosis prior to cardiac catheterization in most instances. This is especially important in planning the work-up of severely ill infants in whom invasive methods carry greater risk.

CYANOSIS

Clinical assessment of cyanosis may not be possible until the arterial oxygen saturation is less than 85 to 90 per cent, making arterial blood gas determination an essential part of the diagnostic evaluation of children with suspected congenital heart disease. Mild to moderate degrees of hypoxemia may result in an increase in hematocrit, a physiologic response that improves arterial oxygen transport.

The cyanosis of congenital heart disease is due to shunting of venous blood into the arterial system. Cyanosis may also occur with normal arterial saturation if the systemic blood flow is sufficiently low owing to left heart failure. In either situation, tissue hypoxemia may ultimately result in metabolic

acidosis, which may be life threatening. For this reason persistent cyanosis in the newborn or young infant is considered a medical emergency. Arterial desaturation depends not only on the magnitude of the right-to-left shunt, but also on the ratio between this shunt and pulmonary blood flow. Any lesion that causes a reduction in pulmonary blood (for example, tetralogy of Fallot) will result in low systemic arterial saturation.

Because arterial desaturation (cyanosis) may be due to noncardiac causes, the following discussion will begin with a consideration of those cardiac lesions that must be

TABLE 7–1. Radiographic Classification of Cyanotic Congenital Heart Disease

---

I. Cyanosis with Normal/Diminished Pulmonary Vascularity
   Associated with a VSD
   A. Tetralogy of Fallot
   B. Tricuspid/Pulmonary Stenosis or Atresia
   C. Single Ventricle with Pulmonary Stenosis*
   D. Complete Transposition with Pulmonary Stenosis*
   E. Double-Outlet Right Ventricle with Pulmonary Stenosis
   Associated with Intact Septum
   F. Ebstein's Anomaly of the Tricuspid Valve
   G. Severe Pulmonary Stenosis or Atresia

II. Cyanosis with Shunt Vascularity
   A. Complete Transposition of the Great Arteries
   B. Single Ventricle
   C. Double-Outlet Right Ventricle
   D. Total Anomalous Pulmonary Venous Return
   E. Persistent Truncus Arteriosus
   F. Tricuspid Atresia (+/− Transposition)

---

*Usually present *without* pulmonary stenosis.

TABLE 7–2. Radiographic-Echocardiographic Approach to Cyanotic Congenital Heart Disease

CYANOTIC
INFANT/CHILD

Chest X-ray
*Echocardiogram

CARDIAC CONDITIONS
Chest X-ray
*Echocardiogram

NORMAL/DIMINISHED VASCULARITY

Tetralogy of Fallot
Tricuspid/Pulmonary Stenosis or Atresia
Single Ventricle with Pulmonary Stenosis
Complete Transposition with Pulmonary Stenosis
Double-Outlet Right Ventricle with Pulmonary Stenosis
Ebstein's Anomaly of the Tricuspid Valve
Severe Pulmonary Stenosis or Atresia

INCREASED VASCULARITY

Complete Transposition of the Great Arteries
Single Ventricle
Double-Outlet Right Ventricle
Total Anomalous Pulmonary Venous Return
Persistent Truncus Arteriosus
Tricuspid Atresia (+/− Transposition)

NONCARDIAC CONDITIONS

Central Hypoventilation
Airway Obstruction
AV Fistulae
Hyperviscosity
Abnormal Hgb
Persistent Fetal
    Circulation

*M-mode and cross-sectional echocardiogram.

TABLE 7–3. Cyanotic Heart Disease
(Yale–New Haven Hospital, 1975–1978)

LESION	PATIENTS	PER CENT	AGE AT PRESENTATION
d-Transposition	27	25.2	Birth–8 months
Tetralogy of Fallot	26	24	Birth–37 years
Single Ventricle ± P.S.	15	14	Birth–3 months
Tricuspid/Pulmonary Atresia	8	7.5	Birth–1 day
Double-Outlet Right Ventricle ± P.S.	8	7.5	Birth–2 months
Ebstein's Anomaly	7	6.5	Birth–2.5 years
Pulmonary Atresia/Intact Ventricular Septum	6	5.4	Birth–8 months
Total Anomalous Pulmonary Venous Return	5	4.7	2 months–8 months
Tricuspid Atresia	3	2.8	3 days–3 months
Persistent Truncus Arteriosus	2	1.9	2 days–6 weeks
	107	100	

differentiated from cyanotic congenital heart defects. This will be followed by a sequential presentation of the radiographic and echocardiographic features of the ten most common cyanotic congenital heart defects.[3-6] The state of the pulmonary vascularity on the chest film can be used to categorize the various lesions into two groups — those presenting with diminished vascularity and those presenting with increased vascularity of the shunt type (Tables 7–1 and 7–2). The latter group will be discussed in Chapter 8. Data presented on the frequency of specific radiographic findings are derived from a retrospective analysis of the chest films in a group of 107 cyanotic children.[5, 6] The frequency of these angiographically and/or surgically proven cases are listed in Table 7–3.

Noncardiac Causes of Cyanosis

The first stage in the evaluation of the cyanotic infant involves distinguishing the noncardiac causes of persistent cyanosis. These are listed in Table 7–2. For the most part, these conditions can be identified by clinical and laboratory means and by echocardiographic findings. One of the more common pulmonary causes of cyanosis is the respiratory distress syndrome (RDS). The chest film findings include a characteristic granular appearance to the lungs,

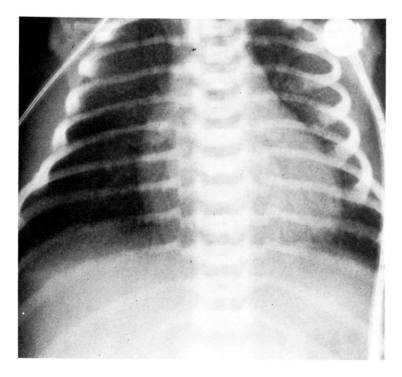

Figure 7–1. Hypoxic infant with typical features of respiratory distress syndrome — granular appearance of lung fields and air bronchograms. Note the lack of thymic tissue in this cyanotic neonate.

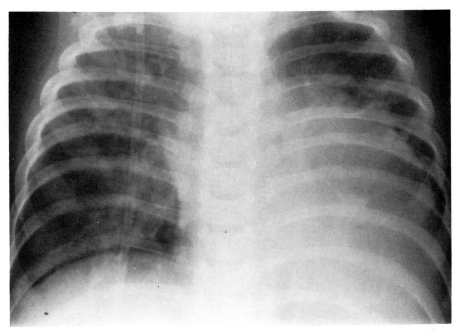

Figure 7–2. Cyanotic six-week-old infant with coarse infiltrates and lucencies throughout both lungs typical of bronchopulmonary dysplasia. Marked cardiomegaly is present secondary to the severe lung disease and pulmonary hypertension.

air bronchograms, and hypoventilation (Fig. 7–1). Children with a more prolonged course of respiratory distress may suffer from bronchopulmonary dysplasia. The chest film demonstrates multiple areas of emphysema and coarse infiltrates (Fig. 7–2).

Prolonged intrauterine stress may result in a syndrome characterized by cyanosis, respiratory distress, polycythemia, congestive failure, and hypoglycemia.[7] Cardiomegaly is often present on the chest film (Fig. 7–3).

Figure 7–3. A cyanotic newborn who suffered prolonged intrauterine stress. Polycythemia, hypoglycemia, and congestive failure were treated medically. Congenital cardiac lesions were ruled out on subsequent echocardiograms.

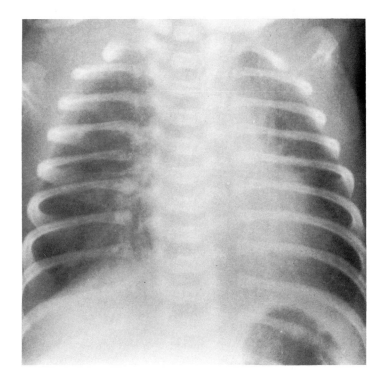

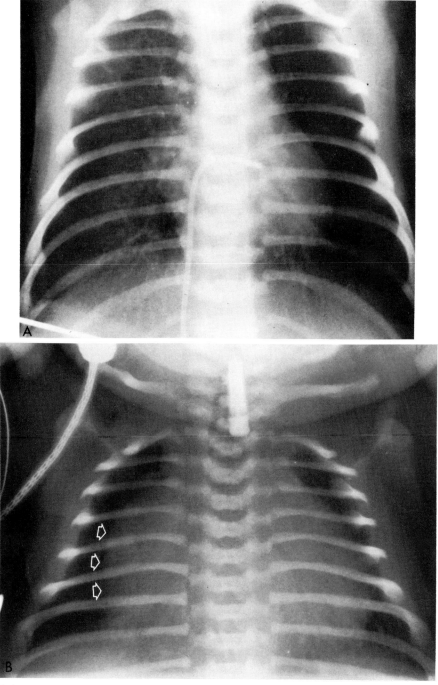

Figure 7–4. *A,* Cyanotic infant with M-mode echocardiographic evidence of elevated pulmonary vascular resistance (RVPEP/RVET > .40). The lung fields are clear and pulmonary vascularity and heart size are normal. This child has the primary form of persistent pulmonary hypertension of the newborn. *B,* Anteroposterior chest radiograph in a cyanotic neonate with persistent pulmonary hypertension and tricuspid regurgitation. The right atrium is significantly enlarged (arrows), reflecting the volume overload lesion.

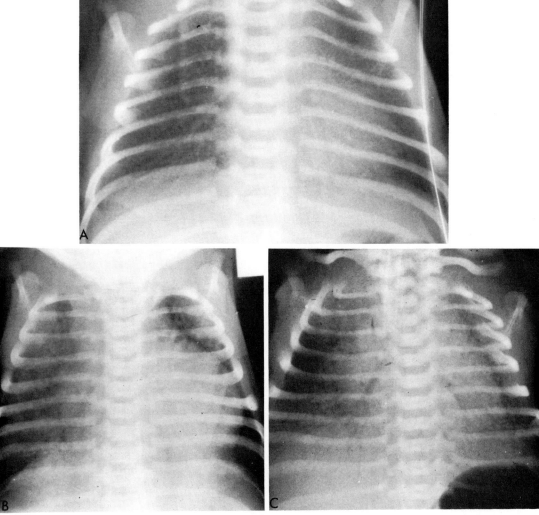

Figure 7–5. Three cyanotic infants with persistent pulmonary hypertension secondary to various pulmonary conditions. The chest radiograph helps to identify these: *A*, respiratory distress syndrome; *B*, meconium aspiration; *C*, neonatal sepsis (streptococcal pneumonia).

A recently recognized entity involving persistent pulmonary hypertension in the newborn (persistent fetal circulation [PFC]) may cause clinical difficulty and must be differentiated from organic congenital heart disease. This condition in the neonate is characterized by persistent cyanosis (unresponsive to oxygen therapy) and elevated pulmonary pressures.[8, 9] Right-to-left shunting at the atrial and/or ductus level occurs. The chest radiograph and M-mode echocardiogram are critical to the diagnosis of this lesion and also help to categorize it into its primary (idiopathic) and secondary forms.[10] The M-mode echocardiogram is helpful in establishing the presence of pulmonary hy-

pertension. This may be suggested by evaluation of the right ventricular systolic time intervals: right ventricular ejection time (RVET) and right ventricular pre-ejection period (RVPEP). An RVPEP/RVET ratio of greater than .40 suggests elevated pulmonary vascular resistance (see Fig. 2–3). In the "primary" form of PFC, the lung fields are clear (Fig. 7–4A). Pulmonary vascularity may vary from diminished to normal (Fig. 7–4A), and heart size generally is normal unless tricuspid regurgitation occurs (Fig. 7–4B). In the "secondary" form, the lung fields are abnormal and a variety of neonatal pulmonary conditions exist. The chest radiograph can distinguish these secondary forms, which include respiratory distress syndrome (Fig. 7–5A), transient tachypnea of the newborn, meconium aspiration (Fig. 7–5B), and neonatal pneumonias (Fig. 7–5C).

After one has excluded noncardiac causes of cyanosis, the next stage in the evaluation of the patient involves classifying the chest film into one that shows either normal to diminished vascularity or increased vascularity. With few exceptions, the ten most common cyanotic congenital heart defects will present in one of these two large categories (Table 7–1). The following chapter will deal with those lesions associated with normal or diminished vascularity. The second category will be dealt with in Chapter 8.

REFERENCES

1. Elliott, L. P., Schiebler, G. L.: Roentgenologic-electrocardiographic approach to cyanotic forms of heart disease. Pediatr Clin North Am 18:1141, 1971.
2. Elliott, L. P., Schiebler, G. L.: X-ray Diagnosis of Congenital Disease in Infants, Children, and Adults. Charles C Thomas, Springfield, 1979.
3. Keith, J. D., Rowe, R. D., Vlad, P.: Heart Disease in Infancy and Adulthood. Macmillan Co., New York, 1979.
4. Krovetz, L. J., Gessner, I. H., Schiebler, G. L.: Handbook of Pediatric Cardiology. Hoeber-Harper, New York, 1981.
5. Shoum, S. M.: Cyanotic Congenital Heart Disease: A Radiographic-Echocardiographic Approach. Senior Thesis, Yale Univ Sch Med, 1978.
6. Kelley, M. J., Jaffe, C., Shoum, S. M., Kleinman, C. S.: A radiographic and echocardiographic approach to cyanotic congenital heart disease. Radiol Clin North Am 18:411, 1980.
7. Cornblath, M., Schwartz, R.: Transient symptomatic hypoglycemia in the neonate. Major Probl Clin Pediatr 3:82, 1966.
8. Hirschfeld, S., Meyer, R., Schwartz, D. C., Korfhagen, J., Kaplan, S.: The echocardiographic assessment of pulmonary pressure and pulmonary vascular resistance. Circulation 52:642, 1975.
9. Levin, D. L., Heymann, K., Kitterman, J. A., Gregory, G. A., Phibbs, R. H., Rudolph, A. M.: Persistent pulmonary hypertension of the newborn. J Pediatr 89:626, 1976.
10. Kelley, M. J., Higgins, C. B., Edwards, D. K., DiSessa, T., Ti, C., Higgins, S. S., Kirkpatrick, S. E., Friedman, W.: Radiographic and echocardiographic features of pulmonary hypertension in the neonate. Abstract presented at the 65th Sci Assembly and Annual Meeting of the Radiol Soc N Am, 1979.

CYANOTIC PATIENT WITH NORMAL OR DIMINISHED VASCULARITY

It should be noted that the child with a suspected cardiac cause for cyanosis may have relatively normal-appearing pulmonary vascularity on the chest film. Subsequent cardiac catheterization and angiographic data may demonstrate diminished pulmonary blood flow in these patients as well as right-to-left shunting. A patent ductus often contributes to pulmonary flow in these patients. Clues to diminished vascularity on the radiograph include the following: diminished number and size of pulmonary vessels (especially in the outer third of the lungs) (Fig. 7–6A); a right descending pulmonary artery that is smaller than the trachea; an overall appearance of the chest film that suggests overpenetrated technique when on closer assessment this is not the case (Fig. 7–6A); and an ill-defined or hypoplastic right pulmonary artery as seen on the lateral chest film (Fig. 7–6B).

Although all the lesions presented in this section have diminished vascularity on the chest radiograph, the heart size may be used to further the differential diagnosis. The heart is generally normal in size in tetralogy of Fallot (Fig. 7–6A) and normal to slightly enlarged in tricuspid atresia (Fig. 7–27), while it is invariably enlarged in pulmonary atresia with intact ventricular septum (Fig. 7–18) and Ebstein's anomaly (Fig. 7–35).

TETRALOGY OF FALLOT

The term *tetralogy of Fallot* should be reserved for those conditions in which a large ventricular septal defect is associated with pulmonary stenosis such that pressures occur in the right ventricle that are at systemic levels, while pulmonary artery pressure is normal to low. Conditions in which a large VSD is associated with pulmonary stenosis and primarily left-to-right shunting at the ventricular level are classified by some as *acyanotic tetralogy of Fallot*. Conditions in which a large ventricular septal defect is associated with pulmonary atresia are best termed *pulmonary atresia with ventricular septal defect*. The term "pseudo–

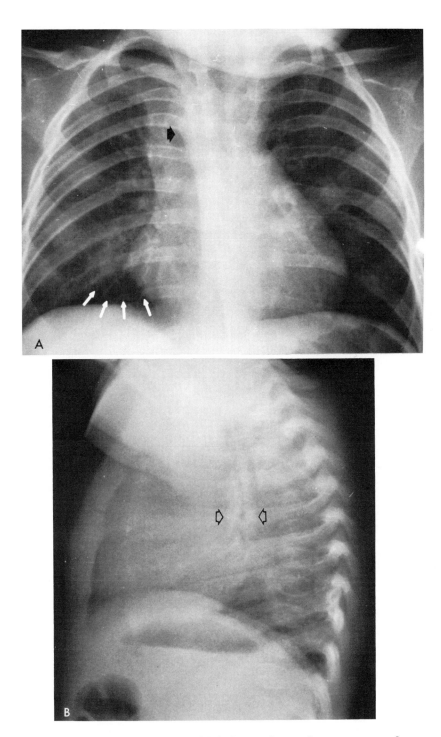

Figure 7–6. Anteroposterior *(A)* and lateral *(B)* chest radiographs in a cyanotic five-month-old boy. Decreased vascularity is reflected in the diminutive lower lobe vessels (arrows) and the hypoplastic hilar vessels (open arrows). There is a right aortic arch (arrow); the heart size is normal with an upturned apex. Note the fused left seventh and eighth ribs (bony abnormalities are more common in cyanotic as opposed to acyanotic lesions). These radiographic features are classic for tetralogy of Fallot.

truncus arteriosus" has been applied to the latter condition but may lead to confusion in that it implies an embryologic basis for the defect that may not be correct.

The physiologic consequences of tetralogy are related to two anatomic defects — namely, a large ventricular septal defect and pulmonic stenosis. A third aspect of tetralogy, dextroposition of the aorta, is of little hemodynamic significance. In fact, these three elements may all arise embryologically owing to malalignment of the conal septum. The fourth element, right ventricular hypertrophy, is a consequence of right ventricular hypertension.

Classic tetralogy of Fallot is associated with a large ventricular septal defect that approximates the size of the aortic orifice. The defect is inferior to the crista supraventricularis and involves an area that includes the region usually occupied by an isolated membranous ventricular septal defect as well as an area slightly anterior to it. The defect is immediately beneath the aortic valve cusp when viewed from the left ventricle. Occasionally, the defect may be in a posterior location — the so-called posterior or cushion type VSD.[1] The aorta straddles the ventricular septal defect, overriding it to a variable degree. The aortic valve maintains anatomic (fibrous) continuity with the anterior leaflet of the mitral valve. This feature distinguishes tetralogy from the dextroposed aorta of double outlet right ventricle.

The pulmonic stenosis may be located at any of four levels, but most commonly it involves the infundibulum and/or the pulmonary valve. Obstruction within the pulmonary trunk or its branches or within the subinfundibular region is unusual.[2] The stenotic pulmonary valve may be bicuspid; tricuspid, but small (hypoplastic); tricuspid, but deformed (dysplastic); or unicuspid.[3] Rarely, the site of stenosis is in the pulmonary trunk or the major branches distal to the pulmonary valve, most commonly the origin of the left pulmonary artery.[3] Subinfundibular stenosis generally involves obstruction by anomalous muscle bundles that may create a double-chambered right ventricle.[4]

Pulmonary atresia with VSD can be thought of as the most severe form of tetralogy of Fallot. In this situation, the right ventricular infundibulum terminates in a rudimentary or atretic pulmonary valve.[5] The pulmonary trunk is a cord-like or funnel-shaped vessel that widens as it approaches the main pulmonary artery bifurcation.[5] All of the blood leaving the right ventricle goes to the systemic circulation (to an enlarged ascending aorta) via a large ventricular septal defect. Commonly, the aortic arch is right sided. Central pulmonary arteries are not well developed, and the entire pulmonary blood flow is through collaterals that reach the pulmonary tree from the transverse and proximal descending thoracic aorta. These may take the form of systemic or bronchial vessels ("systemic collaterals") or of a vertically positioned patent ductus arteriosus. In general, the central right and left pulmonary arteries are patent and confluent at their origins, an important consideration in definitive surgical repair of this condition.[6]

A right aortic arch with a right descending thoracic aorta is relatively common in the classic form of tetralogy of Fallot. The incidence has been reported to be from 20 to 30 per cent.[3] In general, the more severe the degree of pulmonary obstruction, the higher the incidence of right aortic arch. Therefore, the right arch is seen more commonly in patients with pulmonary atresia/VSD than in milder forms of tetralogy.

The condition known as absence of the pulmonary valve occurs commonly in association with other features of tetralogy of Fallot.[7] In this condition, there is no formed valve tissue in the pulmonary valve region, but instead rudimentary valve remnants are present. Pulmonary regurgitation is a common feature of this condition, and tremendous dilatation of the pulmonary trunk to almost aneurysmal proportions has been noted.

Coronary anomalies are not uncommonly associated with tetralogy of Fallot. From a surgical standpoint, the origin of the left anterior descending coronary artery from the right coronary artery is most important. In this situation, the anterior descending coronary artery passes across the infundibulum of the right ventricle — the location for surgical incision and repair of the stenotic infundibulum in tetralogy.[8] A second anomaly is the enlarged conus branch of the right coronary artery that lies across the outflow tract of the right ventricle. When there is a single coronary artery,

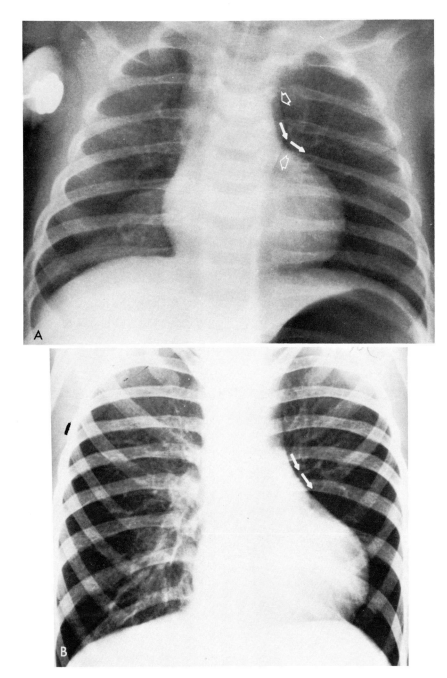

Figure 7-7. Frontal chest radiographs in a cyanotic infant *(A)* and a cyanotic seven year old *(B)*. In both cases the vascularity is diminished and the heart is normal in size with an upturned apex. In the infant, the descending aorta is slightly prominent (open arrows), while in both cases the pulmonary artery segment is concave (arrows).

this conus branch may serve as the functional connection to the right coronary artery; thus the surgeon must be aware of this anomaly as well.[8]

Clinically, patients with tetralogy of Fallot present with obvious cyanosis by the age of three to six months. However, when an infant is born with very severe pulmonary stenosis or pulmonary atresia, cyanosis is present at birth. It has been pointed out that after the age of four years, tetralogy of Fallot is the most common congenital heart disease presenting with cyanosis.[9] In addition, this malformation is the most common among cyanotic *adults* with congenital heart disease.[10] Longevity in tetralogy depends on the development of adequate collateral circulation to the lungs and, to a lesser extent, on the degree of pulmonic stenosis.

Radiographic Features

The chest film in the classic cyanotic tetralogy of Fallot shows diminished vascularity. This is manifested by a reduction in the size and number of pulmonary arteries and veins; diminished size of the hilar vessels on the lateral film, and an overall emphysematous appearance to the lungs (Figs. 7–6 and 7–7). A useful clue to the hypoplastic pulmonary vasculature is an absence of a clearly defined pulmonary trunk density on the frontal chest film. This results in a concavity along the left midheart border (Fig. 7–7). Poststenotic dilatation of the pulmonary trunk and left pulmonary artery as seen in isolated valvar pulmonary stenosis is rare in tetralogy of Fallot.

In the presence of pulmonary atresia with a large VSD, systemic collateral circulation exists and may cause unusual vascular patterns. Commonly there is a stippled or reticular appearance to the lungs that may suggest interstitial lung disease (Fig. 7–8A). The lateral chest film is helpful, showing hypoplastic hilar vessels (Fig. 7–8B). Occasionally, large collaterals will cause impressions on the esophagus that can be detected with a barium swallow (Fig. 7–8B). An additional clue to the nature of abnormal perfusion of the lungs is that the vascular pattern

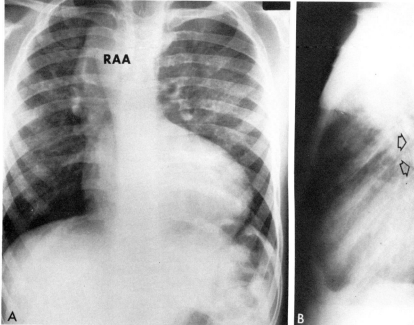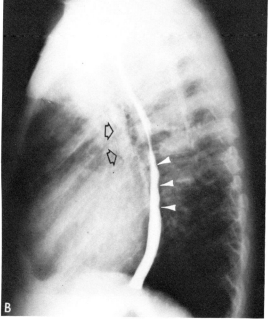

Figure 7–8. Posteroanterior *(A)* and lateral *(B)* chest radiographs in a cyanotic six-year-old with pulmonary atresia/VSD. The lung markings are disorganized and the vascularity appears diminished with small hilar densities on the lateral film (open arrows). There is a large right aortic arch (RAA) and the pulmonary artery segment is absent. As opposed to classic tetralogy, the heart is enlarged. Subtle impressions on the barium-filled esophagus (arrowheads) are due to systemic collaterals.

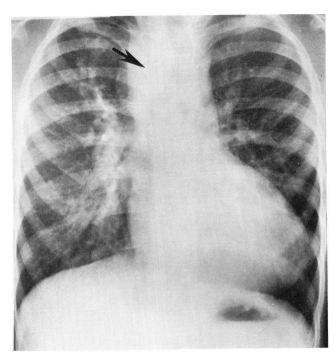

Figure 7–9. Posteroanterior chest radiograph of a cyanotic ten year old. The right pulmonary vascularity appears increased, while the left appears diminished. This nonuniform pattern is typical in pulmonary atresia/VSD and is due to uneven distribution of systemic collateral vessels. Note the right aortic arch (arrow) and the large, "boot-shaped" heart.

is not uniform. Some areas show large tortuous vessels and others demonstrate essentially no vascular markings (Fig. 7–9). The cardiac configuration in pulmonary atresia/VSD is typically the "boot-shaped" heart (Figs. 7–8 and 7–9). A right aortic arch is more common in this severe variety of tetralogy (Figs. 7–8 and 7–9). The incidence approaches 50 per cent.[9]

The ascending aorta and aortic knob are prominent in tetralogy of Fallot (Figs. 7–6 to 7–9). There are three reasons for this: (1) the aorta receives increased blood flow because of the right-to-left shunt and obstruction to pulmonary flow; (2) the ascending aorta is dextroposed; and (3) embryologically, there is maldivision of the truncus in tetralogy, leading to increased tissue to form the aorta and decreased tissue to form the pulmonary trunk. The presence of a right aortic arch has been alluded to, occurring in approximately 25 per cent of patients with classic tetralogy.[11] Clues to the presence of a right aortic arch include a rightward impression on the trachea, deviation of the superior vena cava to the right, the presence of a right descending aorta along the paraspinous region, and absence of the "normal" aortic knob on the left (Figs. 7–6A, 7–8A, and 7–9). The right aortic arch in tetralogy is of the Type I, or mirror-image, variety.

Cardiac size in tetralogy is generally normal (Figs. 7–6 and 7–7), although there may be signs of right ventricular hypertrophy as indicated by an upturned cardiac apex (Figs. 7–6 and 7–7). Generally, the classic "coeur en sabot," or "boot-shaped," heart, is seen in the older child (Fig. 7–7) or in cases of pulmonary atresia/VSD (Figs. 7–8 and 7–9). The infant with tetralogy frequently has a relatively normal cardiac contour.

In our review of 24 patients with tetralogy of Fallot, all but one had diminished vascularity on the chest film.[11] The latter child had pulmonary atresia with a ventricular septal defect and systemic collaterals to the lungs that gave a typical reticular appearance to the vascularity in the chest film. Normal heart size was found in 22 of 24, an upturned apex in 20 of 24, and a prominent aorta in 16 of 24 patients.

The chest x-ray in children with absence of the pulmonary valve associated with tetralogy is quite striking. There is marked dilatation of the pulmonary trunk and its proximal branches, but, often, diminished pulmonary vascularity in the periphery (Fig. 7–10). The left upper lobe bronchus may be compressed by the large pulmonary trunk (Fig. 7–10). The dilated pulmonary trunk and diminished vascularity are due to

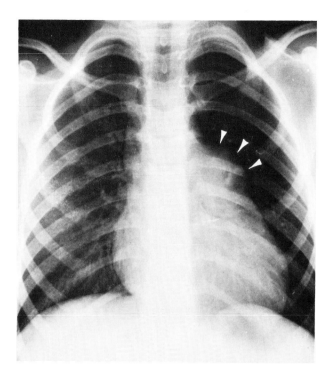

Figure 7–10. Posteroanterior chest radiograph in a child with absence of the pulmonary valve and significant pulmonary regurgitation. The massive pulmonary trunk (arrowheads) has compressed the left upper lobe bronchus, causing air trapping in the left upper lobe. The pulmonary vascularity is decreased and the heart is enlarged.

the significant pulmonary regurgitation that exists. The heart is generally enlarged owing to volume overload of the right ventricle (Fig. 7–10).

Absence of a pulmonary artery in tetralogy of Fallot most frequently involves the left pulmonary artery.[13] The chest film offers significant clues in this situation, in that left lung pulmonary vascularity will be essentially absent, while vascularity on the right will be normal, or even increased. In addition, a right aortic arch is very common in this situation.[14]

Echocardiographic Features

Two-dimensional echocardiographic imaging permits the specific diagnosis of tetralogy of Fallot when combined with the accompanying chest radiograph showing *decreased* pulmonary vascularity. In the long-axis view, septal-aortic discontinuity is demonstrated with the anterior wall of the aorta overriding the ventricular septal defect (Fig. 7–11). The septal defect is a malalignment defect (associated with great vessel override). The presence of a right ventricular outflow tract and the absence of left atrial enlargement in association with a malalignment ventricular septal defect per-

mit the echocardiographer to differentiate this entity from persistent truncus arteriosus. The chest film in the latter condition will demonstrate shunt vascularity and therefore also help to distinguish the two entities. In the apical view, the ventricular septal defect and overriding aorta may be appreciated. Moreover, tetralogy of Fallot can be differentiated from double-outlet right ventricle with pulmonary stenosis, since, in tetralogy, mitral-aortic continuity is easily demonstrated. In double-outlet right ventricle, direct fibrous continuity between the mitral and aortic valve is absent owing to the presence of conal tissue beneath both great arteries.

Angiographic Features

The goals of successful angiography in tetralogy of Fallot should include the following: (1) a complete evaluation of the right ventricular infundibulum, pulmonary valve, pulmonary trunk, and central pulmonary arteries; (2) characterization of the size and location of the VSD, as well as the identification of additional septal defects; (3) an estimation of the size of both ventricles and their relationship to their respective atrioventricular valves; and (4) an as-

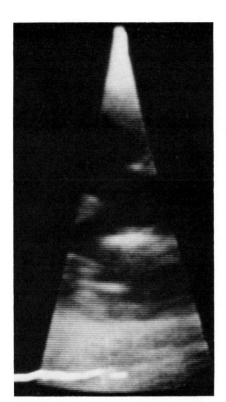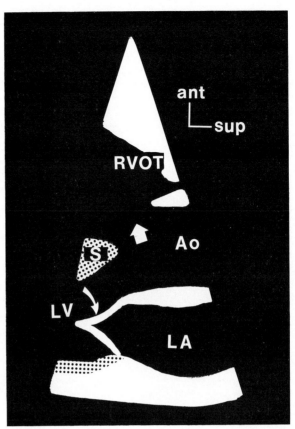

Figure 7–11. Tetralogy of Fallot. Long-axis view of the left ventricle in a patient with tetralogy of Fallot. The right ventricular outflow tract (RVOT) is seen anterior to the aortic root (Ao) and left ventricle (LV). The aorta overrides the interventricular septum (S) by approximately 60 per cent and there is a large ventricular septal defect high in the interventricular septum (bold arrow). The mitral valve (curved arrow) is in continuity with the posterior aspect of the aortic root. The left atrial dimension (LA) is small. The presence of a right ventricular outflow tract anterior to the aortic root and the small left atrial size distinguish this lesion complex from persistent truncus arteriosus.

sessment of the coronary anatomy. In pulmonary atresia/VSD, the origin and extent of systemic-pulmonary collaterals should be enumerated, but, more importantly, the presence and anatomy of a true pulmonary trunk and its branches must be determined.

A right ventriculogram performed in the standard posteroanterior and lateral views (Fig. 7–12) or hepatoclavicular (four-chamber) view (Fig. 7–13) should accomplish the first goal above. Since the left pulmonary artery is frequently stenotic in tetralogy and may not be adequately visualized in standard views, the hepatoclavicular view (Fig. 7–14) or a 45° sitting posteroanterior view may be necessary. The left ventricle and the features of the VSD(s) can

best be studied in the biplane long-axial oblique or hepatoclavicular view (see *Angiography of VSD*, Chapter 6), since standard posteroanterior and lateral projections may miss additional septal defects. An ascending aortogram is usually adequate to assess the coronary anatomy in infants. Selective coronary arteriogram may be required in older patients or in those who have had a previous pericardiotomy.[8] Systemic collaterals may be evaluated from this same aortic injection (Fig. 7–15), although selective injections in the collaterals will better assess their size and course (Fig. 7–16). In the child with pulmonary atresia/VSD, patient positioning for the aortogram is critical in the search for a true pulmonary trunk and confluent pulmonary arteries. The

Text continues on page 358

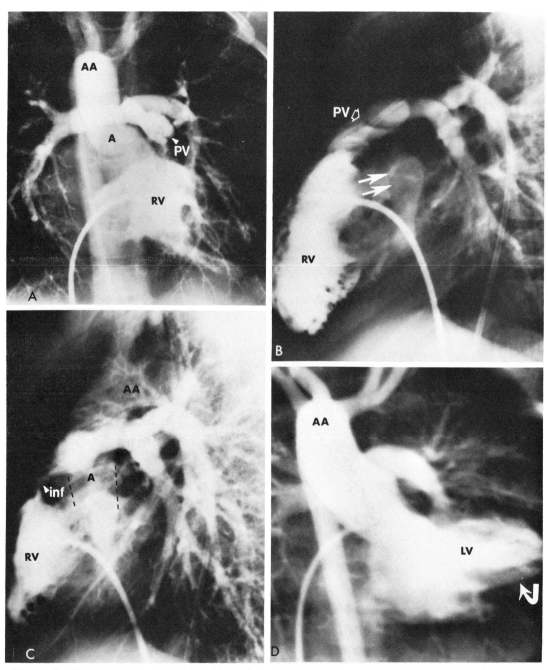

Figure 7–12. Posteroanterior *(A)* and lateral diastolic *(B)* and systolic *(C)* right ventriculograms in a child with tetralogy of Fallot. Note the classic features of tetralogy: the hypertrophied right ventricle (RV); the narrowed infundibulum (inf); the thickened pulmonary valve (PV); the large VSD (double arrows); and the large aorta (A) that overrides the VSD (dotted lines). Posteroanterior left ventriculogram *(D)* shows that the left ventricular apex (LV) is elevated (curved arrow), explaining the chest film appearance of the apex and that there is a mirror-image right aortic arch (AA).

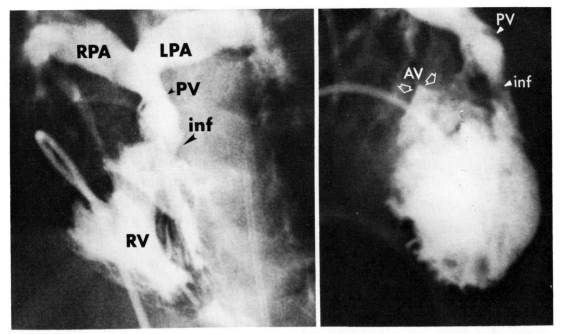

Figure 7–13. Hepatoclavicular (four-chamber) right ventriculogram taken with vertical (*A*) and horizontal (*B*) tubes in a child with tetralogy of Fallot. Certain key features are better visualized than in Figure 7–12: the right ventricular hypertrophy (RV); the narrowed infundibulum (inf); the thickened pulmonary valve (PV). Note that the aortic valve leaflets (AV), not yet opacified by contrast, indicate the aorta's position with respect to the VSD. Note also that both right and left pulmonary arteries (RPA/LPA) are very well delineated.

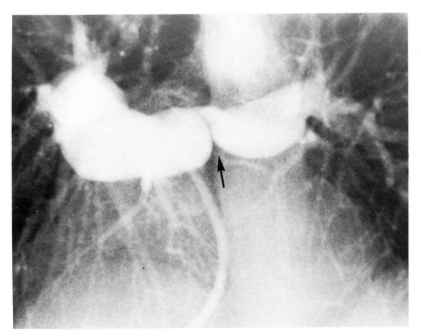

Figure 7–14. Hepatoclavicular view, pulmonary arteriogram in a patient with tetralogy of Fallot shows significant stenosis of the left pulmonary artery (arrow). This lesion could easily be missed using standard (PA/lateral) projections. Complete surgical repair of tetralogy requires the identification of these "hidden" areas of pulmonary stenosis.

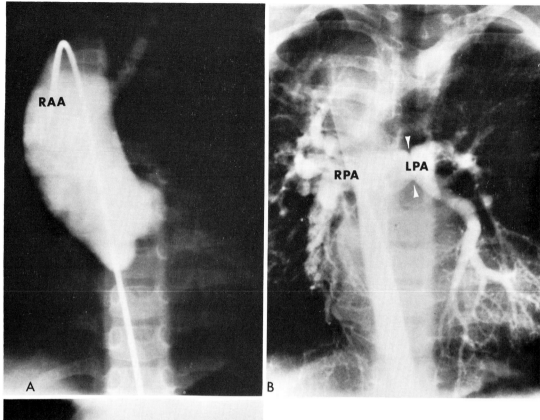

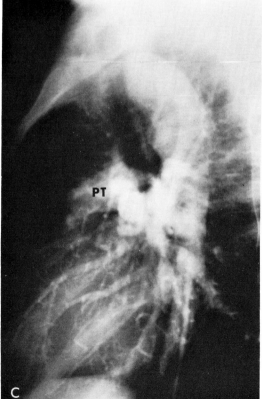

Figure 7–15. Posteroanterior *(A* and *B)* and lateral *(C)* views of an ascending aortogram in a child with pulmonary atresia/VSD. Note the catheter passage into the right aortic arch (RAA). Delayed film *(B)* shows that systemic collateral arteries opacify both right and left pulmonary arteries (RPA, LPA). Note the stenosis of the left pulmonary artery (arrowheads). The lateral view *(C)* demonstrates retrograde flow of contrast into the pulmonary trunk (PT).

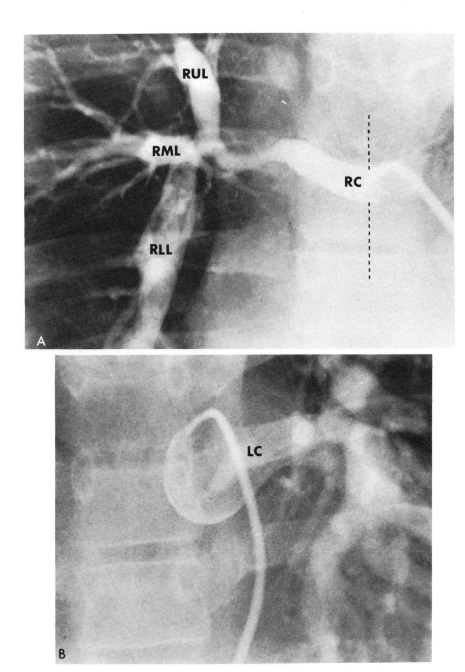

Figure 7–16. Posteroanterior views (A and B) of selective injections into systemic collateral vessels in a child with pulmonary atresia/VSD. In A, the large collateral vessel (RC) arises from the right side of the descending aorta (dotted lines), and communicates with extrahilar pulmonary arteries coursing to the right upper lobe (RUL), right middle lobe (RML), and right lower lobe (RLL). The left collateral vessel (LC) is larger than the right. A selective right coronary (Judkins) catheter was used to enter these collaterals.

latter must be present for successful operative repair of this lesion. The aortogram should be performed in the 45° sitting posteroanterior position, as the standard posteroanterior view may superimpose the systemic collateral arteries on the true pulmonary arteries.[9] Subtraction techniques following thoracic aortography have also been used to detect the pulmonary trunk and pulmonary arteries in patients with pulmonary atresia/VSD.[16] Rarely, the pulmonary arterial bed cannot be visualized by these techniques, and it may be necessary to perform pulmonary venous wedge angiography, which may opacify the pulmonary arteries in a retrograde fashion across the pulmonary capillary bed.

REFERENCES

1. Tandon, R., Moller, J. H., Edwards, J. E.: Tetralogy of Fallot associated with persistent common atrioventricular canal (endocardial cushion defect). Br Heart J 36:197, 1974.
2. Burke, E. C., Kirklin, J. W., Edwards, J. E.: Sites of obstruction to pulmonary blood flow in the tetralogy of Fallot: An anatomic study. Proc Staff Meeting, Mayo Clinic 26:498, 1951.
3. Rao, B. N. S., Anderson, R. C., Edwards, J. E.: Anatomic variations in the tetralogy of Fallot. Am Heart J 81:361, 1971.
4. Gale, G. E., Heimann, K. W., Barlowe, J. B.: Double chambered right ventricle. Br. Heart J 31:291, 1969.
5. Munoz-Armas, S., Anselmi, G., de la Cruz, M. V., Machado, I.: Pulmonary atresia with biventricular aorta. Br Heart J 26:606, 1964.
6. Somerville, J.: Management of pulmonary atresia. Br Heart J 32:641, 1970.
7. Lakier, J. B., Stanger, P., Heymann, M. A., Hoffman, J. I. E., Rudolph, A. M.: Tetralogy of Fallot with absent pulmonary valve; natural history and hemodynamic consideration. Circulation 50:167, 1974.
8. Fellows, K. E., Freed, M. D., Keane, J. F., van Pragg, R., Bernhard, W. F., Castenada, A. C.: Results of routine preoperative coronary angiography in tetralogy of Fallot. Circulation 51:561, 1975.
9. Elliott, L. P., Schiebler, G. L.: The X-ray Diagnosis of Congenital Heart Disease in Infants, Children and Adults. Charles C Thomas, Springfield, 1979.
10. Higgins, C. B., Mulder, D. G.: Tetralogy of Fallot in the adult. Am J Cardiol 29:837, 1972.
11. Lev, M., Echner, F. A.: The pathologic anatomy of tetralogy of Fallot and its variations. Dis Chest 45:251, 1964.
12. Kelley, M. J., Jaffe, C., Shoum, S. M., Kleinman, C. S.: A radiographic and echocardiographic approach to cyanotic congenital heart disease. Radiol Clin North Am 18:411, 1980.
13. Kirklin, J. W., Karp, R. B.: The Tetralogy of Fallot. W. B. Saunders Co., Philadelphia, 1970.
14. Pool, P. E., Vogel, J. H. K., Blount, S. G.: Congenital unilateral absence of the pulmonary artery. Am J Cardiol 10:706, 1962.
15. Caldwell, R. L., Weyman, A. E., Hurwitz, R. A., Girod, D. A., Feigenbaum, H.: Right ventricular outflow tract assessment by cross-sectional echocardiography in tetralogy of Fallot. Circulation 59:395, 1979.
16. Davis, G. D., Fulton, R. E., Ritter, D. C., Mair, D. D., McGoon, D. C.: Congenital pulmonary atresia with ventricular septal defect: angiographic and surgical correlates. Radiology 128:133, 1978.

CRITICAL PULMONARY STENOSIS/PULMONARY ATRESIA WITH INTACT VENTRICULAR SEPTUM

Severe or critical pulmonary stenosis with right-to-left shunting at the atrial level has been termed "trilogy of Fallot."[1] Generally, the pulmonary stenosis is at the valve level, but this is frequently accompanied by subvalvar hypertrophy of the infundibulum.[2] The atrial communication usually exists as a patent foramen ovale, but not infrequently as a true ostium secundum defect.[3] The lack of a VSD suggests that there is no embryologic relationship to tetralogy of Fallot.

When right ventricular outflow obstruction is severe, right ventricular pressures can exceed systemic pressures, and decreased right ventricular compliance and ventricular pump failure may ensue. This leads to right atrial hypertension and right-to-left shunting at the atrial level. Right ventricular failure may be accompanied by tricuspid regurgitation.

Severe pulmonary stenosis with right-to-left shunting at the atrial level usually presents in the newborn period with a conspicuous murmur and intermittent cyanosis. Presentation later in childhood is characterized by persistent cyanosis.[2]

Pulmonary atresia with intact ventricular septum is characterized by complete obstruction to forward outflow from the right ventricle. The pulmonary valve and the infundibular regions are atretic,[4] and the valve consists of an imperforate fibrous membrane.[5] The pulmonary trunk is usually present, but hypoplastic.[5] The size of the right ventricle has been used to classify this defect into two distinct types. In one the right ventricle is small and in the other it is normal in size. In the more common form the right ventricular cavity is diminutive and its wall is thick.[6] In these cases the tricuspid valve is hypoplastic and usually competent. In the minority of cases the ventricle is normal in size, the tricuspid valve orifice is normal, and the valve is incompetent. In the latter situation, the tricuspid valve is usually structurally abnormal. The size of the right atrium varies directly with the size of the right ventricle and the degree of tricuspid regurgitation. A patent foramen ovale usually exists, allowing right-to-left shunting at the atrial level. A patent ductus arteriosus provides the only source of blood to the lungs, and when it closes in the neonatal period death is imminent. Suprasystemic pressures in the right ventricle force blood through intramyocardial sinusoids, and these channels may reach the epicardium, where they communicate with the coronary arteries.[7] This situation is expected when the right ventricular cavity is small and the tricuspid valve is competent.

This lesion presents clinically at birth or shortly thereafter with cyanosis, which progressively deepens as the ductus closes. Without surgical intervention, over half of these infants will die in the first month of life.[5]

Radiographic Features

Severe pulmonary stenosis with right-to-left shunting at the atrial level presents with slightly reduced pulmonary blood flow. This becomes more apparent if right ventricular failure ensues. The pulmonary artery segment may be apparent and even prominent owing to associated poststenotic dilatation. The aorta is normal. The heart size is increased with right heart enlargement (Fig. 7–17). The right atrium may be particularly prominent when tricuspid regurgitation is severe (Fig. 7–17).

Pulmonary atresia with an intact ventricular septum presents in the newborn period with cyanosis, decreased pulmonary vascularity, and cardiomegaly (Fig. 7–18). The heart size is only mildly enlarged in those cases associated with a small right ventricle and a competent tricuspid valve. In this situation cardiomegaly is due to left ventricular enlargement. The pulmonary ar-

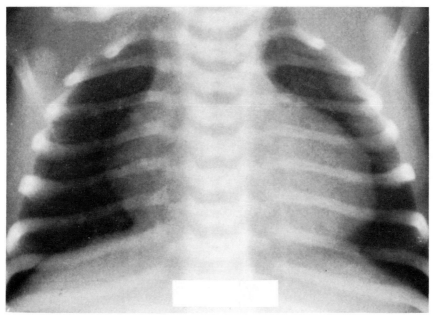

Figure 7–17. Anteroposterior chest radiograph in a six-day-old cyanotic infant. Pulmonary vascularity is diminished and the heart is enlarged with a prominent right atrium. Severe pulmonary stenosis and tricuspid regurgitation were present at cardiac catheterization and angiography.

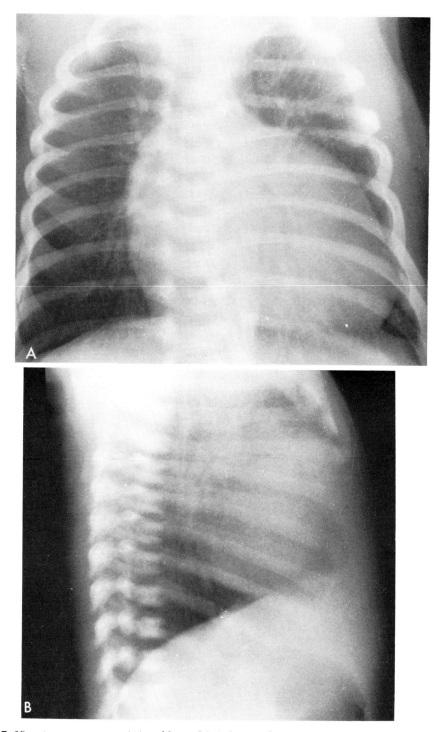

Figure 7–18. Anteroposterior *(A)* and lateral *(B)* chest radiographs in a two-day-old cyanotic infant. Pulmonary vascularity is diminished (note the small right lower lobe vessels), the heart is enlarged, and the pulmonary trunk is inapparent. The narrow mediastinum is due to decreased thymic tissue in this stressed infant. Pulmonary atresia with tricuspid regurgitation was found at cardiac catheterization and angiography.

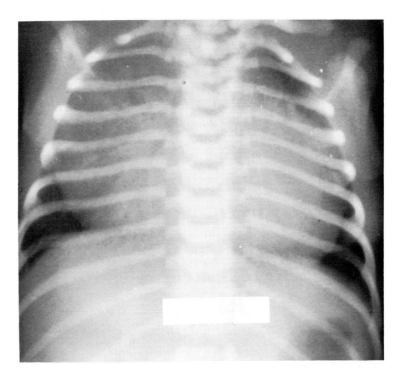

Figure 7–19. Anteroposterior chest radiograph in a six-hour-old cyanotic infant. Vascularity is difficult to assess because of the massive right atrial enlargement. Pulmonary atresia and severe tricuspid regurgitation were present at cardiac catheterization and angiography.

tery segment is usually inapparent (Fig. 7–18) because of the diminutive size of the pulmonary trunk. The aorta may be enlarged and displace the superior vena cava to the right. The right atrium varies in size, depending on the degree of tricuspid regurgitation and may be considerably dilated — often reaching the right chest wall (Fig. 7–19). In these cases, the differential diagnosis must include Ebstein's anomaly of the tricuspid valve or tricuspid regurgitation secondary to transient myocardial dysfunction and neonatal pulmonary hypertension.[8] In our series of 6 patients, all presented with diminished pulmonary vascularity, cardiomegaly, and right atrial enlargement.

Echocardiographic Features

Two-dimensional examination of the cyanotic patient with suspected pulmonary stenosis or atresia can definitively establish the diagnosis.[9] Critical pulmonary stenosis (Fig. 7–20) can usually be differentiated from pulmonary artery atresia (Fig. 7–21). Isolated severe pulmonary stenosis is diagnosed when the longitudinal view of the

pulmonary artery and pulmonary outflow tract or the subxiphoidal view of the right ventricular outflow tract and pulmonary valve visualizes a thickened and domed valve with poststenotic dilatation of the main and/or left pulmonary artery (Fig. 7–20). The two-dimensional echocardiographic examination in pulmonary atresia permits a thorough search for the right ventricular outflow tract and, if the outflow tract is absent or ends blindly (Fig. 7–21), the diagnosis of pulmonary atresia is established.[10]

Angiographic Features

The posteroanterior view of the right ventricle will show the heavy trabecular pattern characteristic of right ventricular hypertrophy (Fig. 7–22). If the patient is elevated 45°, the infundibulum and pulmonary valve region can be more adequately evaluated (Fig. 7–22). A normal-sized ventricle and a domed, thickened pulmonary valve are seen in severe pulmonic stenosis. Poststenotic dilatation beyond the valve is characteristic. Tricuspid regurgitation is usually present (Fig. 7–22). The right-to-left atrial shunt may be demonstrated as con-

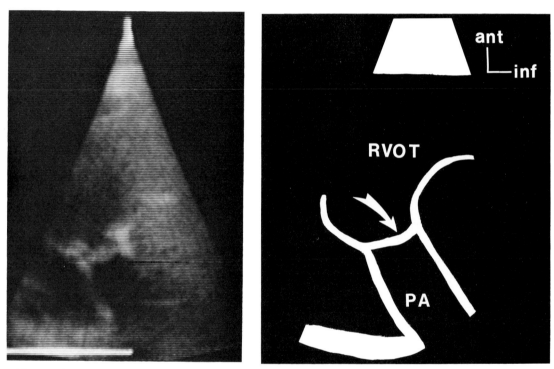

Figure 7–20. Critical pulmonary stenosis. Subxiphoidal view of the right ventricular outflow tract (RVOT). A thickened, domed pulmonic valve (arrow) is seen within the pulmonary artery (PA) and is indicative of severe valvar obstruction of right ventricular outflow.

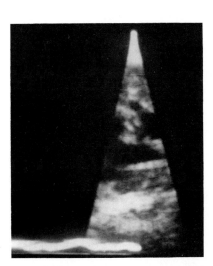
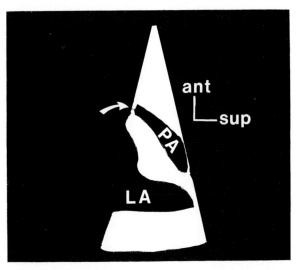

Figure 7–21. Pulmonary atresia with intact ventricular septum. Long-axis view of the pulmonary outflow tract shows that the right ventricular outflow tract is not patent and demonstrates a markedly hypoplastic pulmonary artery (PA). The thickened plate of tissue (arrow) represents an imperforate fibrous membrane in the expected position of the pulmonary valve. The left atrium (LA) is seen posteriorly.

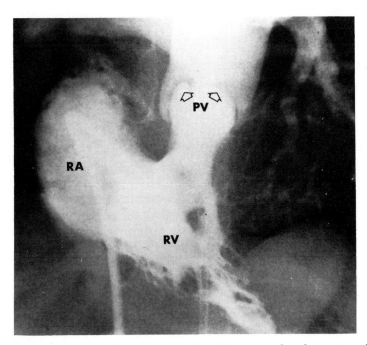

Figure 7–22. Forty-degree sitting posteroanterior (A) view of right ventriculogram. Note the hypertrophied right ventricle (RV), tricuspid regurgitation into the right atrium (RA) and the thickened, domed, pulmonary valve (PV). Although this child was not cyanotic, a more severe deformity of the pulmonary valve would lead to sufficient elevation of right ventricular pressures to produce right-to-left shunting at the atrial level.

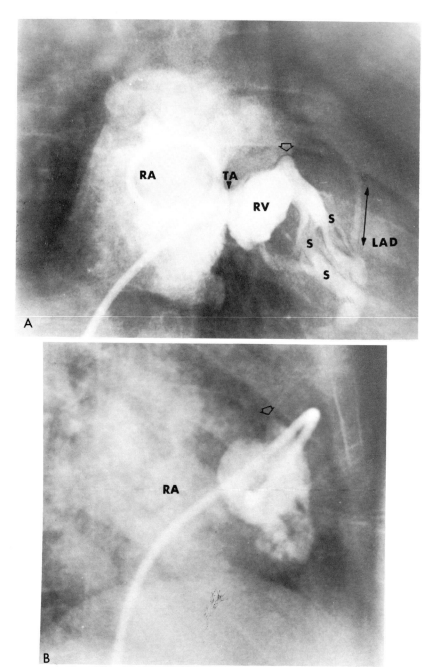

Figure 7–23. Posteroanterior (A) and lateral (B) angiograms in the diminutive right ventricle of a neonate with pulmonary atresia. Filling of right ventricular sinusoids (S) leads to retrograde filling of the left anterior descending coronary artery (LAD — double arrow). Note the atretic right ventricular outflow tract (open arrow), the small tricuspid annulus (TA — arrowhead), and the large right atrium (RA).

trast in the right atrium flows across the atrial septum into the left atrium.

In pulmonary atresia with an intact ventricular septum, the posteroanterior view will demonstrate the size of the right ventricle and tricuspid orifice (Fig. 7–23). The degree of tricuspid regurgitation is difficult to assess, since contrast has no exit except through right ventricular sinusoids or into the right atrium (Fig. 7–23). In this variety

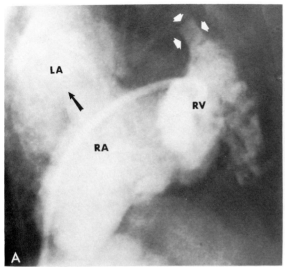

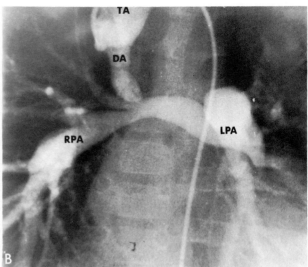

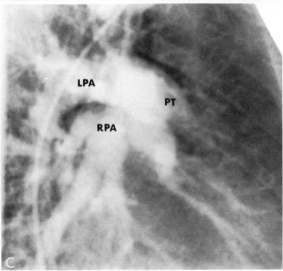

Figure 7–24. Lateral right ventriculogram *(A)* showing hypoplastic right ventricle (RV) and atretic right ventricular outflow tract (arrows) in an infant with pulmonary atresia and an intact ventricular septum. There is tricuspid regurgitation into the right atrium (RA) and right-to-left shunting into the left atrium (arrow — LA). In *(B)* and *(C)*, the catheter in the transverse aorta (TA) opacifies a vertical ductus arteriosus (DA), which provides the only blood flow to the pulmonary arteries (RPA and LPA) and the pulmonary trunk (PT).

of pulmonary atresia the sinusoidal communications that exist between the right ventricle and coronary arteries are readily identified (Fig. 7–23A). Pulmonary blood flow may be visualized only by opacifying the ductus arteriosus (Fig. 7–24B and C).

REFERENCES

1. Joly F., Carlotti, J., Sicot, J. R., Piton, A.: Cardiopathies congenitales, les triologies de Fallot. Arch Mal Coeur 43:687, 1950.
2. Callahan, J. A., Brandenburg, R. O., Swan, H. J. C.: Pulmonary stenosis and interatrial communication with cyanosis: Hemodynamic and clinical study of ten patients. Am J Med 19:189, 1955.
3. Hardy, W. E., Genoj, J., Ayers, S. M., Giannelli, S., Christianson, L. C.: Pulmonic stenosis and associated atrial septal defects in older patients. Am J Cardiol 24:130, 1969.
4. Freedom, R. M., White, R. I., Ho, C. S., Gingel, R. L., Hawker, R. D., Rowe, R. D.: Evaluation of patients with pulmonary atresia and intact ventricular septum by double catheter technique. Am J Cardiol 33:892, 1974.
5. Elliott, L. P., Adams, P., Jr., Edwards, J. E.: Pulmonary atresia with intact ventricular septum. Br Heart J 25:489, 1963.
6. Cole, R. B., Muster, A. J., Lev, M., Paul, M. H.: Pulmonary atresia with intact ventricular septum. Am J Cardiol 21:23, 1968.
7. Freedom, R. M., Harrington, D. P.: Contributions of intramyocardial sinusoids in pulmonary atresia and intact ventricular septum to a right sided circular shunt. Br Heart J 36:1061, 1974.

8. Buciarelli, R. L., Egan, E. A., Gessner, I. H.: Persistence of fetal cardiopulmonary circulation: One manifestation of transient tachypnea of the newborn. Pediatrics 58:192, 1976.
9. Sahn, D. J., Sobol, R. G., Allen, H. D.: Subxiphoid real-time cross-sectional echocardiography for imaging the right ventricle (RV) and right ventricular outflow tract (RVOT). Am J Cardiol 41:354, 1978 (abstract).
10. Neufeld, H. N., Randall, P. A.: Double outlet right ventricle. In Heart Disease in Infants, Children and Adolescents. Moss, A. J., Adams, F. H., Emmanouilides, G. C. (eds.). Williams & Wilkins Co., Baltimore, 1977, p. 335.

TRICUSPID ATRESIA

Tricuspid atresia is a difficult lesion to define because it has some features that are consistently present and others that are variable. The consistent features are (1) an atretic tricuspid valve, (2) a hypoplastic right ventricle, (3) an interatrial defect, and (4) a relatively large left ventricle and mitral valve.[1] The three variable features are (1) the orientation of the great vessels (they may be normally related or transposed), (2) the presence or absence of an obstruction to pulmonary blood flow, and (3) the presence or absence of a ventricular septal defect. It is these latter variations that are the chief determinants of the amount of blood flow reaching the lungs.

In the classic form of the lesion, tricuspid valve tissue is replaced by a dimple in the floor of the right atrium. The intra-atrial communication consists of a patent foramen ovale, although a true atrial septal defect may occur.[2] The defect may not be large enough to permit unobstructed flow from the right atrium, and in these cases the right atrium is enlarged. The right-to-left shunt at the atrial level diminishes the oxygen saturation in the left ventricle and leads to systemic arterial desaturation.

A classification of tricuspid atresia is given in Table 7–4. Tricuspid and pulmonary atresia occur together uncommonly; when they do, the great vessels generally are normally related.[1] In this situation, the right ventricle is rudimentary and the ventricular septum is intact. Blood entering the left ventricle flows into the aorta, and pulmonary blood flow is derived from a patent ductus arteriosus or systemic collaterals.

The most common form of tricuspid atresia is that associated with pulmonary stenosis and normally related great vessels.[1] The ventricular septum has a slit-like opening that allows communication between the left ventricle and the outflow portion of the small right ventricle. This slit constitutes an area of relative subpulmonary stenosis. The pulmonary trunk may be normal or hypoplastic and there may be associated pulmonary valvar stenosis. Blood flow to the lungs is reduced. Tricuspid atresia without pulmonary stenosis and normally related great vessels is an unusual entity.[3] In this situation there is a large ventricular septal defect, a normal pulmonary valve, and a normal-sized pulmonary trunk. The right ventricle may be relatively normal in size as well. In this variety of tricuspid atresia, pulmonary blood flow may be normal or increased owing to the left-to-right shunt.

When tricuspid atresia is associated with transposition of the great vessels, pulmonary atresia as well as valvar and subvalvar pulmonary stenosis is infrequent.[1] The ventricular septal defect is large, and blood flows readily into the transposed aorta. Early in life, resistance in the lungs controls the degree of pulmonary blood flow, but when pulmonary resistance falls, a large amount of pulmonary flow occurs. Tricuspid atresia with increased pulmonary blood flow is relatively uncommon; when it occurs, the great vessels are almost always transposed.[2] Juxtaposition of an atrial appendage (usually of the right appendage to the left side) is relatively frequent with the type of tricuspid atresia associated with transposition of the great vessels.[4]

TABLE 7–4. Classification of Tricuspid Atresia

I. Tricuspid Atresia without Transposition of the Great Arteries
  A. With Pulmonary Atresia and Intact Ventricular Septum
  B. With Pulmonary Stenosis and a Small, Slit-Like Interventricular Communication
  C. With No Pulmonary Stenosis and a Large Ventricular Septal Defect

II. Tricuspid Atresia with Transposition of the Great Vessels
  A. With Pulmonary Atresia and a Large Ventricular Septal Defect
  B. With Pulmonary Stenosis and a Large Ventricular Septal Defect
  C. With no Pulmonary Stenosis and a Large Ventricular Septal Defect

Clinical presentation in tricuspid atresia is variable and depends on the adequacy of the intra-atrial communication and the pulmonary blood flow.[2] Progressive cyanosis typically occurs at the time of birth or shortly thereafter, and the degree of arterial desaturation depends upon the amount of blood flow to the lungs. Mild cyanosis may occur when pulmonary stenosis is absent, and this is most common when the great vessels are transposed.[5] In general, arterial desaturation occurs within the first week of life and almost always by the first month.[5] Since the left ventricle is the only pumping chamber for both circulations, the function of this volume-overloaded chamber takes on great significance. In the presence of increased pulmonary blood flow, there is further left ventricular volume overload. Of the varieties of tricuspid atresia, the lesion that generally presents earliest and has the shortest survival is tricuspid/pulmonary atresia.[6] Longevity is greatest when pulmonary stenosis is of a degree such that pulmonary blood flow to the lungs is close to normal. Patients with tricuspid atresia and transposition of the great vessels and coexisting pulmonary stenosis may survive beyond the first year.[2]

Radiographic Features

When tricuspid atresia presents in its most common form (that is, with normally related great vessels and pulmonary stenosis), the pulmonary vascularity is reduced (Fig. 7–25). The pulmonary artery segment may be concave or flat (Fig. 7–25). The ascending aorta is generally not a prominent feature of the cardiac silhouette. A right aortic arch is rarely seen in tricuspid atresia.[7] In the neonate or young child, the heart size is frequently normal. The development of mild cardiomegaly is due to left ventricular dilatation and hypertrophy (Fig. 7–25). The cardiac apex often shows a rounded appearance (Fig. 7–25). The right heart margin may show a distinct rounded appearance superiorly with a flat inferior margin. This is thought to be due to enlargement of the right atrial appendage together with absence of the right ventricle.[8] In the left anterior oblique or lateral projection, absence of the curvature caused by the right ventricle may be noted (Fig. 7–26).

When tricuspid atresia is associated with pulmonary atresia, the picture resembles the above description except for the presence of a slightly dilated ascending aorta

Figure 7–25. Anteroposterior chest radiograph in a cyanotic infant with tricuspid atresia/pulmonary stenosis. Pulmonary vascularity is severely reduced and the heart is slightly enlarged with a rounded apex. No pulmonary artery segment is identified.

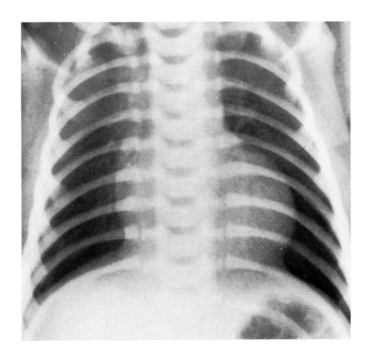

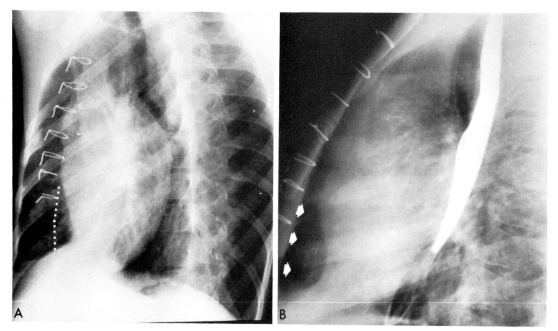

Figure 7–26. Left anterior oblique (A) and lateral (B) chest radiographs in a child who has had palliative surgery for tricuspid atresia. Note the absence of the normal right ventricular density in the LAO view (dotted line). This allows lung tissue to fill in the area of the heart usually occupied by the right ventricle on the lateral film (arrows).

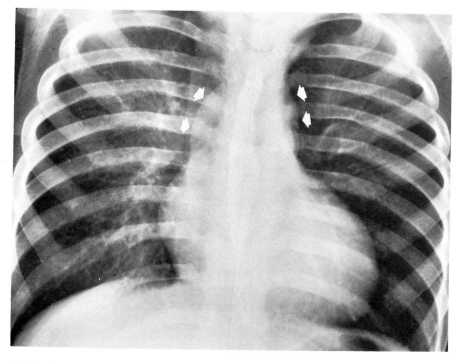

Figure 7–27. Anteroposterior chest radiograph in an infant with tricuspid/pulmonary atresia shows diminished vascularity, normal heart size, and a prominent aorta (arrows).

(Fig. 7–27). When the great vessels are transposed, the radiographic clue resides in the analysis of the mediastinal densities. There is no definable pulmonary artery segment, and the mediastinum is narrow owing to the transposed great vessels (Fig. 7–28). Invariably, the pulmonary vascularity is increased when tricuspid atresia is associated with transposition, since associated pulmonary stenosis is rare (Fig. 7–28). Cardiome-

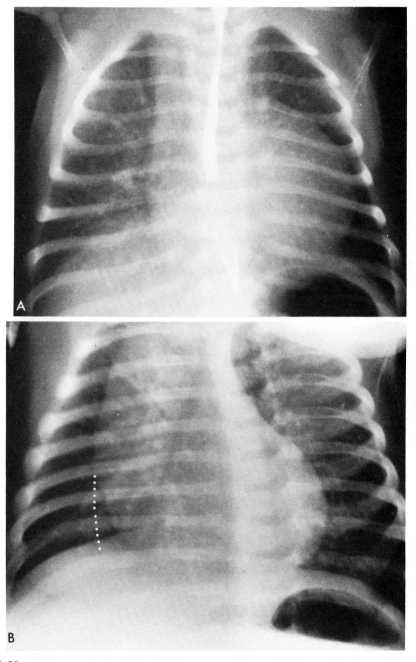

Figure 7–28. Anteroposterior *(A)* and left anterior oblique *(B)* chest radiographs in a one month old infant with tricuspid atresia and transposition of the great vessels. The pulmonary vascularity is increased, the heart enlarged, the pulmonary artery segment is inapparent, and the mediastinum is somewhat narrow. These findings are indistinguishable from transposition without tricuspid atresia. In the LAO view the right ventricular density is absent (dotted lines), suggesting the diagnosis of tricuspid atresia.

galy often accompanies this combination of lesions and is due to left ventricular dilatation (Fig. 7–28). The presence of a juxtaposed right atrial appendage should be considered in any patient who has a flat right atrial border and a bulge along the left heart border (Fig. 7–29). This complex of lesions, therefore, is usually considered in the differential diagnosis of the cyanotic infant with *increased* pulmonary blood flow (see Chapter 8).

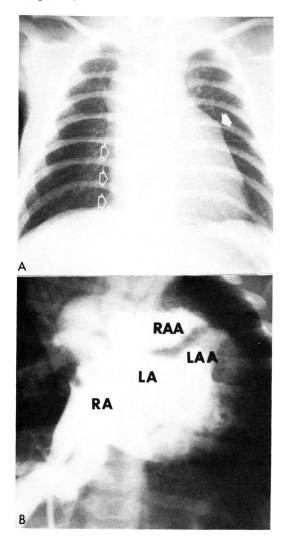

Figure 7–29. Anteroposterior chest radiograph *(A)* and right atriogram in a cyanotic infant. Note the flat right atrial border (arrows) and the bulge along the left mid heart border (arrow). The angiogram demonstrates flow of contrast from right atrium (RA) to left atrium (LA) and a juxtaposed right atrial appendage (RAA) located above the left atrial appendage (LAA). This infant also had d-transposition of the great vessels. (Angiogram courtesy of Dr. Larry P. Elliott.)

In the rare situation in which tricuspid atresia exists with normally related great vessels and a large ventricular septal defect, the chest film may have the appearance of any large right-to-left shunt (Fig. 7–30). Again, this type of tricuspid atresia is usually considered in the cyanotic–*increased* vascularity category (see Chapter 8).

In our patients in whom tricuspid atresia was associated with pulmonary stenosis or atresia, there was diminished vascularity (8 of 8 patients) and increased heart size (7 of 8 patients). The aorta was normal (6 of 8 patients), and absence of the right ventricular density on the LAO chest film was noted in 3 of 8 patients.

Echocardiographic Features

The two-dimensional echocardiogram readily permits diagnosis of tricuspid atresia. In the apical (Fig. 7–31) or subxiphoidal view, the diagnosis is established by demonstrating the presence of a large mitral valve without an accompanying tricuspid valve arising from the right-sided atrioventricular groove.[9] The interatrial septum and both atria are clearly visualized. These patients depend upon an interatrial communication to allow access of systemic venous return to the ventricle. The presence of an interventricular communication may also be identified in these views. In cases of tricuspid atresia with decreased pulmonary vascularity, associated pulmonary valve stenosis or atresia may be detected on the long-axis view.

Angiographic Features

The angiographic examination of tricuspid atresia should (1) establish the diagnosis with a right atrial angiogram; (2) evaluate the left ventricle and the size of ventricular septal defect and right ventricle; and (3) clarify the degree of pulmonary stenosis and the great vessel relationships.

The right atrial angiogram is usually performed in standard posteroanterior and lateral projections (Fig. 7–32). We have found the use of the four-chamber (hepatoclavicular) view useful in demonstrating the atrial septum and the intra-atrial communication (Fig. 7–33). The other goals of the angiographic study can be accomplished by following the contrast injected into the right

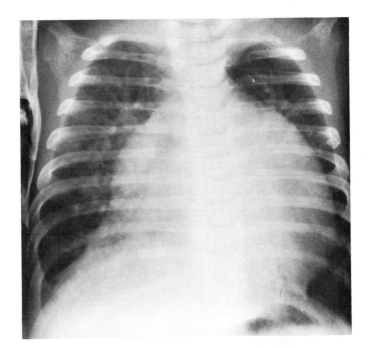

Figure 7–30. Anteroposterior chest radiograph in a cyanotic four month old. There is shunt vascularity and cardiomegaly. This child had tricuspid atresia, a large VSD, and normally related great vessels.

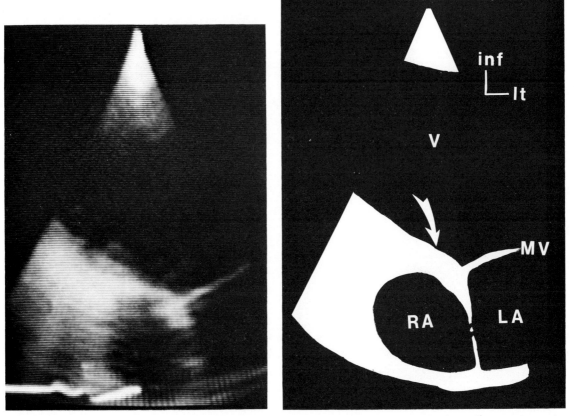

Figure 7–31. Tricuspid/pulmonary atresia. Apical view. Note the dense, thickened region (arrow) in the position normally occupied by the tricuspid valve. The right atrium (RA) does not directly enter the ventricular cavity and it communicates with the ventricle (V) via the left atrium (LA). The communication between the atria is via a secundum atrial septal defect. A large single mitral valve (MV) is seen in the atrioventricular groove. No right ventricular cavity can be visualized in this figure.

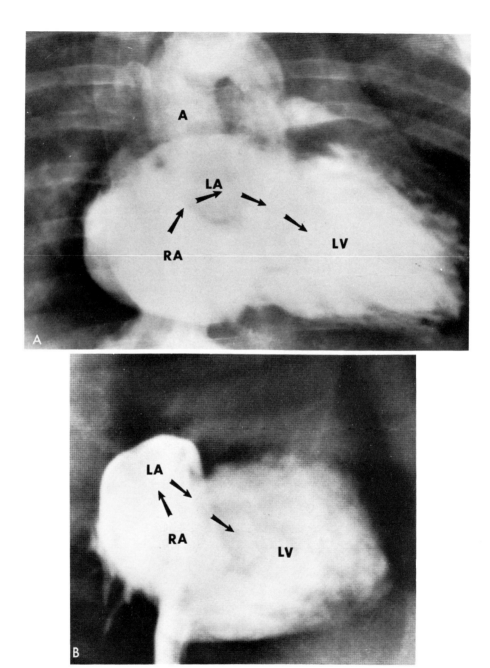

Figure 7–32. Right atrial angiogram in anteroposterior *(A)* and lateral *(B)* projections show flow of contrast from right atrium (RA), to left atrium (LA) to left ventricle (LV) and to aorta (A). This child had tricuspid/pulmonary atresia.

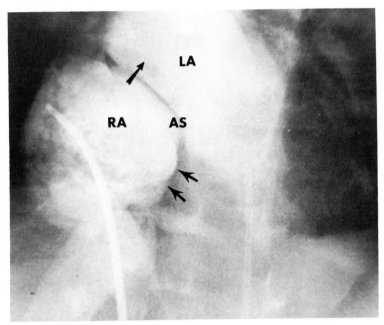

***Figure* 7–33.**   Hepatoclavicular (four-chamber) right atrial angiogram in a child with tricuspid atresia shows right-to-left shunting of contrast from right atrium (RA) to left atrium (LA) across the atrial septum (AS). The atretic tricupsid valve region is indicated (arrows).

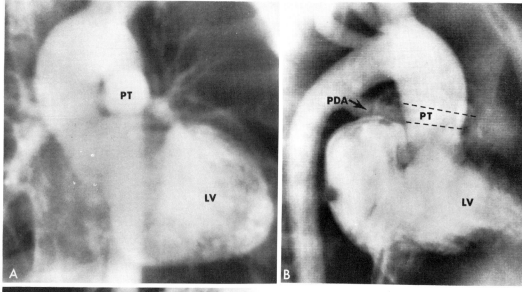

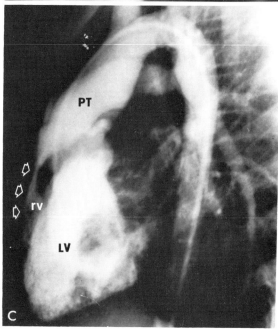

Figure 7–34. Posteroanterior *(A)* and lateral *(B)* views of a left ventriculogram in a child with tricuspid/pulmonary atresia. The left ventricle (LV) is slightly enlarged and the small pulmonary trunk (PT) is filled from a patent ductus arteriosus (PDA). Lateral left ventriculogram *(C)* in a second child with tricuspid/pulmonary stenosis. A restrictive VSD (arrows) is seen filling the diminutive right ventricle (rv) and pulmonary trunk (PT).

atrium as it flows into the left-sided cardiac structures. The source of pulmonary blood flow (through the VSD or from the aorta) should be determined (Fig. 7–34).

REFERENCES

1. Tandon, R., Edwards, J. E.: Tricuspid atresia: A re-evaluation and classification. J Thorac Cardiovasc Surg 67:530, 1974.
2. Dick, M., Fyler, D. C., Nadas, A. S.: Tricuspid atresia: Clinical course of 101 patients. Am J Cardiol 36:327, 1975.
3. Carey, L. S., Edwards, J. E.: Tricuspid atresia: Report of a case without transposition or pulmonary stenosis. Am J Roentgenol 91:321, 1964.
4. Charuzi, Y., Spanos, P. K., Amplatz, K., Edwards, J.

E.: Juxtaposition of the atrial appendage. Circulation 47:620, 1973.
5. Williams, W. G., Rubis, L., Fowler, R. S., Rao, M. K., Trussler, G. A., Mustard, W. T.: Tricuspid atresia: Results of treatment in 160 children. Am J Cardiol 38:235, 1976.
6. Elster, S. K.: Congenital atresia of pulmonary and tricuspid valves. Am J Dis Child 79:692, 1950.
7. Marder, S. N., Seamans, W. P., Scott, W. G.: Roentgenologic considerations in the diagnosis of congenital tricuspid atresia. Radiology 61:174, 1953.
8. Wittenborg, M. H., Neuhauser, E. D., Sprunt, W. H.: Roentgenologic findings in congenital tricuspid atresia with hypoplasia of the right ventricle. Am J Roentgenol 66:712, 1951.
9. Lange, L. W., Sahn, D. J., Allen, H. D., Goldberg, S. J.: Subxiphoid cross-sectional echocardiography in infants and children with congenital heart disease. Circulation 59:513, 1979.

EBSTEIN'S ANOMALY OF THE TRICUSPID VALVE

Ebstein's anomaly involves redundant tricuspid valve tissue that is displaced into the inflow portion of the right ventricle. The anterior leaflet of the tricuspid valve is least affected, while the septal and posterior leaflets characteristically show the greatest deformity.[1] The right atrium is dilated, often massively. The majority of patients have either an incompetent foramen ovale or an ostium secundum atrial septal defect.[2]

The physiologic and hemodynamic consequences of the anomalies associated with Ebstein's anomaly relate to the abnormal tricuspid valve tissue, the atrialized portion of the right ventricle, and the diminished right ventricular pumping capacity. The deformity of the tricuspid valve leads to tricuspid regurgitation. The atrialized portion of the right ventricle contracts poorly, and this leads to diminished forward outflow from the right ventricle. This atrialized segment may in fact act in the same way as an aneurysm in that it distends during atrial contraction and interferes with right ventricular filling.[1] Because of the redundant leaflets and the atrialized segment, there is reduction in volume and capacity of the pumping portion of the right ventricle that contributes to inadequate forward output into the lungs.

The age range for presentation of this lesion is large — in one series extending from less than one year to age 48.[3] An autopsy case of an 85-year-old with Ebstein's anomaly has recently been reported.[4] Palpitations are a frequent complaint and are virtually always related to arrhythmias of various types (usually supraventricular tachycardias). Palpitations in a cyanotic child should always raise the possibility of Ebstein's anomaly.[3] Cyanosis is not an invariable feature of this anomaly — being present in approximately half the patients in one large series.[3]

At cardiac catheterization a *right ventricular electrocardiographic tracing* is obtained from the atrialized portion of the right ventricle while an atrial pressure pulse is being recorded.[5] A spectrum of Ebstein's anomaly may occur with severity depending on the degree of malformation of the leaflets, the size of the atrialized portion of the ventricle, and the size and capacity of the right ventricular pumping chamber.[6-8]

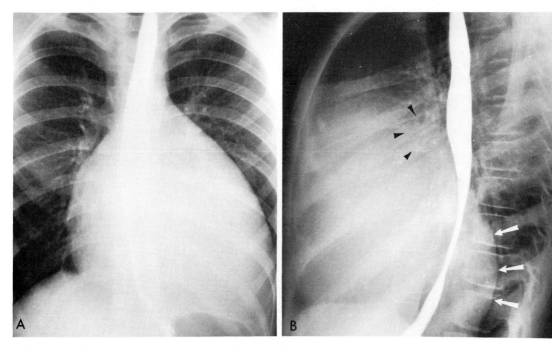

Figure 7–35. Posteroanterior (A) and lateral (B) chest radiographs in a 14-year-old cyanotic boy with Ebstein's anomaly of the tricuspid valve. The vascularity is diminished (note the hypoplastic hilar region [arrowheads]) and there is massive cardiomegaly due primarily to a huge right atrium. The right atrial chamber is so large that it projects behind the left ventricle on the lateral radiograph (arrows).

Radiographic Features

The pulmonary vascularity in patients with Ebstein's anomaly appears normal to diminished (Figs. 7–35 and 7–36). This is often best appreciated in the hilar areas of the lateral film (Figs. 7–35 and 7–36). Diminished pulmonary vascularity correlates with greater degrees of valvar deformity, decreased right ventricular output, and a larger volume right-to-left shunt at the atrial level. The degree of cardiomegaly does not always correlate with the degree of cyanosis.[3] In the more severe forms of this condition, there is massive cardiomegaly due to a markedly dilated right atrium (Figs. 7–35 and 7–36). In some cases, the posterior border of the right atrium may actually project behind the left ventricle on the lateral chest film (Figs. 7–35 and 7–36). In the left an-

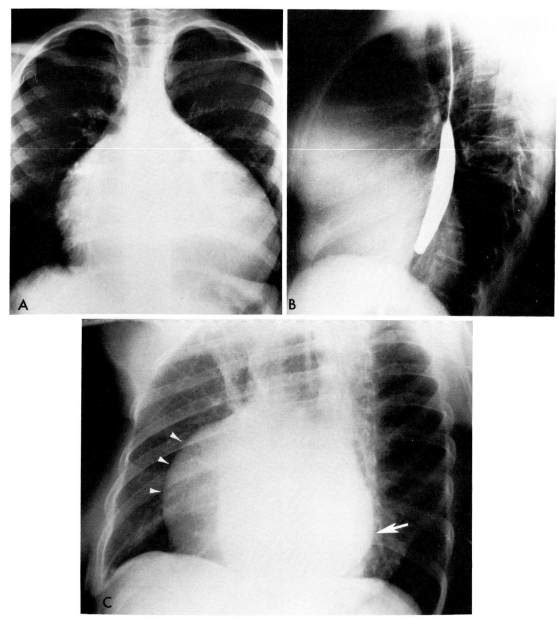

Figure 7–36. Posteroanterior (A), lateral (B), and left anterior oblique (C) chest radiographs in a 30-year-old woman with Ebstein's anomaly. The features are nearly identical to those in Figure 7–35. In the LAO view the left ventricle (arrow) is pushed posteriorly by the dilated right heart (arrowheads).

terior oblique projection, the left ventricle may be displaced posteriorly by the dilated right heart structures (Fig. 7–36). We found cardiomegaly in all seven patients in our group, and all had diminished pulmonary vascularity and right atrial enlargement. When this lesion presents in adulthood with a massive cardiac silhouette, one must consider pericardial effusion in the differential diagnosis (Figs. 7–35 and 7–36).

Echocardiographic Features

The definitive finding on M-mode echocardiography is the presence of a ubiquitous tricuspid valve recorded from several transducer positions (Fig. 7–37). In addition, there may be increased excursion and delayed closure of the valve (> 0.04 seconds after the mitral valve). However, the diagnosis of Ebstein's anomaly can be made with high reliability on the basis of two-dimensional echocardiographic information alone.[9] The apical view, displaying the four chambers simultaneously, permits easy evaluation of the abnormally displaced tricuspid valve leaflets. This displacement can

also be visualized in the subxiphoidal four-chamber view (Fig. 7–38). Downward or apical displacement of the septal leaflet and posterior leaflet insertion into the right ventricular cavity is easily identifiable because it results in an asymmetric relationship when it is compared with the normally aligned mitral valve. The displacement defines the "atrialized" portion of the right ventricle. An interatrial defect may be visualized. Bowing of the interatrial septum toward the left atrium suggests the presence of right-to-left shunting at the atrial level. Such shunting may be further identified by use of peripheral venous contrast echocardiography.

Angiographic Features

The classic angiographic features of Ebstein's anomaly include:[10] (1) aneurysmal dilatation of the right atrium; (2) leftward displacement of the tricuspid valve; (3) tricuspid regurgitation; (4) a right-to-left shunt at the atrial level; (5) an atrialized portion of the right ventricle that distends during atrial contraction; and (6) a small "function-

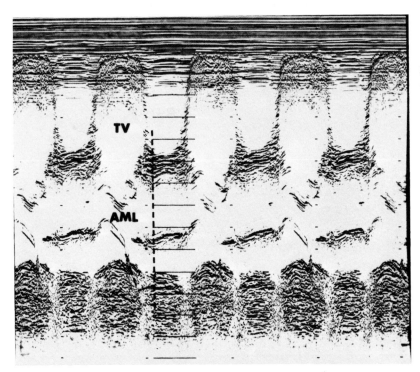

Figure 7–37. M-mode echocardiogram at the level of the anterior leaflet of the mitral valve (AML). The ubiquitous tricuspid valve (TV) shows increased excursion and delayed closure when compared with the mitral valve (dotted line).

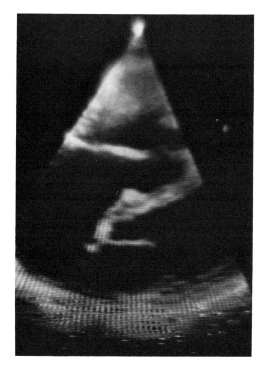
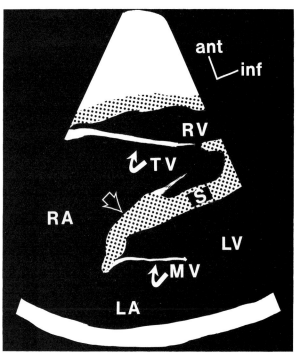

Figure 7–38. Ebstein's anomaly. In the subxiphoidal view, there is enlargement of the right atrium (RA), which includes the "atrialized" portion of the right ventricle (RV) (open arrow). There is marked apical displacement of the posterior and septal leaflets of the tricuspid valve (TV). The normal position of the atrioventricular groove can be estimated from the level of insertion of the anterior mitral leaflet (MV). There is an interatrial communication at the level of the ostium secundum. (LA = left atrium, LV = left ventricle.)

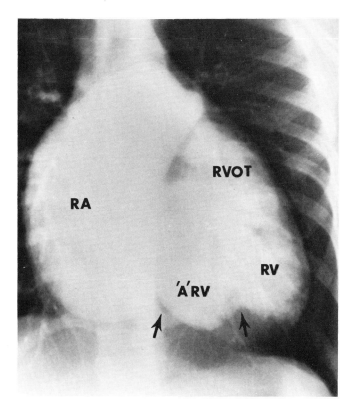

Figure 7–39. Posteroanterior right ventriculogram showing the features of Ebstein's anomaly of the tricuspid valve: a huge right atrium (RA) extending to the tracheal bifurcation; 4+/4+ tricuspid regurgitation; an "atrialized" portion of the right ventricle ('A' RV); and a small functional right ventricle (RV). The right ventricular outflow tract forms the left upper heart border.

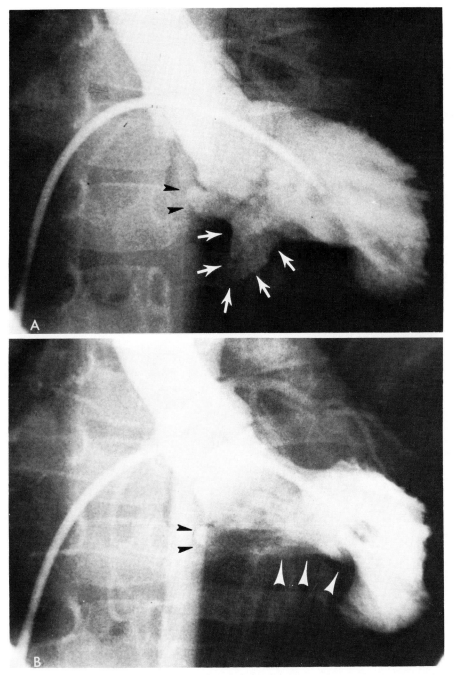

Figure 7–40. Left ventricular angiograms in a child with Ebstein's anomaly of the tricuspid valve. These posteroanterior views (*A* and *B*) show superior displacement of the left ventricular diaphragmatic wall (white arrowheads) and a slender projection (white arrows) extending from the left ventricular posterobasal wall. Mitral valve prolapse (black arrowheads) is also demonstrated.

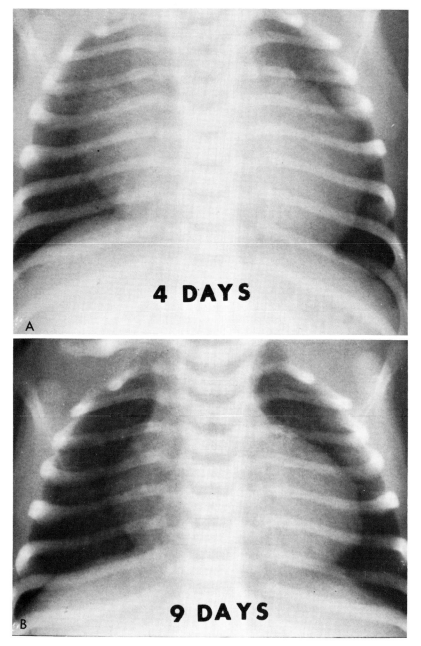

Figure 7–41. *A*, Anteroposterior chest radiographs in a four-day-old cyanotic infant with pulmonary hypertension and tricuspid regurgitation. Decreased vascularity and right atrial enlargement are present. The radiographic differential diagnosis would include pulmonary atresia with intact ventricular septum and Ebstein's anomaly. *B*, Follow-up anteroposterior chest radiograph at age nine days shows considerable reduction in heart size. The tricuspid regurgitation murmur has subsided.

al" right ventricle with decreased ventricular filling and reduction of flow to the lungs. These findings are illustrated in Figure 7–39. An interesting feature of this anomaly is that the left ventricle may show a variety of angiographic abnormalities. These include (1) superior displacement of the left ventricular diaphragmatic wall with accentuated septal contractility (Fig. 7–40B); (2) a slender projection extending from the left ventricular posterobasal wall in systole (Fig. 7–40A); and (3) mitral valve prolapse (Fig. 7–40). These abnormalities likely relate to the absence of normal right ventricular counterforces to left ventricular contraction and the abnormal insertion of the septal leaflet of the tricuspid valve near the diaphragmatic surface of the left ventricle.

REFERENCES

1. Hardy, K. L., May, I. A., Webster, C. A., Kimball, K. G.: Ebstein's anomaly: a functional concept in successful definitive repair. J Thorac Cardiovasc Surg 48:927, 1964.
2. Edwards, J. E.: Pathologic features of Ebstein's malformation of the tricuspid valve. Proc Staff Meeting, Mayo Clinic 28:89, 1953.
3. Bialostozky, D., Horwitz, S., Espino-Vela, J.: Ebstein's malformation of the tricuspid valve. Review of 65 cases. Am J Cardiol 29:826, 1972.
4. Seward, J. B., Tajik, A. J., Feist, D. J., Smith, H. C.: Ebstein's anomaly in an 85 year old man. Mayo Clin Proc 54:193–196, 1979.
5. Perloff, J. K.: Cardiac catheterization. A clinical discipline illustrated by a study of Ebstein's anomaly of the tricuspid valve. Med Ann D.C. 31:342, 1962.
6. Kumar, A. E., Fyler, D. C., Mitteten, O. S., Nadas, A. S.: Ebstein's anomaly: Clinical profile and natural history. Am J Cardiol 28:84, 1971.
7. Giuliani, E. R., Fuster, V., Brandenburg, R. O., Mair, D. D.: Ebstein's anomaly. Mayo Clin Proc 54:163–173, 1979.
8. Anderson, K. R., Zuberbuhler, J. R., Anderson, R. H., Becker, A. E., Lie, J. T.: Morphologic spectrum of Ebstein's anomaly of the heart. Mayo Clin Proc 54:174–180, 1979.
9. Ports, T. A., Silverman, N. H., Schiller, N. B.: Two-dimensional echocardiographic assessment of Ebstein's anomaly. Circulation 58:336, 1978.
10. Ellis, K., Griffiths, S. P., Burris, J. O., et al.: Ebstein's anomaly of the tricuspid valve. Angiocardiographic considerations. Am J Roentgenol 92:1338, 1964.

TRANSIENT TRICUSPID INSUFFICIENCY

Radiographic Echocardiographic Features

Some cyanotic infants with decreased pulmonary blood flow may be found to have tricuspid insufficiency. This is caused by myocardial dysfunction and is often secondary to pulmonary hypertension.[1] The dysfunction may be transient. Chest film findings are variable in this syndrome, but cardiomegaly with right atrial enlargement is the rule with gradual return to normal (Fig. 7–41). M-mode echocardiography suggests the presence of pulmonary hypertension (see discussion this chapter and Chapter 2). The apical and subxiphoid views of the tricuspid valve can be used to provide indirect information about tricuspid insufficiency. A large right ventricle and right atrium, with bowing of the interatrial septum toward the left atrium, is suggestive evidence of this entity. Definite confirmation can be provided by contrast techniques.[2] Injection of indocyanine-green dye or saline into a peripheral arm vein generates a cloud of contrast within the right atrium. Two-dimensional echo examination of the right atrium from the subxiphoid view along the inferior vena cava can be used to detect reflux of the microbubbles into the inferior vena cava. When present, this is considered strong evidence for tricuspid insufficiency. One can also detect the presence of right-to-left atrial shunting, if present, by noting the passage of these microbubbles from the right to the left atrium and then into the left ventricle and left ventricular outflow tract.

REFERENCES

1. Buciarelli, R. L., Egan, E. A., Gessner, I. H.: Persistence of fetal cardiopulmonary circulation: One manifestation of transient tachypnea of the newborn. Pediatrics 58:192, 1976.
2. Lieppe, W., Behar, V. S., Scallion, R., Kisslo, J. A.: Detection of tricuspid regurgitation with two-dimensional echocardiography and peripheral vein injections. Circulation 57:128, 1978.

Chapter 8

CYANOTIC PATIENT WITH INCREASED VASCULARITY

The increased vascularity that accompanies the cyanotic lesions in this category is due to increased pulmonary blood flow. All of the lesions presented here are characterized by an intracardiac defect (or in the case of total anomalous pulmonary venous return, an extracardiac defect) that allows excess blood to reach the lungs. Shunt vascularity is characterized by an increase in size and number of lung vessels and by dilated hilar vessels. Some element of interstitial edema may accompany this pattern. The clinical presentation in these cases may be one of congestive heart failure as well as cyanosis. Three of the defects in this category may be associated with pulmonary stenosis: complete transposition, single ventricle, and double-outlet right ventricle. The chest film in these instances may demonstrate diminished vascularity, leading to a differential diagnosis of the lesions presented in Table 7–1, category I. These three defects, however, most commonly present *without* pulmonary stenosis, and therefore they will be discussed here in their classic form.

Complete transposition of the great arteries is the first consideration in the infant or child who presents with cyanosis and increased vascularity of the shunt type on the chest film. In our own series of 107 patients, this was the most common cyanotic congenital heart defect (Table 7–3), although in other larger series it is second to tetralogy of Fallot in occurrence.[1-3] The other lesions in the differential diagnosis are listed in Table 7–1, category II. As a mnemonic, one may remember the "four T's": transposition, total anomalous pulmonary venous return,

truncus arteriosus, and tricuspid atresia. Tricuspid atresia is included in this differential because in two instances (when it is associated with a large VSD and no pulmonary stenosis, or when the great vessels are transposed) the chest film demonstrates increased pulmonary vascularity.

An analysis of the pulmonary artery segment on the chest radiograph may prove helpful in this group of patients. Patients with transposition of the great arteries do not have a well-defined pulmonary artery segment, since the pulmonary trunk is medially situated and no longer border forming.[4] In persistent truncus arteriosus, the pulmonary artery segment is absent because the pulmonary arteries arise from the truncus itself. A well-defined pulmonary artery segment may be expected in three cyanotic lesions presenting with increased pulmonary vascularity: total anomalous pulmonary venous return, double-outlet right ventricle, and tricuspid atresia with normally related great vessels.

COMPLETE TRANSPOSITION OF THE GREAT ARTERIES

A definition of transposition of the great arteries should take into account the relationship between the great arteries and the ventricles from which they arise[5-7] and the relationships of the great arteries to each other regardless of the ventricle of origin.[8, 9] Since the physiologic consequences and, therefore, the clinical manifestations of the deranged anatomy are to create two circulations in parallel, stress should be placed on the relationship between the great arteries and their ventricles of origin. We shall employ the following definition of complete transposition of the great arteries: (1) there is a reversed position of the aorta and the pulmonary trunk relative to the ventricles; (2) the aortic valve is anterosuperior and arises from the morphologic right ventricle; (3) the pulmonary valve is posteroinferior and arises from the morphologic left ventricle; (4) the aorta is anterior and to the right and the pulmonary trunk is posterior and to the left in 85 per cent of cases (d-[dextro] transposition), directly anteroposterior in 15 per cent of cases (a-transposition), or rarely to the left (l-transposition); and (5) a communication exists between the pulmonary and systemic circuits — at either the atrial, the ventricular, or the great vessel level. This definition assumes that the right and left atria connect to the morphologic right and left ventricle — that is, that there is atrioventricular concordance. The course of blood flow is systemic veins → right atrium → right ventricle → aorta → systemic arteries → back to systemic veins; and pulmonary veins → left atrium → left ventricle →

pulmonary trunk → pulmonary arteries → back to pulmonary veins. This parallel arrangement of the systemic and pulmonary circulations requires that communications previously mentioned must exist between the two circuits in order for blood to exchange between them (via bidirectional shunting) and for the infant to survive. In neonates with an intact ventricular septum, it is thought that there is an admixture of systemic and pulmonary venous shunting via the ductus arteriosus.[10] When these anatomic communications are inadequate, the presentation is usually that of a severely cyanotic neonate.

There are several other features of transposition that bear mentioning. Since the pulmonary trunk arises from the anatomic left ventricle, the pulmonary valve is in fibrous continuity with the anterior leaflet of the mitral valve. The coronary arteries take origin from the transposed aorta, most commonly with the right coronary, or with the right coronary and left circumflex coronary artery arising from the posterior aortic sinus.[11] Obstruction to left ventricular outflow leading to pulmonary stenosis occurs

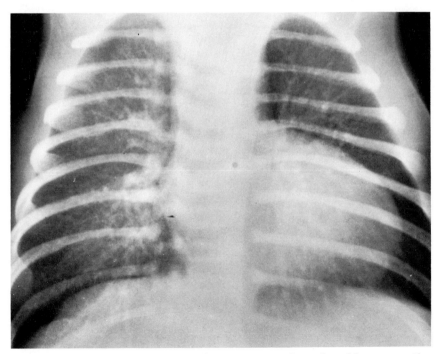

Figure 8–1. Anteroposterior chest radiograph in a cyanotic three-day-old neonate. Shunt vascularity, cardiomegaly, and a narrow mediastinum lead to the classic radiographic picture of transposition of the great arteries. The oval ("egg") shape of the heart is due to combined right atrial and left ventricular dilatation. The narrow mediastinum is due to decreased thymic tissue in this stressed infant and the lack of a pulmonary artery segment. Note that the vascularity in the right lung is somewhat greater than that in the left lung.

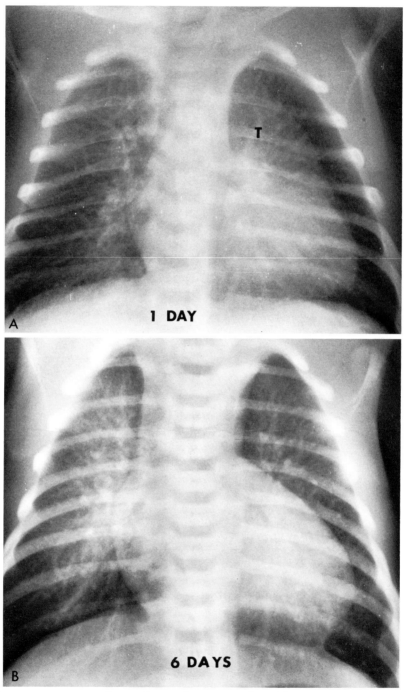

Figure 8–2. Anteroposterior chest radiographs in a one-day-old neonate *(A)* with follow-up film at six days *(B),* when cyanosis was clinically evident. Note that the pulmonary vascularity has increased and that the mediastinum has narrowed. The former is due to a drop in pulmonary resistance and the latter to a regression of the thymus (T) present at birth in this neonate with transposition of the great arteries.

in forms similar to those occurring in the normal left ventricle—namely, membranous subpulmonary stenosis;[12] fibromuscular tunnel stenosis;[13] and systolic anterior mitral leaflet motion abutting the interventricular system in a manner similar to idiopathic hypertrophic subaortic stenosis.[12] These varieties of pulmonary stenosis may occur with or without a ventricular septal defect. There is strong association between transposition and juxtaposition of the atrial appendages (most commonly juxtaposition of the right appendage to the left[14]). This entity is usually diagnosed only after angiography.[15] Finally, a right aortic arch occurs in 10 to 15 per cent of patients with transposition, especially when there is a VSD and pulmonary stenosis.[16]

Radiographic Features

In the absence of pulmonary stenosis and in the presence of low pulmonary vascular resistance, the communications between the systemic and pulmonary circulations lead to an increase in pulmonary vascularity (Figs. 8–1 to 8–3). This, however, may not be manifest until after the first few days of life. The degree of increased pulmonary flow depends on the size of the communication(s) between the systemic and pulmonary circulations. The density created by the thymus is invariably absent or transient in transposition (Fig. 8–2) (probably because of the stress imposed upon the infant by the cardiac lesion).[7] This allows one to analyze the mediastinum without interference from the thymus. The transposed pulmonary trunk leads to two radiographic features typical of transposition. First, the transposed pulmonary trunk changes the orientation of the right pulmonary artery so that it lines up with the right ventricular outflow tract. This arrangement allows blood to preferentially flow into the right lung.[18] In the older child, this difference in flow (right greater than left) may be appreciated on the chest film (Figs. 8–1 and 8–2B). Second, because of the posterior and medial position of the trunk, it is no longer border forming as a convex density along the left upper heart border (Figs. 8–1, 8–2B and 8–3).[4] This "negative" finding is further emphasized by the presence of increased pulmonary vascularity, since the latter situation is usually associated with a well-defined, if

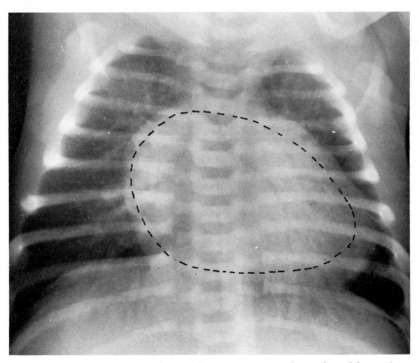

Figure 8–3. Anteroposterior chest radiograph in a cyanotic three-day-old. In this neonate with transposition the right atrium is particularly prominent. The "egg" is indicated by dotted lines.

not enlarged, pulmonary trunk. The narrow mediastinum or narrow "waist" of the cardiomediastinal silhouette typical of transposition is due primarily to the abnormal position of the pulmonary trunk and the lack of thymic tissue (Figs. 8–1, 8–2B, and 8–3). The heart is usually mildly enlarged and appears oval or egg-shaped owing to combined right atrial and left ventricular dilatation (Figs. 8–1 to 8–3). If the atrial septum is intact, the left atrium will be enlarged. The narrow mediastinum and the shape of the heart have led to the radiographic findings in transposition being called the "egg on a string." In our group of 27 patients with complete transposition, the pulmonary trunk was inapparent in 20 and cardiomegaly was present in 18. Only four patients had diminished pulmonary vascularity and all had subpulmonary stenosis.

Echocardiographic Features

Two-dimensional echocardiography permits the diagnosis of transposition to be firmly established by demonstrating an ab-normal cross-sectional relationship of the great arteries at their origins.[19, 20] In the short-axis view, the transposed great arteries are seen as two circles unlike the normal circle-sausage configuration (Fig. 8–4). Identification of the individual arteries may be accomplished by evaluating the systolic time intervals from the semilunar valve leaflets on M-mode echocardiography. The pulmonary valve is the valve with the longest interval between the onset of electrical systole and semilunar valve closure.[21] Since this does not hold in the presence of elevated pulmonary vascular resistance, we have found that the most accurate and reliable method for determining the identity of the arteries (and thus classifying the type of transposition) is to orient the transducer along the long axis of each great artery once malposition has been demonstrated in the short-axis view. In the long axis, it is possible to determine which great artery ascends toward the head (the aorta) and which artery dives posteriorly and bifurcates (the pulmonary artery) (Fig. 8–5). In the various forms of transposition, the aorta may be positioned

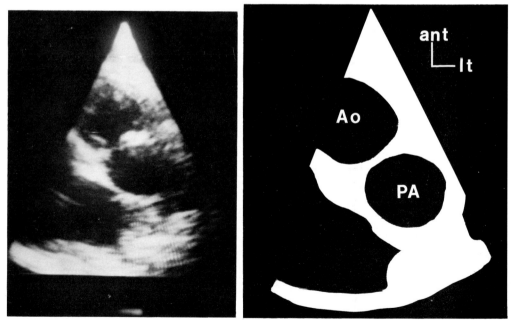

Figure 8–4. D-transposition of the great arteries. Short-axis view of the great arterial roots in d-transposition of the great arteries. In contrast to the normal circle and sausage arrangement (see Chapter 2), the great vessels form two circles with the anterior aorta (Ao) lying to the patient's right (d-transposition of the great arteries) and the pulmonary artery (PA) lying posteriorly and to the left.

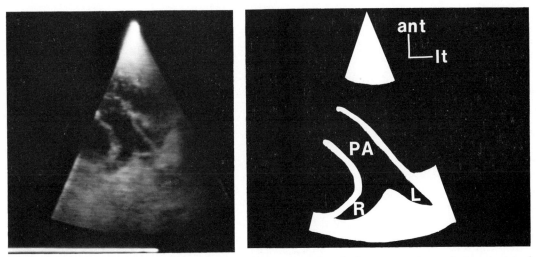

Figure 8–5. Transposition of the great arteries. Angulated short-axis view of the ventricular outflow tract in patient with transposition of the great arteries. The posterior great artery can easily be identified as the pulmonary artery (PA) because it can be followed to its point of bifurcation. (R = right pulmonary artery; L = left pulmonary artery.)

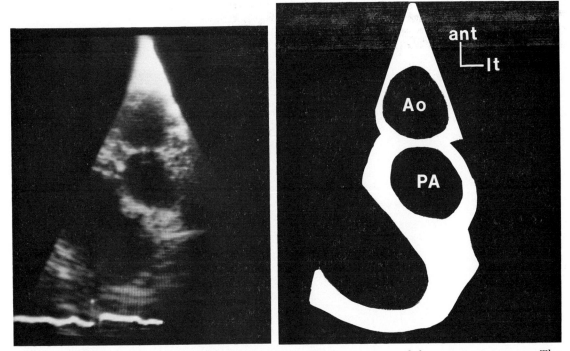

Figure 8–6. A-transposition of the great arteries. Short-axis view of the great artery roots. The transposed great arteries are oriented in a direct anteroposterior relationship. This is referred to as "a" transposition of the great arteries, with the aorta (Ao) originating from the right ventricular cavity in a position directly anterior to the posterior pulmonary artery (PA).

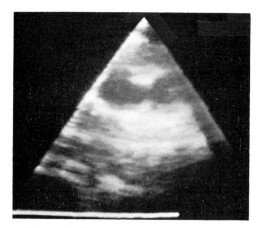
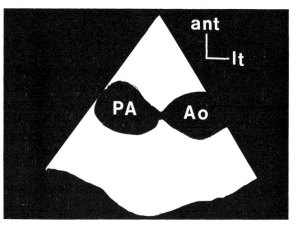

Figure 8–7. L-transposition of the great arteries. The short-axis view at the level of the great arteries in l-transposition of the arteries demonstrates the side-by-side interrelationship with aorta (Ao) to the left of the pulmonary arterial (PA) origin. (Ao = aorta; PA = pulmonary artery.)

to the right of the pulmonary trunk ("d"-transposition) (Fig. 8–4); directly anterior to the pulmonary trunk ("a"-transposition) (Fig. 8–6); or to the left of the pulmonary trunk ("l"-transposition) (Fig. 8–7). The integrity of the interventricular septum may be evaluated in both the long-axis view of the left ventricle and the subxiphoidal four-chamber view. The integrity of the inter-

atrial septum may be evaluated both before diagnostic procedures are performed and following cardiac catheterization to evaluate the adequacy of balloon atrial septostomy (Fig. 8–8).[22] An additional method for identifying a great artery at the aortic root involves the identification of the origin of the coronary arteries. In the post-operative state, the surgically created interatrial baf-

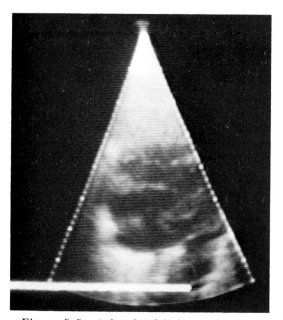
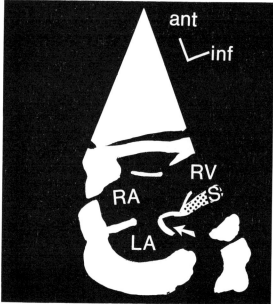

Figure 8–8. Subxiphoidal short-axis view of the interatrial septum. This patient with complete transposition of the great arteries has recently undergone balloon atrial septostomy (Rashkind procedure). Note that the inferior rim of the foramen ovale has been torn and prolapses into the left atrial cavity during this phase of the cardiac cycle (arrow). This indicates that there is a large interatrial communication and a successful balloon septostomy procedure. (LA = left atrium; RA = right atrium.)

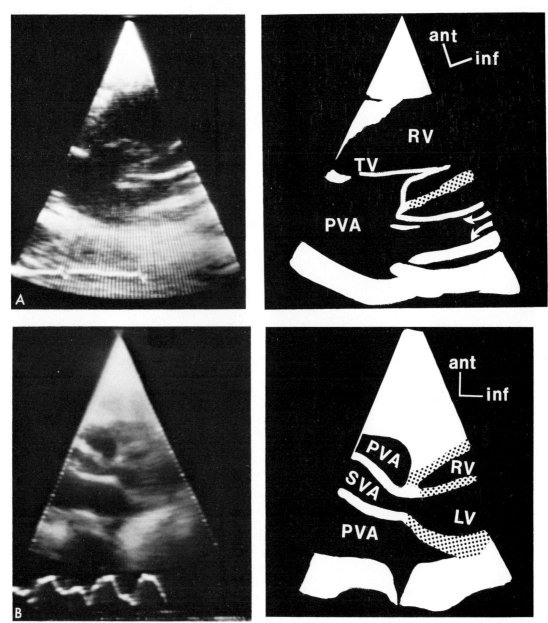

Figure 8–9. *A*, Transposition of the great arteries, postoperative Mustard baffle. Subxiphoid view of a patient with transposition of the great arteries who has undergone creation of a Mustard intra-atrial baffle (arrows), which returns oxygenated blood to the pulmonary venous atrium (PVA). (RV = right ventricle; TV = tricuspid valve; stippled area = interventricular septum.) *B*, Transposition of the great arteries — post-op Senning procedure. Subxiphoidal view showing the left ventricle (LV) and right ventricle (RV). The atrial region has been restructured so that the systemic venous atrium (SVA) drains into the left ventricle and the pulmonary venous atrium (PVA) drains into the right ventricle (RV).

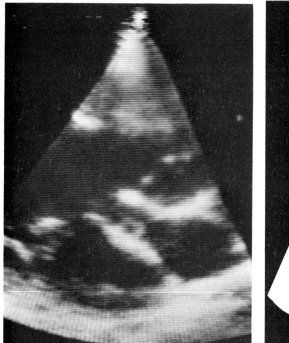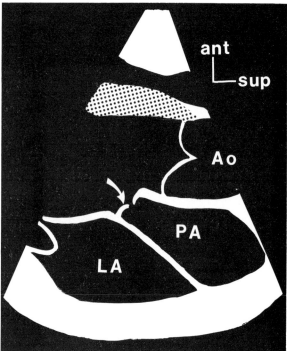

Figure 8–10. Transposition, ventricular septal defect, and pulmonary stenosis. Long-axis view of the ventricle in a patient with a large interventricular septal defect and d-transposition of the great arteries. The aorta (Ao) is seen anterior to a posterior pulmonary artery (PA). In addition, the pulmonary valve (arrow) is thickened and domed, indicating valvar pulmonary stenosis. Note the characteristic appearance of the posterior great artery in continuity with the mitral valve. When the posterior great artery is followed into the supravalvar region, it dives posteriorly and branches in a manner characteristic of the pulmonary artery. Note the absence of septal tissue beneath the great arteries, suggesting the presence of a large VSD. (LA = left atrium.)

fle may be examined in the short axis, subxiphoidal, and apical views (Fig. 8–9A and B).[23] The presence of pulmonary venous or systemic venous atrial obstruction may also be evaluated in such studies.

The physiology of the combination of complete transposition of the great vessels, ventricular septal defect, and pulmonary stenosis is quite similar to that of tetralogy of Fallot. In these cases, the two-dimensional short-axis view of the great arteries permits diagnosis of transposition with high certainty and reliability.[24] The identity of each of the great arteries is established by the methods outlined above. If the pulmonary vessel is small, or if the pulmonary valve is thickened and domed, or if the subpulmonary region is narrow or obstructed, the associated presence of pulmonary stenosis can be inferred (Fig. 8–10). Large interventricular septal defects are visible in

the apical or subxiphoidal view (Fig. 8–10).

Angiographic Features

Both ventricles should be studied angiographically in transposition. The goals should be to (1) establish the diagnosis and classify the type of transposition (d,a, or l); (2) identify the size and location of systemic to pulmonary communications (especially a ventricular septal defect); and (3) evaluate the left ventricular outflow tract for possible subpulmonary obstruction. The right ventriculogram will establish the diagnosis and classify the type of transposition as d (Fig. 8–11), a (Fig. 8–12), or l (Fig. 8–13). Although standard posteroanterior and lateral left ventriculography may allow adequate visualization of the left ventricular outflow tract and pulmonary valve region (Figs. 8–14 and 8–15), we have found the hepa-

Text continues on page 395

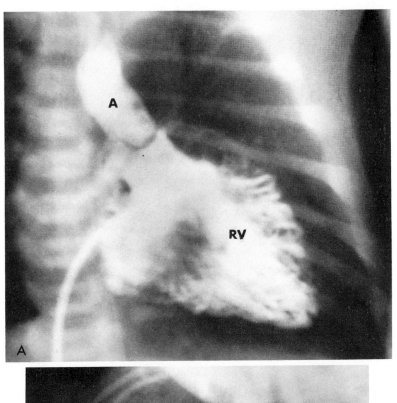

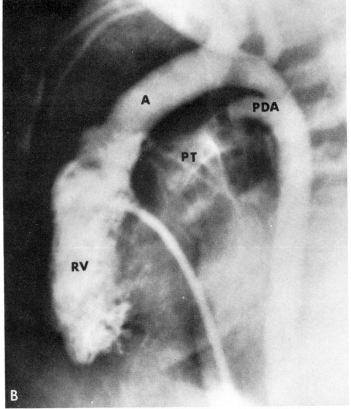

Figure 8–11. Posteroanterior *(A)* and lateral *(B)* right ventriculograms showing the morphologic right ventricle (RV) giving rise to an anterior and rightward-positioned aorta (A). The pulmonary trunk (PT) arose from the left ventricle posterior to and slightly to the left of the aorta (A). This is the aortic position in d-(dextro) transposition of the great vessels. Note the patent ductus arteriosus (PDA) filling the pulmonary trunk (PT).

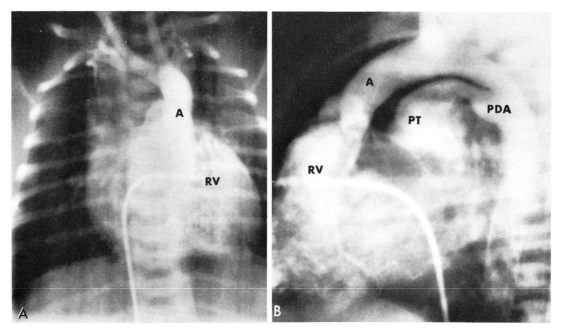

Figure 8–12. Posteroanterior *(A)* and lateral *(B)* right ventriculogram demonstrates that the morphologic right ventricle (RV) gives rise to an aorta (A) that is directly anterior to the posterior pulmonary trunk (PT). The pulmonary trunk (PT) is filled from a patent ductus arteriosus (PDA). This is the aortic position in a-(anterior) transposition of the great vessels.

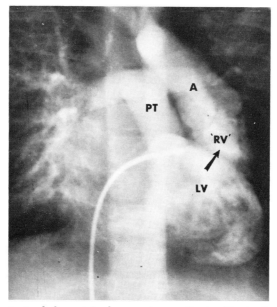

Figure 8–13. Posteroanterior left ventriculogram in a patient with single ventricle and l-transposition of the great vessels. The morphologic left ventricle (LV) gives rise to the pulmonary trunk (PT) and communicates with the small right ventricle (RV) through a large VSD (arrow). Note that the aorta (A) arises above the rudimentary chamber ('RV') and to the *left* of the pulmonary trunk (PT).

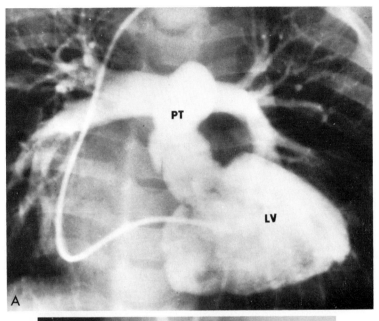

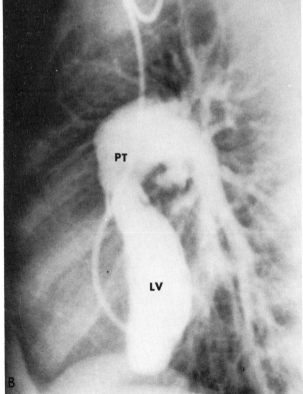

Figure 8–14. Posteroanterior (*A*) and lateral (*B*) views of a left ventriculogram in a child with d-transposition of the great vessels. The morphologic left ventricle (LV), posteriorly displaced ("pancaked") by dilated right heart structures, gives rise to the pulmonary trunk (PT). There is no evidence of subvalvar or valvar pulmonary stenosis.

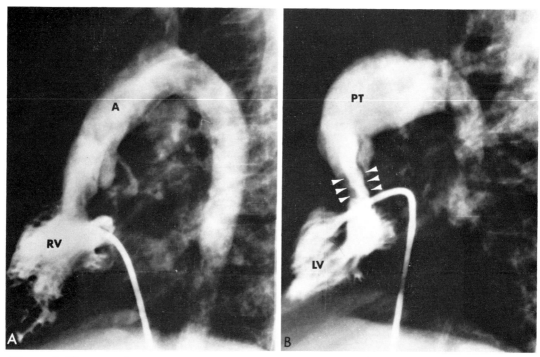

Figure 8–15. Lateral view right ventriculogram (*A*) and left ventriculogram (*B*) in a child with complete transposition of the great vessels. Note the ventricular–great vessel relationships: right ventricle (RV) → anterior aorta (A); left ventricle (LV) → posterior pulmonary trunk (PT). Note also the elongated, narrowed left ventricular outflow region (arrowheads) just beneath the pulmonary valve. There is poststenotic dilatation of the pulmonary trunk.

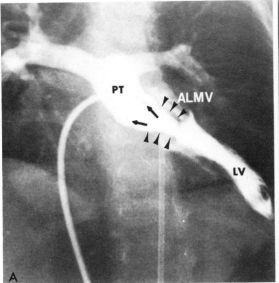

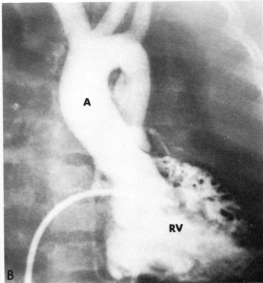

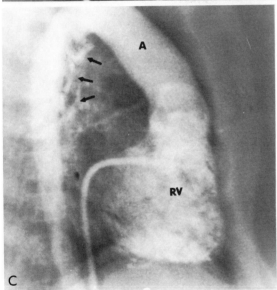

Figure 8–16. A, Hepatoclavicular (four-chamber) view left ventriculogram readily demonstrates an elongated, narrowed region (arrowheads) between the left ventricle (LV), pulmonary valve (arrows), and pulmonary trunk (PT). The obstruction is due to an abnormal systolic motion of the anterior leaflet of the mitral valve (ALMV). Note the normal appearance of the pulmonary valve leaflets (arrows). Posteroanterior *(B)* and lateral *(C)* right ventriculogram performed in the child shown in Figure 8–16A. The anterior aorta (A) arises from the right ventricle (RV) as expected in this case of d-transposition. Note the bronchial collateral vessels (arrows) arising from the proximal descending aorta.

toclavicular (four-chamber) view to be ideal for demonstrating the size and location of a ventricular septal defect and the presence and type of subpulmonary stenosis (Fig. 8–16). The subpulmonary stenosis may involve a tubular narrowing of the outflow tract (Fig. 8–15) or an abnormal attachment of the anterior leaflet of the mitral valve onto the left ventricular outflow tract (Fig. 8–16A).

REFERENCES

1. Keith, J. D., Rowe, R. D., Vlad, P.: Heart Disease in Infancy and Childhood. Macmillan Co., New York, 1979.

2. Gasul, B. M., Arcilla, R. A., Lev, M.: Diagnosis and Treatment. Lippincott, Philadelphia, 1966.

3. Krovetz, L. J., Gessner, I. H., Schiebler, G. L.: Handbook of Pediatric Cardiology. Hoeber-Harper, New York, 1981.

4. Tonkin, I. L., Kelley, M. J., Bream, P. R., Elliott, L. P.: The frontal chest film as a method of suspecting transposition complexes. Circulation 53:1016, 1976.

5. Elliott, L. P., Neufeld, H. N., Anderson, R. C., Adams, P., Jr.: Complete transposition of the great vessels. I. An anatomic study of sixty cases. Circulation 27:1105, 1963.

6. Lev, M., Rimoldi, H. J. A., Paiva, R., Arcilla, R. A.: The quantitative anatomy of simple complete transposition. Am J Cardiol 23:409, 1969.

7. Van Praagh, R.: Transposition of the great arteries. Am J Cardiol 28:739, 1971.

8. Goor, D. A., Edwards, J. E.: The spectrum of

transposition of the great arteries: with specific reference to developmental anatomy of the conus. Circulation 48:406, 1973.

9. Van Mierop, L. H. S.: Transposition of the great arteries. Am J Cardiol 28:735, 1971.

10. Jarmakani, J. M. M., Edwards, S. B., Spach, M. S., Canent, R. V., Capp, M. P., Hagan, M. J., Barr, R. C., Jain, V.: Left ventricular pressure volume characteristics in cyanotic congenital heart disease. Circulation 37:879, 1968.

11. Elliott, L. P., Amplatz, K., Edwards, J. E.: Coronary arterial patterns in transposition complexes. Anatomic and angiocardiographic studies. Am J Cardiol 17:362, 1966.

12. Shrivastava, S., Tadavarthy, S. M., Fukuda, T., Edwards, J. E.: Anatomic causes of pulmonary stenosis in complete transposition. Circulation 54:154, 1976.

13. Shaher, R. M., Puddu, G. C., Khoury, G., Moes, F., Mustard, W. T.: Complete transposition of the great vessels with anatomic obstruction of the outflow tract of the left ventricle. Am J Cardiol 19:658, 1967.

14. Charuzi, Y., Spanos, P. K., Amplatz, K., Edwards, J. E.: Juxtaposition of the atrial appendages. Circulation 47:620, 1973.

15. Deutsch, V., Shemtov, A., Yahini, J. H., Neufeld, H. N.: Juxtaposition of atrial appendages: Angiographic observations. Am J Cardiol 34:240, 1974.

16. Mathew, R., Rosenthal, A., Fellows, K.: The significance of right aortic arch in D-transposition of the great arteries. Am Heart J 87:314, 1974.

17. Carey, L. S., Elliott, L. P.: Complete transposition of the great vessels. Roentgenographic findings. Am J Roentgenol 91:529, 1964.

18. Muster, A. J., Paul, M. H., van Grondelle, A., Conway, J. J.: Asymmetric distribution of the pulmonary blood flow between the right and left lungs in D-transposition of the great arteries. Am J Cardiol; 38:352, 1976.

19. Bierman, F. Z., Williams, R. G.: Prospective diagnosis of d-transposition of the great arteries in neonates by subxiphoid, two-dimensional echocardiography. Circulation 60:1496, 1976.

20. Sahn, D. J., Allen, H. D., Lange, L. W., Goldberg, S. J.: Cross-sectional echocardiographic diagnosis of the sites of total anomalous pulmonary venous drainage. Circulation 60:1317, 1979.

21. Solinger, R., Elbl, F., Minhas, K.: Deductive echocardiographic analysis in infants with congenital heart disease. Circulation 50:1072, 1974.

22. Bierman, F. Z., Williams, R. G.: Subxiphoid two-dimensional imaging of the interatrial septum in infants and neonates with congenital heart disease. Circulation 60:80, 1979.

23. Silverman, N. H., Schiller, N. B.: Apex echocardiography. A two-dimensional technique for evaluating congenital heart disease. Circulation 57:503, 1978.

24. Henry, W. L., Maron, B. J., Griffith, J. M., Redwood, D. R., Epstein, S. E.: Differential diagnosis of anomalies of the great arteries by real-time two-dimensional echocardiography. Circulation 51:283, 1975.

SINGLE VENTRICLE

The vast majority of cases classified as a single ventricle are included in the following definition: A single ventricle exists when a ventricular chamber (usually the anatomic left ventricle) receives both atrioventricular valves or a common atrioventricular valve. At the base of this ventricle is a rudimentary chamber that represents the outlet portion of the anatomic right ventricle. The single ventricle communicates with the outlet chamber through a bulboventricular foramen (VSD) and the outlet chamber gives rise to the aorta. The pulmonary trunk arises from the main ventricular compartment. The outlet chamber is most commonly on the left in an inverted position (l-loop) and the great vessels are situated in l-transposition (anterior leftward aortic valve; posterior rightward pulmonary valve). Although the great vessel positions are identical to those in corrected transposition, the term l-"malposition" has been used to describe this great vessel arrangement, in which only one ventricular chamber or an incomplete ventricular septum exists. Infrequently, the outlet chamber is on the right (d-loop) and the great vessels are arranged in d-malposition. The single ventricle has been associated with valvar or subpulmonary stenosis and anomalies of the left AV valve (stenosis, atresia, Ebstein's anomaly).

Another, less frequent form of single ventricle exists in which the ventricular morphology presents features of *both* right and left ventricle or of *neither* ventricle. This variety of single ventricle has been termed the "primitive ventricle."[1] An additional anomaly, "double-inlet left ventricle," also requires definition. In this rare defect, there are two distinct ventricular inflow sinuses that communicate through a VSD. The left ventricle receives the mitral valve and part of the tricuspid apparatus that straddles the VSD ("straddling tricuspid valve"). The morphologic right ventricle is usually hypoplastic but normally formed.[2]

The degree of cyanosis associated with single ventricle largely depends upon the amount of intraventricular mixing and upon pulmonary blood flow. In the classic variety of this lesion, complete mixing of venous and arterial blood is unusual owing to favorable streaming of right atrial blood into the pulmonary trunk and left atrial blood across the bulboventricular foramen and into the aorta. Cyanosis may therefore be mild or even absent.[3] With the typical large increase in pulmonary blood flow the first clinical presentation is frequently characterized by congestive heart failure. The deeply cyanotic patient with single ventricle may have either pulmonary vascular obstructive disease or pulmonary stenosis. The chest film may be helpful in predicting which of these exists, showing a pulmonary arterial hypertensive pattern in the former and diminished pulmonary vascularity in the latter.

Radiographic Features

In the absence of pulmonary stenosis, the pulmonary vascularity is increased of the shunt type. In the 15 patients in our series, 10 showed increased vascularity (Fig. 8–17A and B) and 5 showed diminished vascularity (Fig. 8–18). The latter group all had pulmonary stenosis. Elevation or dilatation of the right pulmonary artery may be noted in association with single ventricle (Fig. 8–17A and B). This has been termed the "waterfall" right hilum.[4] Cardiomegaly is expected because of the volume overload of the single ventricle and was present in 14 of 15 patients in our series. Left atrial enlargement is present when the atrial septum is intact.[5] Because of its transposed and, therefore, medial position, the density normally produced by the pulmonary trunk is absent (Fig. 8–17A and B). It is replaced by an obliquely running, straight or slightly concave density (Fig. 8–18). This density is created by the l-transposed ascending aorta (see Figs. 8–20 to 8–22 for angiographic correlation). Because of the unusual position occupied by the ascending aorta, the densities normally created by the ascending aorta, aortic knob, and descending aorta continuum are inconspicuous or absent (Fig. 8–17A and B).[5] This appearance is identical to that seen in corrected transposition (see Chapter 5). A discrete bulge below the straight density of the ascending aorta represents the rudimentary right ventricular outlet chamber (Fig. 8–17A and B)

(see Figs. 8–21 and 8–22 for angiographic correlation). The above findings were present in 11 of our 15 patients with single ventricle. In patients with single ventricle and pulmonary stenosis, the ascending aorta may become quite dilated (since it carries excess blood flow) and gives a "box-shaped" appearance to the cardiomediastinal silhouette (Fig. 8–18).

Echocardiographic Features

The presence of a single ventricle is suggested by lack of demonstrable interventricular septum[6] on either parasternal, apical (Fig. 8–19), or subxiphoidal two-dimensional imaging. The interrelationship of the great arteries is easily determined from the short-axis view of the great arterial roots[7] (see Figs. 8–4, 8–6, and 8–7). In patients with single ventricle and malposed great arteries, the anteriorly located circular cross section of the aorta is usually to the left of the pulmonary trunk (l-malposition), but it may be located to the right (d-malposition) or directly anterior (a-malposition). Associated pulmonary valvar or subvalvar obstruction and atrioventricular abnormalities can also be demonstrated on two-dimensional echocardiography.

Angiographic Features

Angiography of this complex of anomalies can be greatly aided by foreknowledge of associated lesions. Ideally, one should have a clear understanding of (1) the great vessel relationships; (2) the status of the atrioventricular valves; (3) the size of the ventricular septal defect and residual septum; and (4) the presence of any associated anomalies (for example, pulmonary stenosis). Abnormalities of the atrioventricular valves (especially the left) or of the pulmonary valve or subvalvar region may be diagnosed readily by real-time echocardiography. Although the echocardiogram may also suggest the presence or absence of ventricular septal tissue, this is perhaps best evaluated angiographically (Figs. 8–20A and 8–21C). This holds true for establishing the size of the rudimentary anatomic right ventricle (Fig. 8–21C) and the size of the ventricular septal defect (bulboventricular foramen) (Figs.

Text continues on page 402

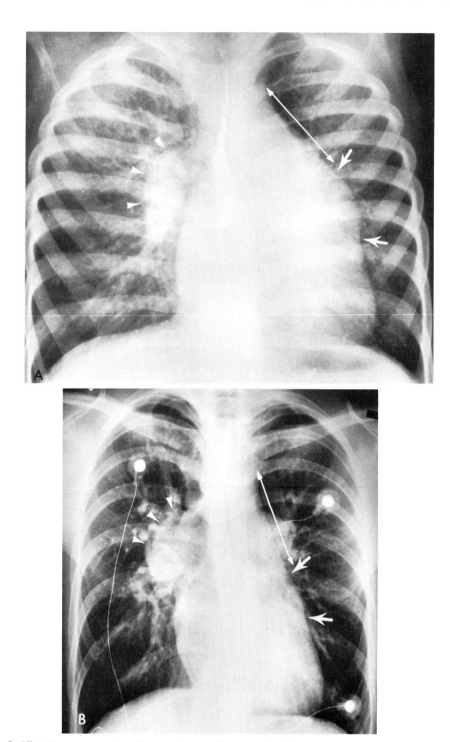

Figure 8–17. Posteroanterior chest radiographs in a child *(A)* and a teenager *(B)* with a single ventricle/l-transposition. Shunt vascularity is present in the child and a pulmonary arterial hypertensive pattern in the teenager. Note the prominent ("waterfall") right pulmonary artery in both cases (arrowheads). Despite the prominent pulmonary vascularity, the pulmonary trunk is inapparent. It is replaced by an oblique straight density (double arrow) created by the l-transposed ascending aorta. A discrete bulge (arrows) below the aortic density represents the rudimentary right ventricular outlet chamber.

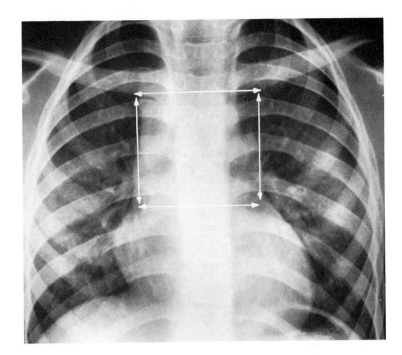

Figure 8–18. Posteroanterior chest radiograph in a cyanotic child with single ventricle/l-transposition and pulmonary stenosis. The pulmonary vascularity is decreased and the prominent aorta gives a "box" shape to the mediastinal silhouette.

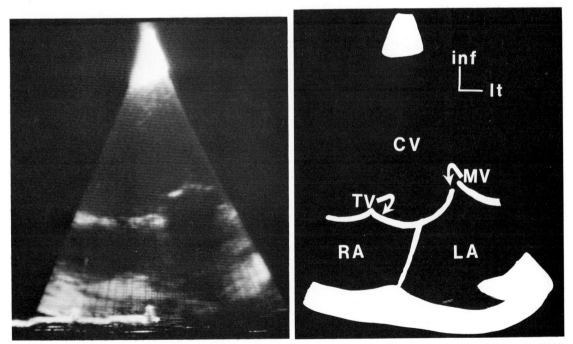

Figure 8–19. Single ventricle. In this apical view, the interatrial septum separates the right (RA) and left atria (LA). Note that the two atrioventricular valves (MV and TV) enter the large common (single) ventricular chamber (CV) with no evidence of interventricular septal tissue. The great arteries are not visualized in this study, but in most cases they are located with the aorta anterior and to the left of the pulmonary artery (l-malposition) (see Fig. 8–7).

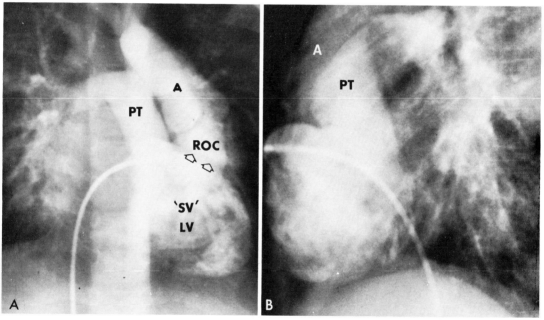

Figure 8–20. Posteroanterior *(A)* and lateral *(B)* ventriculograms in a child with congestive failure and mild cyanosis. The smooth-walled "single" ventricle has the anatomic characteristics of a left ventricle ('SV,' LV). It communicates with the rudimentary right ventricular outlet chamber (ROC) via a large septal defect (arrows). The pulmonary trunk (PT) arises from the single ventricle, and the aorta (A) arises above the outlet chamber and to the left of the pulmonary trunk. The relationship of the great vessels is well depicted in the lateral view *(B)* with the aorta (A) slightly anterior to the pulmonary trunk (PT). There is no evidence of pulmonary stenosis.

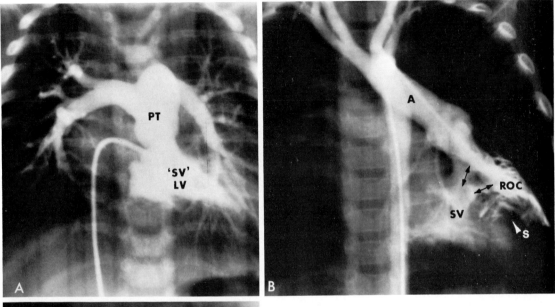

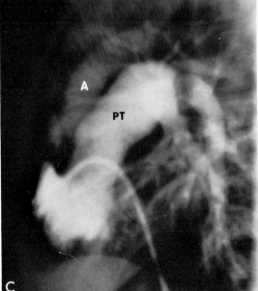

Figure 8–21. Posteroanterior *(A and B)* and lateral *(C)* selective ventriculograms in child with single ventricle/l-transposition. The ventricular anatomy and great vessel relationships are identical to the case illustrated in Figure 8–20, except that the right ventricular outlet chamber (ROC) appears somewhat larger. Note the position and size of the septum (S) and the size of the defect in the bulboventricular foramen (double arrows). (A = aorta; LV = left ventricle; PT = pulmonary trunk; 'SV' = single ventricle.)

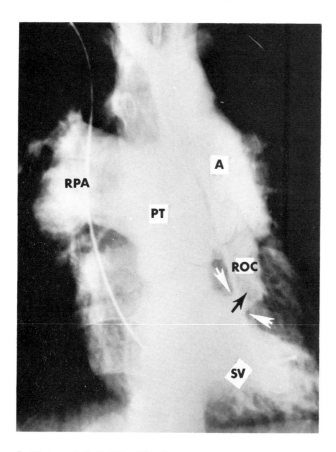

Figure 8–22. Anteroposterior angiogram in a teenager with single ventricle and l-transposition. There are two significant differences from the previous two cases: (1) There is narrowing of the communication (arrow) between the single ventricle (SV) and the right ventricular outflow chamber (ROC). This creates a "bottleneck" (arrowheads) and relative obstruction to flow into the aorta (A). (2) The pulmonary trunk (PT) and right pulmonary artery (RPA) are massively dilated owing to severe pulmonary arterial hypertension.

8–20A and 8–21C). The latter may create a relative obstruction to systemic flow (Fig. 8–22). Standard posteroanterior and lateral angiographic projections are generally adequate for these evaluations.

REFERENCES

1. Anderson, R. H., Becker, A. E., Wilkinson, J. L., Gerlis, L. M.: Morphogenesis of univentricular hearts. Br Heart J 38:558, 1976.
2. Tandon, R., Becker, A. E., Moller, J. H., Edwards, J. E.: Double inlet left ventricle. Straddling tricuspid valve. Br Heart J 36:747, 1974.
3. Rahmitoola, S. H., Ongley, P. A., Swan, H. J. C.: The hemodynamics of common (or single) ventricle. Circulation 34:14, 1966.
4. Elliott, L. P., Gedgaudas, E.: The roentgenologic findings in common ventricle with transposition of the great vessels. Radiology 82:850, 1964.
5. Tonkin, I. L., Kelley, M. J., Bream, P. R., Elliott, L. P.: The frontal chest film as a method of suspecting transposition complexes. Circulation 53:1016, 1976.
6. Sahn, D. J., Goldberg, S. J., Allen, H. D., Friedman, W. F.: The utility of real-time cross-sectional echocardiography for the noninvasive evaluation of single ventricle. Pediatr Res 10:316, 1976 (abstract).
7. Henry, W. L., Maron, B. J., Griffith, J. M., Redwood, D. R., Epstein, S. E.: Differential diagnosis of anomalies of the great arteries by real-time two-dimensional echocardiography. Circulation 51:283, 1975.

DOUBLE-OUTLET RIGHT VENTRICLE

In double-outlet right ventricle (DORV) both great arteries arise from the morphologic right ventricle and there is discontinuity between the fibrous rings of the semilunar valves and the atrioventricular valves. A ventricular septal defect provides the only outlet from the left ventricle and is present in one of three locations: (1) below the crista supraventricularis in close relationship to the aortic valve (infracristal, subaortic VSD); (2) above the crista in close relationship to the pulmonary valve (supracristal, subpulmonary VSD); or (3) in a position uncommitted to either semilunar valve. The lack of atrioventricular valve to semilunar valve continuity in this lesion is due to the presence of conal tissue beneath both arteries. The great arteries usually lie side by side with the aorta to the right of the pulmonary trunk. The semilunar valves tend to lie in the same transverse plane. The clinical spectrum of double-outlet right ventricle is varied and depends upon both the location of the ventricular septal defect and the presence of pulmonary stenosis. In patients with a subaortic ventricular septal defect and pulmonary stenosis, the clinical presentation is similar to that of tetralogy of Fallot. When the VSD is subpulmonic and no pulmonary stenosis exists, the clinical presentation is similar to that of d-transposition. In this situation (the Taussig-Bing anomaly), the aorta arises directly from the right ventricle and receives mainly venous blood and the pulmonary trunk straddles the VSD and receives mainly arterial blood from the left ventricle.[1] This group of patients has a high incidence of aortic coarctation.[2] A third group of patients has a subaortic ventricular septal defect and no pulmonary stenosis, with a presentation similar to that of children with a large ventricular septal defect. In a small group of patients, the ventricular septal defect is not committed to either great vessel. This group also resembles children with large ventricular septal defects.[2]

Radiographic Features

This lesion has variable radiographic features. In DORV with either an infracristal or a supracristal VSD, the chest film may demonstrate findings similar to those seen with a large VSD with shunt vascularity and left atrial and left ventricular enlargement (Fig. 8–23). Since the pulmonary trunk is in its normal location, it reflects the presence of increased flow and appears dilated (Fig. 8–23). In the cyanotic child, this appearance should help to distinguish DORV from complete transposition, since the malpositioned pulmonary trunk is not apparent in the latter condition. Since the pulmonary vascularity depends on the presence or absence of pulmonary stenosis, it is not surprising that it was diminished in four of eight patients in our group with DORV and pulmonary stenosis (Fig. 8–24). In these patients the chest film may be identical to that seen with classic tetralogy of Fallot (diminished vascularity, absent pulmonary trunk and prominent aorta [Fig. 8–24]). A helpful differential point is the fact that cardiomegaly is quite common in DORV (six of eight patients in our series) but rare in tetralogy (Fig. 8–24).

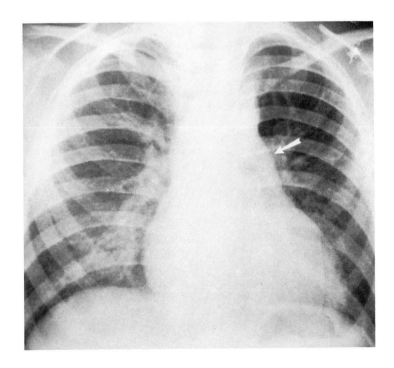

Figure 8–23. Posteroanterior chest radiograph in a cyanotic child. There is shunt vascularity and mild cardiomegaly. The density of the pulmonary trunk is well defined (arrow). This appearance should rule out transposition of the great vessels. This child had double-outlet right ventricle and large VSD.

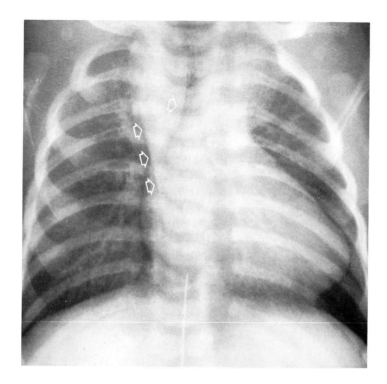

Figure 8–24. Anteroposterior chest radiograph in a cyanotic infant. The pulmonary vascularity is diminished, and there is a right aortic arch (arrows). The pulmonary artery segment is inapparent and there is an upturned cardiac apex. Although these features are typical of tetralogy, the enlarged heart should suggest another diagnosis. This infant had double-outlet right ventricle with severe pulmonary stenosis.

Another, more subtle difference is the rounded cardiac apex seen in DORV, as opposed to the upturned apex typical of tetralogy. This is thought to be related to the relatively large left ventricle associated with DORV.[3]

Echocardiographic Features

Two-dimensional echocardiography demonstrates the lack of atrioventricular valve to semilunar valve continuity due to the presence of conal tissue beneath both arteries (Fig. 8–25). In addition, serial cross-sectioning in the short-axis view of the ventricular body and ventricular outflow tracts, when superimposed, shows both great arteries to originate from the right ventricular side of the interventricular septum (Fig. 8–26).[4, 5] The great arteries of these patients are frequently side by side (Fig. 8–26), with the semilunar valves in approximately the same transverse plane. Other great vessel arrangements are possible — for example, aorta to the right of and anterior to the pulmonary artery (as in d-transposition) or aorta to the left of and anterior to the pulmonary artery (as in l-transposition). These are characterized in the manner previously described.

Angiographic Features

The typical angiographic features of double-outlet right ventricle include (1) the absence of fibrous continuity between the mitral valve and either semilunar valve (Figs. 8–27D and 8–28B) and (2) the presence of both semilunar valves at approximately the same horizontal level (Fig. 8–27A). The second feature usually exists when the great vessels are side by side (Fig. 8–27A). When the aorta is to the right and anterior to the pulmonary artery (the d-transposed position) the aortic valve is frequently more cephalic than the pulmonary valve (Fig. 8–28B). The presence of muscular tissue (conal tissue) dividing the outflow tracts ("infundibula") of both ventricles may be appreciated in the posteroanterior view (Fig. 8–27A).

Pulmonary stenosis is frequently part of the DORV complex (Figs. 8–27A and 8–28A), being present in 17 of 34 patients in one series.[6] Other associated anomalies that angiography may uncover include subaortic stenosis, atrial septal defect, endocardial cushion abnormalities, patent ductus arteriosus, and right aortic arch (Fig. 8–28A). Demonstration of the position of the ventricular septal defect is best accomplished

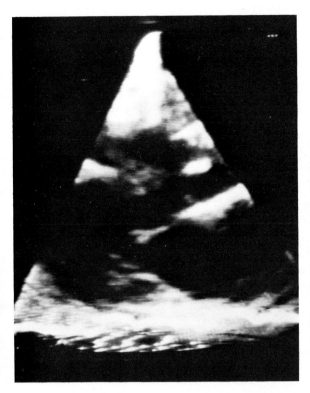
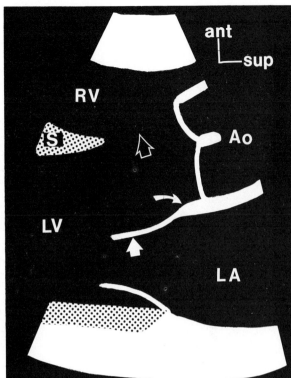

Figure 8–25. Double-outlet right ventricle with pulmonary stenosis. Long-axis view of the outflow tract. Note the large overriding aorta (Ao) and the large interventricular communication (open arrow). There is discontinuity between the mitral valve (straight arrow) and the aortic valve owing to the presence of conal tissue (curved arrow) between the atrioventricular valve and the posterior root. This patient had a subaortic ventricular septal defect and pulmonary stenosis. The clinical presentation was quite similar to that of tetralogy of Fallot. (LV = left ventricle; S = septum; LA = left atrium.)

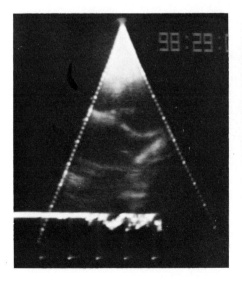
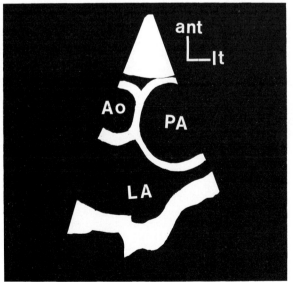

Figure 8–26. Double-outlet right ventricle. Short-axis view demonstrates that the great arteries originate from a similar level. With serial short-axis views, one can demonstrate that both great arteries arise from the right ventricular side of the interventricular septum. The pulmonary artery (PA) is large and to the left of the aorta (Ao). The abnormal arrangement is depicted as two circular cross sections of these vessels.

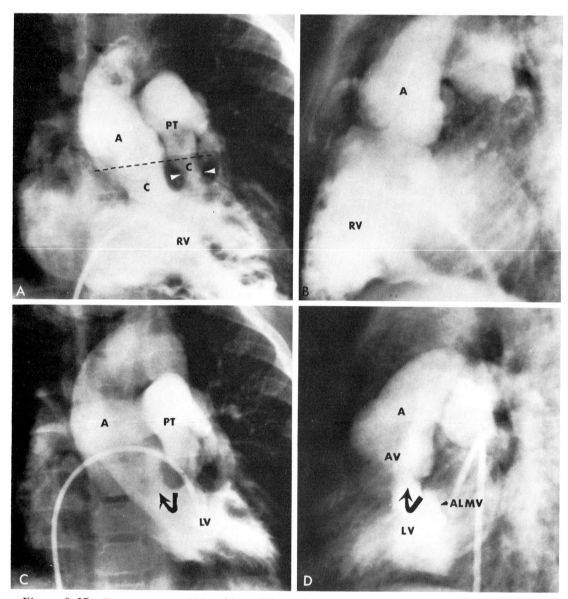

Figure 8–27. Posteroanterior *(A)* and lateral *(B)* right ventriculograms and posteroanterior *(C)* and lateral *(D)* left ventriculograms in a child with double-outlet right ventricle. The right ventriculogram shows that both the aorta (A) and pulmonary trunk (PT) arise above conal tissue (C) from the right ventricle (RV). The aorta is located to the right and anterior to the pulmonary trunk and the semilunar valves are at the same level (dotted line). Subvalvar pulmonary stenosis (arrowheads) is present. Because of the anterior position of the aorta and the subaortic conal tissue, there is lack of continuity between the anterior leaflet of the mitral valve (ALMV) and the aortic valve (AV). The VSD (curved arrow) provides the only outlet for the left ventricle (LV) into the aorta (A).

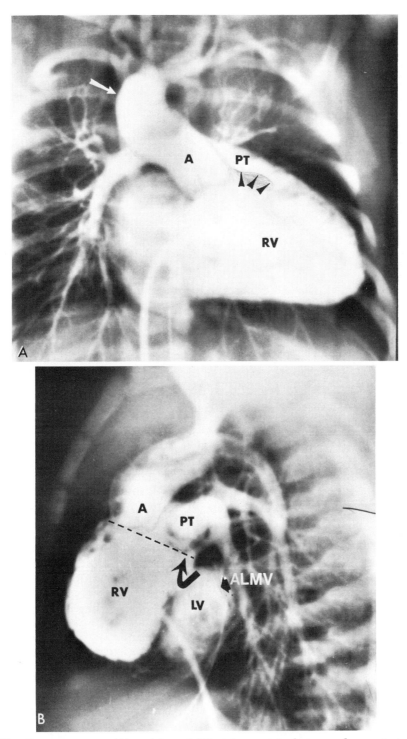

Figure 8–28. Posteroanterior *(A)* and lateral *(B)* right ventriculograms demonstrate the origin of both aorta (A) and pulmonary trunk (PT) from the right ventricle (RV). Note the right aortic arch (white arrow) and the narrow subpulmonary region (arrowheads). The aorta and pulmonary trunk are located anteroposterior (as in d-transposition) and the aortic valve is slightly cephalad to the pulmonic valve. Note that the VSD is committed primarily to the pulmonary trunk (curved arrow) and that there is lack of continuity between the anterior leaflet of the mitral valve (ALMV) and the pulmonary valve.

with a left ventriculogram performed in biplane posteroanterior and lateral or long-axial oblique projections. The VSD is located posteroinferior to the crista supraventricularis. Its relationship to the great arteries should be sought. Generally, when the great arteries are side by side the defect relates to the aortic valve (Fig. 8–27D).[6] When the great vessels are positioned as in d-transposition the VSD is closer to the origin of the posteriorly positioned pulmonary valve (Fig. 8–28B).

REFERENCES

1. Sridaromont, S., Feldt, R. H., Ritter, D. G., Davis, G. D., Edwards, J. E.: Double outlet right ventricle: Hemodynamic and anatomic correlations. Am J Cardiol 38:85, 1976.
2. Sondheimer, H. M., Freedom, R. M., Olley, P. M.: Double outlet right ventricle: Clinical spectrum and prognosis. Am J Cardiol 39:709, 1977.
3. Van Praagh, R., Perez-Trevino, C., Reynolds, J. L., Moes, C. A. F., Keith, J. D., Roy, D. L., Belcourt, C., Weinberg, T. M., Parisi, L. F.: Double outlet right ventricle with subaortic ventricular septal defect and pulmonary stenosis. Am J Cardiol 35:42, 1975.
4. Henry, W. L., Maron, B. J., Griffith, J. M., Redwood, D. R., Epstein, S. E.: Differential diagnosis of anomalies of the great arteries by real-time two-dimensional echocardiography. Circulation 51:283, 1975.
5. DiSessa, T. G., Hagan, A. D., Pope, C., Samtoy, L., Friedman, W. F.: Two-dimensional echocardiographic characteristics of double outlet right ventricle. Am J Cardiol 44:1146, 1979.
6. Hallerman, F. J., Kincade, O. W., Ritter, D. G., Ongley, P. A., Titus, J. L.: Angiocardiographic and anatomic findings in origin of both great arteries from the right ventricle. Am J Roentgenol 109:51, 1970.

TOTAL ANOMALOUS PULMONARY VENOUS CONNECTION

In total anomalous pulmonary venous connection (TAPVC), all of the pulmonary veins leave the lungs and unite to form a "confluence" behind the heart. From there, blood is conducted via a second vascular channel in one of three directions: (1) supracardiac level via the left vertical vein to the innominate vein or superior vena cava; (2) cardiac level to the coronary sinus or right atrium; or (3) infradiaphragmatic level to the portal vein. In the infradiaphragmatic type of connection, the vascular channel leaves the confluence and enters the abdominal cavity through the esophageal hiatus and connects with the portal vein or its branches. Because venous return must flow through the hepatic capillary bed there is resultant severe pulmonary venous obstruction and diminished left heart output. Obstruction to venous return is much less common in the supracardiac variety of TAPVC.[1] When it occurs, it is usually due to compression of the vertical vein and the left mainstem bronchus — the so-called "hemodynamic vise."[2]

In the most common variety of TAPVC, pulmonary venous blood enters the vertical vein (persistent left superior vena cava) and is conducted through the innominate vein and right superior vena cava to the right atrium. Thus, there is an obligatory right-to-left shunt at the atrial level (through a patent foramen ovale or a true atrial septal defect), since all of the blood from the systemic and pulmonary venous circulations directly or indirectly enters the right atrium. When pulmonary vascular resistance is low, a large portion of right atrial blood enters the right ventricle and the pulmonary arteries. Thus there is a large amount of pulmonary venous blood flow through the right heart. Because of this the right-to-left shunt results in only mild systemic desaturation and cyanosis. The clinical presentation is therefore commonly one of congestive failure and mild cyanosis with increased pulmonary blood flow.

Radiographic Features

This lesion illustrates well how the chest x-ray and echocardiogram complement each other. In the nonobstructive variety of TAPVC, the chest radiograph nearly always demonstrates signs of significant shunt vascularity and features closely resembling those of an isolated atrial septal defect (normal left atrium, dilated right heart structures) (Figs. 8–29 and 8–30). In the older child with the supracardiac type of this anomaly, the density of the vertical vein and dilated right superior vena cava often form a mediastinal density that gives a "figure 8" or "snowman" configuration on the frontal chest film (Fig. 8–29). In the younger child, these venous structures may be rather subtle and may be mistaken for the normal thymic density (Fig. 8–30A). The lateral

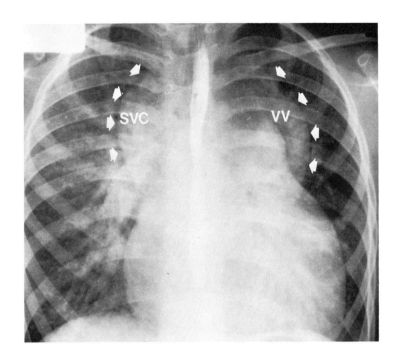

Figure 8–29. Posteroanterior chest radiograph in a mildly cyanotic child with congestive heart failure. There is shunt vascularity (note the large, distinct lower lobe vessels). The pulmonary trunk is prominent and the heart is enlarged. The mediastinal silhouette shows a biconvex density (arrows), giving the cardiomediastinal silhouette a "figure 8" or "snowman" appearance. At cardiac catheterization and angiography this child had total anomalous pulmonary venous connection to the vertical vein (VV) and a markedly dilated superior vena cava (SVC).

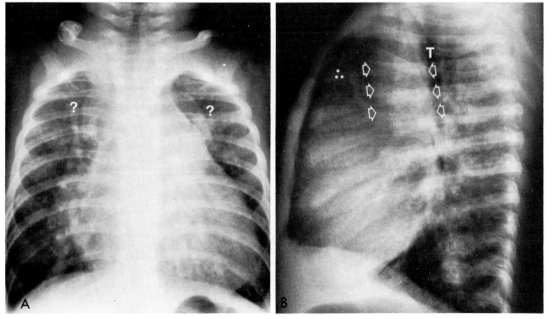

Figure 8–30. Anteroposterior *(A)* and lateral *(B)* chest radiographs in a mildly cyanotic infant with congestive heart failure. There is shunt vascularity, the pulmonary trunk is well defined, and the heart is enlarged. There are densities (?) in the upper mediastinal regions that could represent thymic tissue. The lateral view demonstrates a clear retrosternal space ($_o*_o$) (which the thymus should occupy) and a broad vertical density (arrowheads) anterior to the trachea (T). This infant had total anomalous pulmonary venous connection to the vertical vein. The vertical density on the lateral film represents the superimposed superior vena cava and vertical vein.

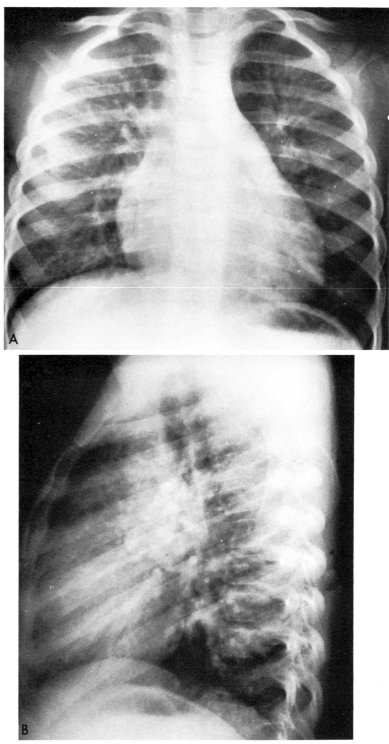

Figure 8–31. Anteroposterior *(A)* and lateral *(B)* chest radiographs in a mildly cyanotic child. The chest film appearance of shunt vascularity and mild cardiomegaly is indistinguishable from that of any moderate left-to-right shunt. This child had total anomalous pulmonary venous connection to the right atrium.

chest film may show the straight density of the dilated right superior vena cava and the vertical vein anterior to the trachea (Fig. 8–30B). The sign is especially useful in the infant prior to the appearance of the classic "snowman" configuration in the frontal projection.[3] When TAPVC occurs directly to the superior vena cava or azygous vein, these structures may be asymmetrically enlarged. When TAPVC involves cardiac structures, the chest film appearance is similar to that seen with an isolated atrial septal defect (Fig. 8–31). Prominence in the region of the coronary sinus may suggest that this is the final venous drainage site. In our series, four of five patients demonstrated the classic "snowman" appearance (Fig. 8–29). One patient in whom the total return was directly through the coronary sinus to the right atrium showed shunt vascularity and cardiomegaly (Fig. 8–31).

The radiographic and clinical picture of TAPVC below the diaphragm is distinctly different from TAPVC of the cardiac or supracardiac type and has been discussed in Chapter 5.

Echocardiographic Features

There are no definitive M-mode echocardiographic findings. Right ventricular volume overload results in increased right ventricular dimension in association with paradoxical septal motion (Fig. 8–32). The left atrial dimension is usually small but may be normal (Fig. 8–32). An echo-free space posterior to the left atrium may suggest the presence of a common chamber posterior to the left atrium.

The two-dimensional long-axis (Fig. 8–33) and subxiphoidal views (Fig. 8–34) will demonstrate large right heart structures. In the apical view, which normally demonstrates insertion of the left lower pulmonary vein into the left atrium, one cannot identify such insertion. The left atrial cavity is usually smaller than normal, and the interatrial septum appears to bow toward the left atrial cavity. An interatrial septal defect may be identified in both the apical and subxiphoidal views. The confluence of the pulmonary veins into a common pulmonary vein may, on occasion, be identified posteri-

Text continues on page 416

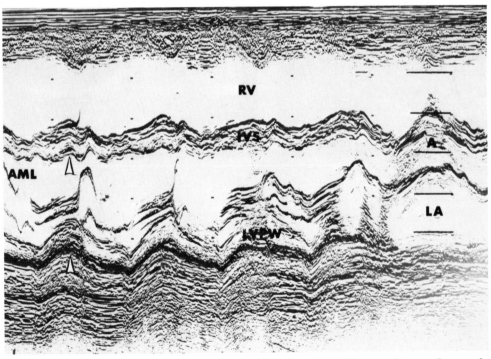

Figure 8–32. M-mode echocardiogram in a child with supracardiac total anomalous pulmonary venous connection. There is right ventricular (RV) dilatation, paradoxical septal motion (arrowheads) indicating right ventricular volume overload, and a small left atrium (LA). These findings are indistinguishable from those of a common atrial septal defect. (AML = anterior leaflet mitral valve; LVFW = left ventricular free wall.)

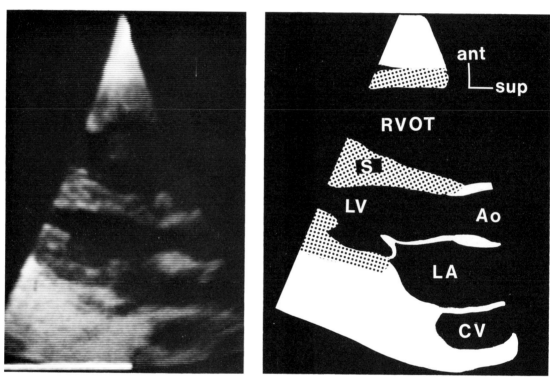

Figure 8–33. Total anomalous pulmonary venous return, supradiaphragmatic. Long-axis view of the left ventricle. Note the small left atrium (LA) and left ventricle (LV) and the enlarged right ventricular outflow tract (RVOT) anteriorly. The cavity lying posterior to the left atrial posterior wall is the common pulmonary vein (CV). (S = septum; Ao = aorta.)

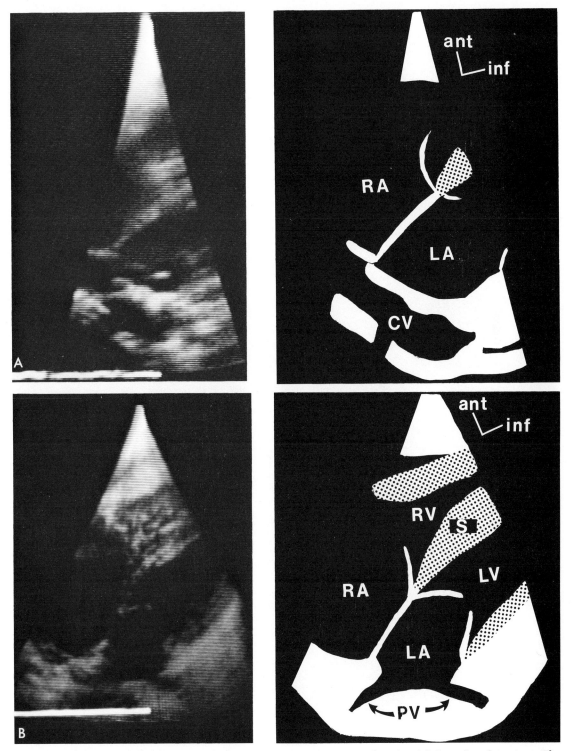

Figure 8–34. A, Total anomalous pulmonary venous return. Subxiphoidal four-chamber view. The left atrium (LA) is smaller than the right atrium (RA). Posterior to the left atrium is a large channel representing the common pulmonary vein (CV). B, Total anomalous pulmonary venous return, postoperative. Subxiphoidal four-chamber view. Note the change in the appearance from the images in A. The left atrial cavity (LA) has been enlarged by the addition of the common pulmonary vein into the posterior aspect of the chamber. The individual pulmonary veins (PV) can be seen entering the posterior aspect of this atrial chamber. (RA = right atrium; S = septum; LV = left ventricle.)

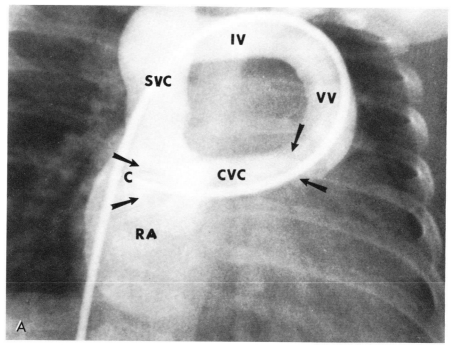

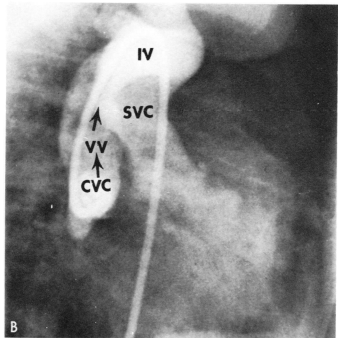

Figure 8–35. Posteroanterior *(A)* and lateral *(B)* angiograms performed through a catheter *(C)* located in the common venous canal (CVC) showing washout of contrast from blood returning from the pulmonary veins (arrows). The dilated vertical vein (VV), innominate vein (IV), and superior vena cava (SVC) are well visualized as they conduct the blood to the right atrium (RA). The lateral view demonstrates no obstruction in the vertical vein (VV).

Illustration continued on opposite page

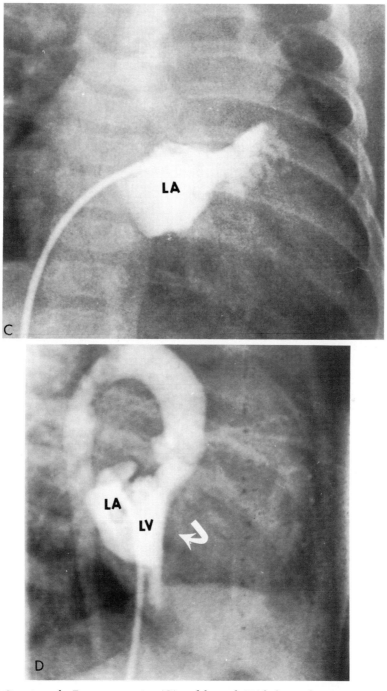

Figure 8–35 Continued Posteroanterior *(C)* and lateral *(D)* left atrial angiogram in the same child shows a small left atrium (LA) and a left ventricle (LV) "pancaked" by dilated right heart structures.

or to the left atrial wall in both the subxiphoidal (Fig. 8–34) and short-axis views of the left atrium.[4] In circumstances in which the drainage is into the coronary sinus, an enlarged coronary sinus may be visualized posterior to the left atrium, along the atrioventricular groove.[4, 5] Peripheral vein contrast injections in these patients show right-to-left shunting at the atrial level, since these patients are dependent upon right-to-left atrial communications in order to maintain systemic ventricular output.

Angiographic Features

The most common variety of total anomalous pulmonary venous connection is associated with pulmonary venous drainage into a common venous channel that courses in a relatively horizontal fashion posterior to, but near the roof of, the left atrium. Although this anomalous drainage pattern may be visualized on the levophase of a pulmonary angiogram, it is best studied by selective retrograde catheter placement into the anomalous channels. This allows clear visualization of the common venous chamber, the ascending vertical vein, and the dilated native systemic venous structures (Fig. 8–35A). The lateral view of a biplane posteroanterior angiogram will also help one to rule out obstruction between the vertical vein and the bronchus (Fig. 8–35B). Small left heart structures are associated with this lesion (Fig. 8–35C and D).

REFERENCES

1. Delisle, G., Ando, M., Calder, A. L., Zuberbuhler, J. R., Rochenmacher, S., Alday, L. E., Mangini, O., Van Praagh, S., Van Praagh, R.: Total anomalous pulmonary venous connection. Am Heart J 91:99, 1976.
2. Elliott, L. P., Edwards, J. E.: The problem of pulmonary venous obstruction in total anomalous pulmonary venous connection to the left innominate vein. Circulation 25:913, 1962.
3. Weaver, M. D., Chen, J. T. T., Anderson, P. A. W., Lester, R. G.: Total anomalous pulmonary venous return to the left vertical vein. Radiology 118:679, 1976.
4. Sahn, D. J., Allen, H. D., Lange, L. W., Goldberg, S. J.: Cross-sectional echocardiographic diagnosis of the sites of total anomalous pulmonary venous drainage. Circulation 60:721, 1979.
5. Snider, A. R., Ports, T. A., Silverman, N. H.: Venous anomalies of the coronary sinus: detection by M-mode, two-dimensional and contrast echocardiography. Circulation 60:721, 1979.

PERSISTENT TRUNCUS ARTERIOSUS

Truncus arteriosus is characterized by a single great vessel (the truncus) leaving the heart. This great artery gives rise to the coronary, pulmonary, and systemic circulations. The truncal valve is seated astride a large ventricular septal defect (malalignment VSD) and receives the blood from both ventricles. The truncal valve may have from two to six cusps[1] and is frequently incompetent.[2] The pulmonary arteries arise from the ascending portion of the truncus. A distinct pulmonary trunk may arise from the left lateral wall of the truncus and branch into right and left pulmonary arteries (type I truncus).[1] Separate right and left pulmonary arteries may arise from the posterior truncal wall (type II truncus) or from the lateral walls (type III truncus).

Generally, patients with truncus arteriosus present in infancy with congestive heart failure, recurrent respiratory infections, and mild cyanosis. The first is due to volume overload of the left heart and the last to mixing at the ventricular level and to pulmonary edema with right-to-left intrapulmonary shunting. In the presence of increased pulmonary vascular resistance, however, these patients may become increasingly cyanotic.

Radiographic Features

Radiographically, this condition may mimic other admixture lesions, especially transposition of the great arteries (Fig. 8–36A). A pertinent differential point is the presence of right aortic arch in approximately 30 per cent of patients with truncus arteriosus[2] (Fig. 8–36B). There is increased vascularity of the shunt type, and there may be superimposed interstitial edema (Fig. 8–36B). In the rare instance in which one pulmonary artery branch is hypoplastic or atretic, the pulmonary vascularity will demonstrate unilateral prominence (Fig. 8–

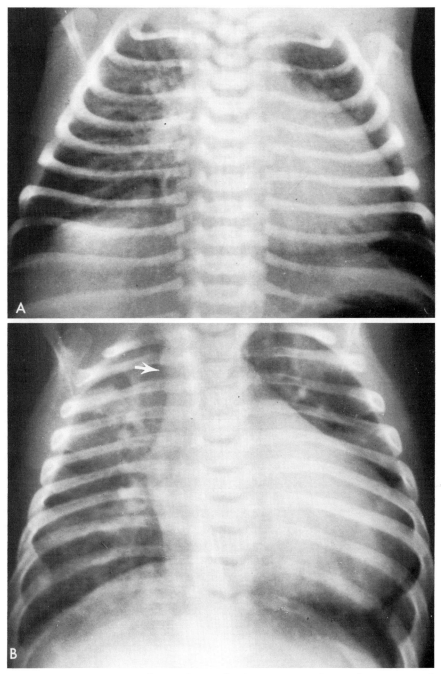

Figure 8–36. A, Anteroposterior chest radiograph of a cyanotic infant with congestive failure. The presence of shunt vascularity, a narrow mediastinum, and cardiomegaly makes this radiograph indistinguishable from that of transposition of the great arteries. This infant had truncus arteriosus type I. *B,* Anteroposterior chest radiograph in another cyanotic infant with congestive heart failure. The lung fields show interstitial edema (as well as shunt vascularity) and there is marked cardiomegaly. The presence of a right aortic arch (arrow) should help to distinguish this case of truncus arteriosus from transposition.

Illustration continued on following page

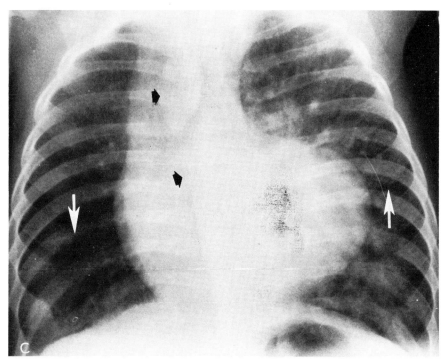

Figure 8–36 Continued C, Anteroposterior chest radiograph of another cyanotic infant. The vascularity is decreased in the right lung (↓) and increased in the left (↑). The upturned apex and right aortic arch are apparent (arrows). This infant had a "hemitruncus" with an atretic right pulmonary artery.

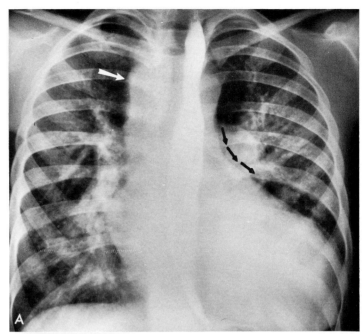

Figure 8–37. Posteroanterior (A) and lateral (B) chest radiographs in a four-year-old cyanotic boy. There is shunt vascularity and the pulmonary artery segment is concave (arrows). There is a right aortic arch (arrow) and marked cardiomegaly with biventricular enlargement. This child had truncus arteriosus type I with elevated pulmonary vascular resistance.

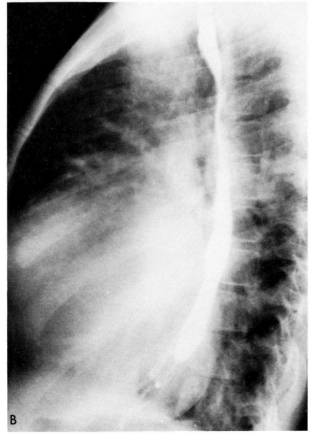

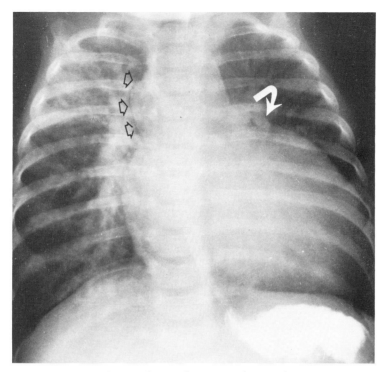

Figure 8–38. Anteroposterior chest radiograph in an infant with type I truncus arteriosus. Note the prominence in the pulmonary trunk region (curved arrow)—the "hilar comma." This density represents the left pulmonary artery, not the pulmonary trunk. Note the dilated ascending portion of the truncus (arrows) in this infant.

36C). There is cardiomegaly involving all chambers (Fig. 8–37), and the region usually occupied by the pulmonary trunk is flat or concave (since this structure is absent) (Figs. 8–36 and 8–37). The left main pulmonary artery may be particularly distinct as a curved density in the left upper lobe (Fig. 8–38). This has been called the left "hilar comma."[3] This prominent left pulmonary artery may simulate the pulmonary trunk in type I truncus arteriosus, in which the pulmonary arteries arise from the left lateral wall of the truncus (Fig. 8–38). The dilated truncus may give a prominent concave appearance to the right upper heart border (Fig. 8–38).

Echocardiographic Features

The two-dimensional echocardiographic findings include the presence of a defect in the truncal or conal interventricular septum best identified in the long-axis view of the left ventricle (Fig. 8–39). In addition, the large overriding truncus arteriosus can be seen straddling the defect.[4] The right ventricle has no outflow tract (Fig. 8–40). From the subxiphoidal view, the ventricular outflow tract is identified and the presence of truncal override of the ventricular septal defect is seen. This view may provide imaging of the origin of the pulmonary artery from the base of the truncus arteriosus (in type I truncus arteriosus).[5]

Angiographic Features

The diagnosis of truncus arteriosus should generally be derived from clinical information and noninvasive imaging techniques. The angiographic evaluation should include an assessment of the type of truncus present (I, II, or III) (Fig. 8–41) and should diagnose unexpected lesions or pulmonary artery hypoplasia (Fig. 8–42). The degree of truncal valve insufficiency should also be

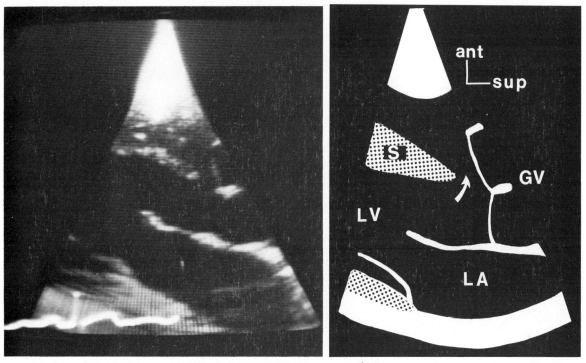

Figure 8–39. Truncus arteriosus. Long-axis view of the left ventricle. The enlarged great vessel root (GV) overrides the interventricular septum (S) by 50 per cent. There is no evidence of a discrete right ventricular outflow tract anteriorly. The interventricular septal defect (arrow) is high in the ventricular septum and represents a malalignment or conal interventricular septal defect. (LV = left ventricle; LA = left atrium.)

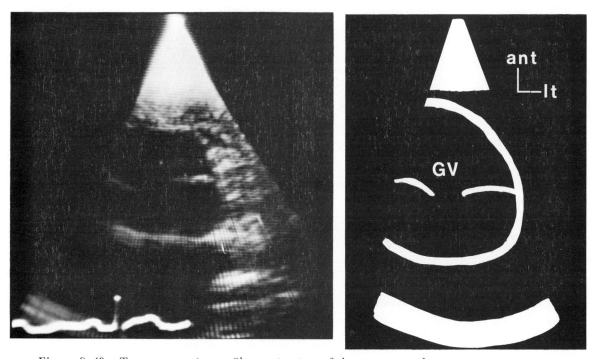

Figure 8–40. Truncus arteriosus. Short-axis view of the great vessel root in persistent truncus arteriosus. Only a single, large great vessel (GV) arises from the ventricle. The semilunar valve leaflets are redundant. There is no anterior outflow tract visible.

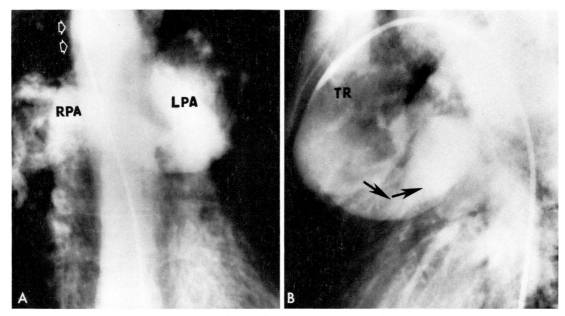

Figure 8–41. Posteroanterior (A) and lateral (B) angiograms in the truncus (TR). This massively enlarged great vessel gives rise to the pulmonary arteries (RPA, LPA) from its posterolateral wall (straight arrows). This patient had severe pulmonary hypertension and elevated pulmonary vascular resistance. Note the right arch (open arrows).

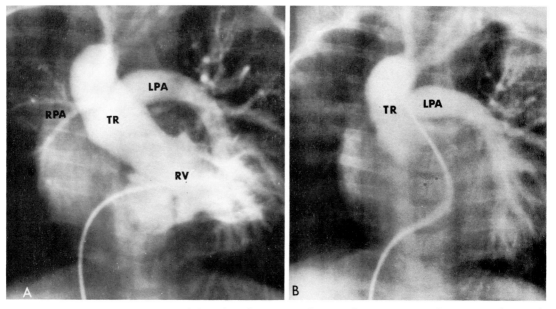

Figure 8–42. Anteroposterior (A) and right ventriculogram demonstrating the origin of a single great vessel (the truncus — TR) arising from the right ventricle (RV) and giving rise to a large left pulmonary artery (LPA) and a hypoplastic right pulmonary artery (RPA). Selective injection of contrast in the mid portion of the truncus demonstrates the origin of the left pulmonary artery from the posterolateral wall (Type II).

estimated. Direct injections in the truncus or in the left ventricle in standard projections are usually adequate for this evaluation (Fig. 8–42).

REFERENCES

1. Collett, R. W., Edwards, J. E.: Persistent truncus arteriosus: Classification according to anatomic types. Surg Clin North Am 29:1245, 1949.
2. Calder, L., Van Praagh, R., Van Praagh, S., Sera, S. W.P., Corwin, R., Levy, A., Keith, J. D., Paul, M. H.: Truncus arteriosus communis: Clinical angiographic and pathologic findings in 100 patients. Am Heart J 92:23, 1976.
3. Abrams, H. L., Kaplan, H. S.: Angiocardiographic Interpretation in Congenital Heart Disease. Charles C Thomas, Springfield, Illinois, 1956.
4. Henry, W. L., Maron, B. J., Griffith, J. M., Redwood, D. R., Epstein, S. E.: Differential diagnosis of anomalies of the great arteries by real-time two-dimensional echocardiography. Circulation 51:283, 1976.
5. Bierman, F. Z., Williams, R. G.: Prospective diagnosis of d-transposition of the great arteries in neonates by subxiphoid, two-dimensional echocardiography. Circulation 60:1496, 1979.

Chapter 9

FETAL ECHOCARDIOGRAPHY

M-mode and two-dimensional echocardiographic imaging techniques are uniquely capable of being applied to the study of the developing heart of the human fetus during the late second and throughout the third trimester of pregnancy.[1-3]

B-mode and abdominal real-time scans are used to orient the position of the fetus within the uterus and amniotic sac. The position of the fetal heart with respect to the maternal anterior abdominal wall is determined, and a two-dimensional echocardiographic study is performed with an effort made to simulate the standard precordial and four-chamber views usually performed

in postnatal studies (see Chapter 2). Occasionally, the fetus may be positioned with limbs or spine interposed between the maternal anterior abdomen and the fetal heart. In this situation it is often helpful to have the mother reposition herself on the examining couch or to have her take a short walk. An alternate approach is to have the obstetrician gently apply external version techniques. Such methods allow successful imaging of the fetal heart to be performed in 90 to 95 per cent of cases. Visualization is facilitated by the fact that the fetus is immersed in the fluid-filled amniotic cavity and the lungs are also fluid-filled (Fig. 9–1).

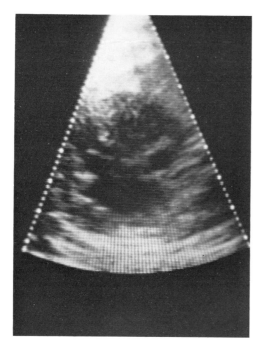
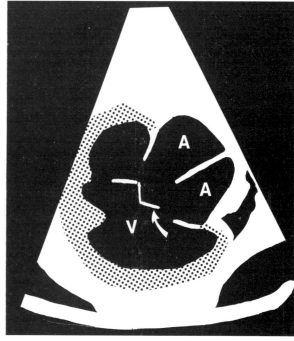

Figure 9–1. Four-chamber apical view of a 28-week gestational fetus demonstrating a large endocardial cushion defect with a common atrioventricular valve (arrow) opening into a large single ventricular chamber (V). (A = atrial chamber.)

TABLE 9–1. Profile of Obstetric Risk Factors

RISK FACTOR	NUMBER OF PATIENTS	PER CENT
Fetal Risk Factors		
Intrauterine growth retardation	87	16
Fetal cardiac dysrhythmia	48	9
Abnormal amniocentesis (trisomies)	2	0.4
Somatic anomalies (ultrasound)	6	1.1
Maternal Risk Factors		
Heart disease		
Congenital	46	8
Acquired	23	4
Drug ingestion		
Alcohol	23	4
Narcotics (opiates)	13	2
Amphetamines	6	1.1
Anticonvulsants	19	3
Lithium	4	1
Birth control pills	17	3
Other sex hormones	19	3
Polyhydramnios	7	1
Oligohydramnios	2	0.4
Rh sensitization	26	5
Diabetes mellitus	52	9
Pre-eclampsia	7	1
Collagen vascular disease	19	3
Familial Risk Factors		
Congenital heart disease		
Previous offspring	109	20
Paternal	19	3
TOTAL	554	100

Since images are easy to obtain in "unorthodox" planes rather than solely through the usual limited number of "echocardiographic windows," it is important to use certain landmarks as clues to the identification of examining planes and intracardiac structures. It is, for example, often useful to identify the interatrial septum and foramen ovale in order to determine the specific identity of the atria. Since fetal blood flows from the inferior vena cava right-to-left across the patent foramen ovale, the tissue of the atrial septum secundum can be visualized pointing toward the left atrium. The sinus venosus portion of the right atrium may be identified by the insertions of the venae cavae. The aorta is identified by following the artery's sweep to the arch and the branching of the arch vessels.

By applying fetal echocardiography to the evaluation of a population of patients deemed to be at "high risk" for the occurrence of congenital cardiac malformation (see Table 9–1), two-dimensional fetal echocardiography may be used to diagnose certain major cardiac malformations prenatally.

Our experience at Yale–New Haven Medical Center over the past three years has included the imaging of almost 600 "high-risk" pregnancies between 16 and 41 weeks' gestation. To date, eight major structural cardiac abnormalities have been accurately diagnosed (see Table 9–2).

Using echocardiographic systems that have the capacity for either simultaneous (phased array systems) or sequential (mechanical scanners) M-mode recording during two-dimensional echo imaging, it is possible to obtain hard copy M-mode studies that are spatially oriented with reference to an accompanying two-dimensional scan (Fig. 9–2). The M-mode study provides an excellent means to study the electromechanical patterns of cardiac motion and is particularly useful for fetal rhythm disturbances. Using M-mode scans, the atrioventricular contraction sequence may be evaluated by studying motion of the inter-

TABLE 9–2. Congenital Cardiac Malformations Diagnosed in Utero

GESTATIONAL AGE	DIAGNOSIS
34	Pulmonary atresia with intact interventricular septum; hypoplastic right ventricle
34	Tricuspid atresia; hypoplastic right ventricle
28	Univentricular heart°
28	Tetralogy of Fallot; complex dysrhythmia; hydrops fetalis
32	Massive septal rhabdomyoma; hydrops fetalis
28	Isolated levocardia; AV canal defect; polysplenia syndrome; complete heart block; hydrops fetalis
32	Large membranous ventricular septal defect
36	"Acardiac" monster (twin pregnancy)

°See Figure 9–2.

ventricular septum, the atrial and ventricular walls, and the atrioventricular and semilunar valve leaflets. These observations and the study of postectopic intervals are of great assistance in the analysis of fetal cardiac dysrhythmias (Fig. 9–3).

We have evaluated 34 dysrhythmias in 48 fetuses referred with suspected rhythm disturbances (see Table 9–3).[4] The majority have been isolated ectopic beats, and all but the most recently encountered of these have proved to be benign, self-limited disturbances of rhythm that have spontaneously resolved during the remainder of pregnancy or within the first five days of life. A single case of isolated atrial ectopic activity has been documented to result in atrial bigeminy and eventually (presumably through reentry) to multiple episodes of sustained supraventricular tachycardia. Fetal digitalis therapy administered transplacentally via maternal ingestion of the medication has successfully controlled this rhythm disturbance.

Three cases of sustained supraventricular tachycardia have been encountered, and all three have been associated with varying degrees of fetal congestive heart failure (hy-

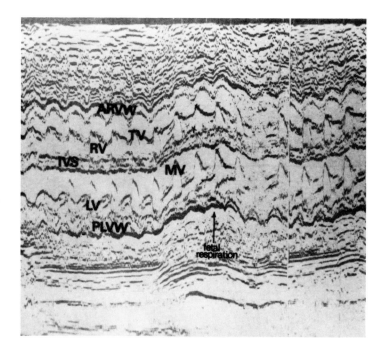

Figure 9–2. M-mode echocardiogram at midventricular level in a 33-week fetus. (ARVW = anterior right ventricular wall; IVS = interventricular septum; LV = left ventricular cavity; MV = mitral valve; RV = right ventricular cavity; TV = tricuspid valve.)

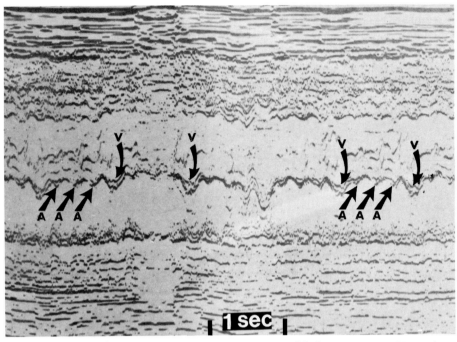

Figure 9–3. M-mode tracing at the level of the aorta and left atrium in a 34-week gestational fetus. Note rapid regular undulations of the atrial wall at a rate of 360/minute (A). Ventricular responses cause more pronounced motion (V) and occur regularly—every fourth beat. The study was consistent with atrial flutter with 4:1 AV block.

drops fetalis). Echocardiography can then be used as a noninvasive means of monitoring fetal antidysrhythmic therapy following the administration of digitalis to the pregnant mother.

The association of severe fetal hydrops with sustained dysrhythmias and/or congenital cardiac malformations with sustained dysrhythmias has been found to have an ominous portent (three of six cases resulted in in utero or neonatal demise).

Using M-mode echocardiographic imaging of semilunar valve motion in association with simultaneous transabdominal fetal electrocardiography permits calculation of fetal systolic time intervals. Preliminary

TABLE 9–3. Fetal Dysrhythmias Analyzed Echocardiographically

DYSRHYTHMIA	NUMBER ENCOUNTERED	PER CENT
Self-Limited Disturbances		
Isolated supraventricular ectopy	21	62
Isolated ventricular ectopy	1	3
Sinus bradycardia (<100 beats/min)	6	18
Subgroup Total	28	82
Sustained Disturbances		
Supraventricular tachycardias		
Atrial flutter*	2	6
Paroxysmal atrial tachycardia	1	3
Complex dysrhythmia (atrial and		
ventricular)	1	3
Complete heart block	2	6
Subgroup Total	8	18
TOTAL	34	100

*See Figure 9–3.

data appear to suggest that in utero myocardial dysfunction influences these intervals in a manner similar to the alteration seen postnatally (see Chapter 2). These studies may also be useful for evaluating the effects of cardioactive medications on fetal myocardial function — such as the beta-mimetics, currently being used to arrest premature labor.

In utero echocardiographic study of the fetus, therefore, is a tool that can provide important information concerning the structural and functional integrity of the developing heart. This information may be invaluable for counseling prospective parents at risk for bearing children with heart disease and for allowing the obstetric-pediatric team to lay plans for the psychologic and medical management of the remainder of pregnancy, delivery, and the neonatal period.

REFERENCES

1. Winsberg, F.: Echocardiography of the fetal and newborn heart. Invest Radiol 3:152, 1972.
2. Kleinman, C. S., Hobbins, J. C., Jaffe, C. C., Lynch, D. C., Talner, N. S.: Echocardiographic studies of the human fetus: Prenatal diagnosis of congenital heart disease and cardiac dysrhythmias. Pediatrics 65:1059, 1980.
3. Lange, L. W., Sahn, D. J., Allen, H. D., Goldberg, S. J., Anderson, C., Giles, H.: Qualitative real-time cross-sectional echocardiographic imaging of the human fetus during the second half of pregnancy. Circulation 62:799, 1980.
4. Kleinman, C. S., Hobbins, J. C., Lynch, D. C., Donnerstein, R., Jaffe, C. C., Talner, N. S.: The use of fetal echocardiography in the diagnosis and management of antenatal arrhythmias. Am J Cardiol 47:457, 1981.

INDEX